# Management of Obesity, Part I: Overview and Basic Mechanisms

*Editor*

## LEE M. KAPLAN

# GASTROENTEROLOGY CLINICS OF NORTH AMERICA

www.gastro.theclinics.com

*Consulting Editor*
## ALAN L. BUCHMAN

June 2023 • Volume 52 • Number 2

**ELSEVIER**

1600 John F. Kennedy Boulevard • Suite 1800 • Philadelphia, Pennsylvania, 19103-2899
http://www.theclinics.com

**GASTROENTEROLOGY CLINICS OF NORTH AMERICA Volume 52, Number 2**
**June 2023 ISSN 0889-8553, ISBN-13: 978-0-323-94025-2**

Editor: Kerry Holland
Developmental Editor: Hannah Almira Lopez

*Gastroenterology Clinics of North America* (ISSN 0889-8553) is published quarterly by Elsevier Inc., 360 Park Avenue South, New York, NY 10010-1710. Months of issue are March, June, September, and December. Business and Editorial Offices: 1600 John F. Kennedy Blvd., Suite 1800, Philadelphia, PA 19103-2899. Customer Service Office: 6277 Sea Harbor Drive, Orlando, FL 32887-4800. Periodicals postage paid at New York, NY and additional mailing offices. Subscription prices are $379.00 per year (US individuals), $100.00 per year (US students), $849.00 per year (US institutions), $407.00 per year (Canadian individuals), $100.00 per year (Canadian students), $1041.00 per year (Canadian institutions), $482.00 per year (international individuals), $220.00 per year (international students), and $1041.00 per year (international institutions). Foreign air speed delivery is included in all *Clinics* subscription prices. All prices are subject to change without notice. **POSTMASTER**: Send address changes to *Gastroenterology Clinics of North America*, Elsevier Health Sciences Division, Subscription Customer Service, 3251 Riverport Lane, Maryland Heights, MO 63043. **Telephone: 1-800-654-2452 (U.S. and Canada); 314-447-8871 (outside U.S. and Canada). Fax: 314-447-8029. E-mail: journalscustomerservice-usa@elsevier.com (for print support); journalsonlinesupport-usa@elsevier.com (for online support)**.

*Reprints*. For copies of 100 or more, of articles in this publication, please contact the Commercial Reprints Department, Elsevier Inc., 360 Part Avenue South, New York, New York 10010-1710. Tel. 212-633-3874, Fax: 212-633-3820, E-mail: reprints@elsevier.com.

*Gastroenterology Clinics of North America* is also published in Italian by Il Pensiero Scientifico Editore, Rome, Italy; and in Portuguese by Interlivros Edicoes Ltda., Rua Commandante Coelho 1085, 21250 Cordovil, Rio de Janeiro, Brazil.

*Gastroenterology Clinics of North America* is covered in *MEDLINE/PubMed (Index Medicus)*, *Excerpta Medica*, *Current Contents/Clinical Medicine*, *Science Citation Index*, *ISI/BIOMED*, and *BIOSIS*.

# Contributors

## CONSULTING EDITOR

**ALAN L. BUCHMAN, MD, MSPH, FACP, FACN, FACG, AGAF**
Professor of Clinical Surgery, Medical Director, Intestinal Rehabilitation and Transplant Center, The University of Illinois at Chicago/UI Health, Chicago, Illinois, USA

## EDITOR

**LEE M. KAPLAN**
Director, Boston Course in Obesity Medicine, The Obesity and Metabolism Institute, Boston, Massachusetts, USA

## AUTHORS

**NAJI ALAMUDDIN, MD, MTR, Diplomate ABOM**
RCSI Bahrain, King Hamad University Hospital, Al Sayh, Bahrain

**NASREEN ALFARIS, MD, MPH**
King Fahad Medical City, Riyadh, Saudi Arabia

**ALI MOHAMMED ALQAHTANI, MBBS**
King Fahad Medical City, Riyadh, Saudi Arabia

**CAROLINE M. APOVIAN, MD, FACN, FACP, DABOM**
Co-Director, Center for Weight Management and Wellness, Brigham and Women's Hospital, Member of the Faculty, Harvard Medical School, Boston, Massachusetts, USA

**JASON P. BLOCK, MD, MPH**
Associate Professor, Department of Population Medicine, Harvard Pilgrim Health Care Institute, Harvard Medical School, Boston, Massachusetts, USA

**CAROLINE E. COLLIS, BA**
Department of Population Medicine, Harvard Pilgrim Health Care Institute, Boston, Massachusetts, USA

**DONALD GOENS, MD**
Division of Gastroenterology, University of California San Diego, La Jolla, California, USA

**STEVEN B. HEYMSFIELD, MD**
Professor, Pennington Biomedical Research Center, Louisiana State University System, Baton Rouge, Louisiana, USA

**SOPHIA V. HUA, PhD, MPH**
Postdoctoral Research Fellow, Department of Nutrition, Harvard T.H. Chan School of Public Health, Boston, Massachusetts, USA

**AWAB ALI IBRAHIM, MD**
Pediatric Gastroenterology, Massachusetts General Hospital, Harvard Medical School,
Boston, Massachusetts, USA

**PRIYA JAISINGHANI, MD**
Division of Endocrinology, Diabetes and Metabolism, NYU Grossman School of Medicine,
New York, New York, USA

**VERONICA R. JOHNSON, MD**
Department of Medicine, Division of General Internal Medicine and Geriatrics,
Northwestern University Feinberg School of Medicine, Chicago, Illinois, USA

**SARAH E. JUNG, MA**
Veterans Affairs San Diego Health Sciences, San Diego, California, USA

**KARLA KENDRICK, MD, MPH**
Beth Israel Deaconess Medical Center, Harvard Medical School, Boston, Massachusetts,
USA

**REKHA KUMAR, MD**
Division of Endocrinology, NewYork-Presbyterian Hospital, Weill Cornell Medical Center,
New York, New York, USA

**SONALI MALHOTRA, MD**
MGH Weight Center, Massachusetts General Hospital, Harvard Medical School, Rhythm
Pharmaceuticals, Boston, Massachusetts, USA

**EMILY OKEN, MD, MPH**
Division of Chronic Disease Research Across the Lifecourse, Department of Population
Medicine, Instructor of Pediatrics, Harvard Medical School, Harvard Pilgrim Health Care
Institute, Boston, Massachusetts, USA

**REBECCA M. PUHL, PhD**
Deputy Director, Rudd Center for Food Policy and Health, University of Connecticut,
Hartford, Connecticut, USA; Professor, Department of Human Development and Family
Sciences, University of Connecticut, Storrs, Connecticut, USA

**JONATHAN Q. PURNELL, MD, FTOS**
Professor of Medicine, Knight Cardiovascular Institute, Division of Endocrinology,
Diabetes, and Clinical Nutrition, Professor, Department of Medicine, Oregon Health &
Science University, Portland, Oregon, USA

**GEORGIA RIGAS, MBBS, FRACG**
St George Private Hospital, Kogarah, New South Wales, Australia

**MICHAEL ROSENBAUM, MD**
Division of Molecular Genetics, Departments of Pediatrics and Medicine, Columbia
University Irving Medical Center, New York, New York, USA

**THOMAS R. RUTLEDGE, PhD**
Veterans Affairs San Diego Health Sciences, San Diego, California, USA

**JESSICA E.S. SHAY, MD, PhD**
Gastroenterology Clinical and Research Fellow, Massachusetts General Hospital,
Postdoctoral Researcher, Koch Institute at MIT, Cambridge, Massachusetts, USA

**AMANDEEP SINGH, MD, PhD**
Assistant Professor, Harvard Medical School, Associate Medical Director of Endoscopy,
Massachusetts General Hospital, Boston, Massachusetts, USA

**RAMYA SIVASUBRAMANIAN, MD**
Department of Pediatrics, SUNY Downstate Medical Center, Brooklyn, New York, USA

**GITANJALI SRIVASTAVA, MD**
Department of Medicine, Division of Diabetes, Endocrinology and Metabolism, Departments of Surgery and Pediatrics, Vanderbilt University School of Medicine, Vanderbilt Weight Loss Center, Vanderbilt University Medical Center, Nashville, Tennessee, USA

**FATIMA CODY STANFORD, MD, MPH, MBA, MPA**
Department of Medicine - Neuroendocrine Unit, Pediatric Endocrinology, MGH Weight Center, Nutrition Obesity Research Center at Harvard, Massachusetts General Hospital, Harvard Medical School, Boston, Massachusetts, USA

**PRIYA SUMITHRAN, MBBS, PhD**
Associate Professor, Department of Medicine (St Vincent's), University of Melbourne, St Vincent's Hospital, Fitzroy, Victoria, Australia; Department of Endocrinology, Austin Health

**KRISTEN SUN, BA**
Boston University School of Medicine, Boston, Massachusetts, USA

**LUCY TU**
Departments of Sociology and Molecular and Cellular Biology, Harvard College, Cambridge, Massachusetts, USA

**AMANDA VELAZQUEZ, MD, DABOM**
Director of Obesity Medicine, Acting Assistant Professor, Departments of Medicine and Surgery, Cedars-Sinai Medical Center, Los Angeles, California, USA

**NICOLE E. VIRZI, MS**
Department of Clinical Psychology, San Diego State University/University of California, San Diego Joint Doctoral Program, San Diego, California, USA

**TIFFANI BELL WASHINGTON, MD, MPH**
Harvard T.H. Chan School of Public Health, Boston, Massachusetts, USA

**GUNTHER WONG, BS**
Department of Medicine, Division of Diabetes, Endocrinology and Metabolism, Departments of Surgery and Pediatrics, Vanderbilt University School of Medicine, Vanderbilt Weight Loss Center, Vanderbilt University Medical Center, Nashville, Tennessee, USA

**ALLISON J. WU, MD, MPH**
Division of Gastroenterology, Hepatology and Nutrition, Boston Children's Hospital, Instructor of Pediatrics, Harvard Medical School, Boston, Massachusetts, USA

**MICHELE M.A. YUEN, MBBS (HK), MRCP (UK), FRCP (Edin), FHKCP, FHKAM (Medicine), MPH (HK)**
Department of Medicine, Obesity, Metabolism and Nutrition Institute, Massachusetts General Hospital, University of Hong Kong, Pok Fu Lam, Hong Kong

**AMIR ZARRINPAR, MD, PhD**
Division of Gastroenterology, UC San Diego, La Jolla, California, USA; VA San Diego Health Sciences, San Diego, California, USA

# Contents

> Advances in the understanding of weight regulation provide the framework for the recognition of obesity as a chronic disease. Lifestyle approaches are foundational in the prevention of obesity and should be continued while weight management interventions, including antiobesity medications and metabolic-bariatric procedures, are offered to eligible patients. Clinical challenges remain, however, including overcoming obesity stigma and bias within the medical community toward medical and surgical approaches, ensuring insurance coverage for obesity management (including medications and surgery), and promoting policies that reverse the upward worldwide trend in obesity and adiposity complications in populations.

> The prevalence of preobesity and obesity is rising globally, multiple epidemiologic studies have identified preobesity and obesity as predisposing factors to a number of noncommunicable diseases including type 2 diabetes (T2DM), cardiovascular disease (CVD), and cancer. In this review, we discuss the epidemiology of obesity in both children and adults in different regions of the world. We also explore the impact of obesity as a disease not only on physical and mental health but also its economic impact.

> Disturbances in body weight and adiposity in both humans and animals are met by compensatory adjustments in energy intake and energy expenditure, suggesting that body weight or fat is regulated. From a clinical viewpoint, this is likely to contribute to the difficulty that many people with obesity have in maintaining weight loss. Finding ways to modify these physiologic responses is likely to improve the long-term success of obesity treatments.

> At usual weight, energy intake and expenditure are coupled and covary to maintain body weight (energy stores). A change in energy balance, especially weight loss, invokes discoordinated effects on energy intake and output that favor return to previous weight. These regulatory systems reflect physiological changes in systems regulating energy intake and expenditure rather than a lack of resolve. The biological and behavioral

physiology of dynamic weight change are somewhat different from those of attempts at static weight maintenance of an altered body weight. This suggests that optimal therapeutic approaches to losing or gaining vs. sustaining weight changes are different for most individuals.

## Genetic Contributors to Obesity

Ramya Sivasubramanian and Sonali Malhotra

Genetic forms of obesity contribute to ∼7% of severe obesity in children and adolescents. The exact global prevalence of monogenic and syndromic forms of obesity is not well established, most likely due to missed or delayed diagnosis. The challenge in determining the prevalence can be attributed to the lack of consensus on identifying and evaluating symptoms of genetic defects in a timely manner and hence a vastly undertested patient population. Further large-scale and long-term studies are needed to advance the understanding of this unique phenotype of obesity and effective treatment options.

## Developmental Contributions to Obesity: Nutritional Exposures in the First Thousand Days

Allison J. Wu and Emily Oken

Obesity is prevalent and continuing to rise across all age groups, even children. As obesity is challenging to manage and treat, prevention is critical. Here, we highlight nutritional influences during periods of early developmental plasticity, namely the prenatal period and infancy, that have been shown to contribute to the development of obesity into childhood and beyond. We review recent research that examines maternal nutritional factors including dietary patterns and quality, as well as the infant diet, such as complementary foods and beverages, that influence long-term obesity risk. We end with recommendations for clinicians.

## Obesity, Chronic Stress, and Stress Reduction

Donald Goens, Nicole E. Virzi, Sarah E. Jung, Thomas R. Rutledge, and Amir Zarrinpar

The obesity epidemic is caused by the misalignment between human biology and the modern food environment, which has led to unhealthy eating patterns and behaviors and an increase in metabolic diseases. This has been caused by the shift from a "leptogenic" to an "obesogenic" food environment, characterized by the availability of unhealthy food and the ability to eat at any time of day due to advances in technology. Binge Eating Disorder (BED) is the most commonly diagnosed eating disorder, characterized by recurrent episodes of binge eating and a sense of loss of control over eating, and is treated with cognitive-behavioral therapy-enhanced (CBT-E). Shift work, especially night shift work, can disrupt the body's natural circadian rhythms and increase the risk of obesity and other negative health consequences, such as cardiovascular disease and metabolic syndrome. One dietary approach to address circadian dysregulation is time-restricted eating (TRE), which involves restricting food intake to specific periods of the day to synchronize the body's internal clock with the external environment. TRE has been found to cause modest weight loss and improve metabolic outcomes such as insulin sensitivity and blood pressure, but the extent to which it is beneficial may depend on adherence and other factors such as caloric restriction.

## Health Complications of Obesity: 224 Obesity-Associated Comorbidities from a Mechanistic Perspective                    363
Michele M.A. Yuen

Obesity is associated with a wide range of comorbidities that transverse multiple specialties in clinical medicine. The development of these comorbidities is driven by various mechanistic changes including chronic inflammation and oxidative stress, increased growth-promoting adipokines, insulin resistance, endothelial dysfunction, direct loading and infiltrative effect of adiposity, heightened activities of the renin-angiotensin-aldosterone system and sympathetic nervous system, impaired immunity, altered sex hormones, altered brain structure, elevated cortisol levels, and increased uric acid production, among others. Some of the comorbidities might develop secondary to one or more other comorbidities. Considering the obesity-associated comorbidities in the context of the mechanistic changes is helpful in understanding these conditions and in guiding treatment and future research.

## The Effects of Obesity on Health Care Delivery                    381
Amanda Velazquez and Caroline M. Apovian

The rates of obesity continue to rise among adults and children in the United States; hence, it is natural that obesity is reshaping health care delivery. This is seen in numerous ways, including physiologic, physical, social, and economic impacts. This article reviews a broad range of topics, from the effects of increased adiposity on drug pharmacokinetics and pharmacodynamics to the changes health care environments are making to accommodate patients with obesity. The significant social impacts of weight bias are reviewed, as are the economic consequences of the obesity epidemic. Finally, a patient case that demonstrates the effects of obesity on health care delivery is examined.

## Obesity and Viral Infections                    393
Priya Jaisinghani and Rekha Kumar

The 2019 novel coronavirus disease (COVID-19) triggered a rapidly expanding global pandemic. The presence of obesity in patients with COVID-19 has been established as a risk factor for disease severity, hospital admission, and mortality. Thus, it is imperative those living with obesity be vaccinated against COVID-19. Although there is a timeframe COVID-19 vaccines are efficacious in those living with obesity, more studies need to be conducted to ensure that those long-lasting protection is maintained, as obesity has implications on the immune system.

## The Effect of Obesity on Gastrointestinal Disease                    403
Jessica E.S. Shay and Amandeep Singh

Obesity exerts both direct and indirect effects on gastrointestinal function. From physical effects of central adiposity on intragastric pressure resulting in higher incidence of reflux to dyslipidemia and effects on gallstone disease, the gastrointestinal manifestations of obesity are wide-ranging. Of particular emphasis is the identification and management of non-alcoholic fatty liver disease including non-invasive assessment and lifestyle and pharmacologic interventions for patients with non-alcoholic steatohepatitis. Additional focus is on the impact of obesity and western diet on intestinal disorders and colorectal cancer. Bariatric interventions involving the gastrointestinal tract are also discussed.

Rebecca M. Puhl

Weight stigma is prevalent with negative consequences for health and well-being. This problem is present in health care; stigmatizing attitudes toward patients with obesity are expressed by medical professionals across diverse specialties and patient care settings. This article summarizes the ways in which weight stigma creates barriers to effective care, including poor patient-provider communication, reduced quality of care, and healthcare avoidance. Priorities for stigma reduction in healthcare are discussed, with a clear need for multifaceted approaches and inclusion of people with obesity whose perspectives can inform strategies to effectively remove bias-related barriers to patient care.

Tiffani Bell Washington, Veronica R. Johnson, Karla Kendrick, Awab Ali Ibrahim, Lucy Tu, Kristen Sun, and Fatima Cody Stanford

Obesity is a chronic disease and a significant public health threat predicated on complex genetic, psychological, and environmental factors. Individuals with higher body mass index are more likely to avoid health care due to weight stigma. Disparities in obesity care disproportionately impact racial and ethnic minorities. In addition to this unequal disease burden, access to obesity treatment varies significantly. Even if treatment options are theoretically productive, they may be more difficult for low-income families, and racial and ethnic minorities to implement in practice secondary to socioeconomic factors. Lastly, the outcomes of undertreatment are significant. Disparities in obesity foreshadow integral inequality in health outcomes, including disability, and premature mortality.

Gunther Wong and Gitanjali Srivastava

Obesity in the pediatric population is increasing in the United States and globally. Childhood obesity is associated with cardiometabolic and psychosocial comorbidities and decreased overall life span. The cause of pediatric obesity is multifactorial and includes genetic predisposition, lifestyle, behavioral patterns, and consequences of social determinants of health. Routine screening of BMI and comorbid conditions is essential to identifying patients who require treatment. The AAP recommends immediate Intensive Health Behavior and

Lifestyle Treatment for children with obesity, encompassing lifestyle changes, behavioral changes, and mental health treatments. Pharmacologic interventions and metabolic and bariatric surgery are also available when indicated.

The Federal Drug Administration has approved, following rigorous testing, 6 pharmacologic agents and one drug in device form for the management of overweight and obesity. Myriad products that purport to act on physiological mechanisms leading to weight loss also pervade the market with minimal regulatory oversight. Systematic reviews and meta-analyses of these products and their ingredients fail to establish any as meaningfully effective at the clinical level. Moreover, safety concerns prevail with adulteration, hypersensitivity reactions, and recognized adverse reactions. Lifestyle, pharmacologic, and bariatric surgical treatments are increasingly available, effective, and safe management tools for practitioners who should council patients, many of whom are susceptible to misinformation, on the lack effective and safe dietary supplements for weight loss.

Nutrition policies can work with clinical treatments to address the obesity epidemic. The United States has passed beverage taxes at the local level and calorie labeling mandates at the federal level to encourage healthier consumption. Nutritional changes to federal nutrition programs have been either implemented or suggested; evidence shows that the changes that have been implemented have resulted in improvements in diet quality and are cost-effective in decreasing the increase in obesity prevalence. A comprehensive policy agenda that addresses risk of obesity on multiple levels of the food supply will have meaningful long-term effects on obesity prevalence.

# GASTROENTEROLOGY
# CLINICS OF NORTH AMERICA

**SERIES OF RELATED INTEREST**

*Clinics in Liver Disease*
(Available at: http://www.liver.theclinics.com/)
*Gastrointestinal Endoscopy Clinics of North America*
(Available at: http://www.www.giendo.theclinics.com/)

**THE CLINICS ARE AVAILABLE ONLINE!**
Access your subscription at:
www.theclinics.com

# Foreword

# Fat Forward—What We've Learned About Obesity, Where We Are, and Where We Need to Go

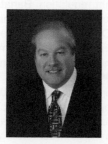

Alan L. Buchman, MD, MSPH
*Consulting Editor*

Fat has become a "big" public health issue. It's treated like a four-letter word, even though it is only three. As parodized by Weird Al Yankovic in his song, "Fat," numerous health consequences of what we now understand is a serious chronic disease, obesity, have been exposed as we understand more and more about the impact of fat mass. Obesity has become a global epidemic. We are now growing to understand the genetic and environmental contributions to obesity and its resultant effect on multiple organs.

We know that obesity may lead to or worsen diseases that affect nearly every organ system: endocrine (diabetes), gastrointestinal (nonalcoholic fatty liver disease, GERD, and gallstones), musculoskeletal (knee and hip weight-bearing issues), cardiovascular (atherosclerosis), neurologic (mild cognitive impairment), hematologic (increased risk for venous thrombosis), renal (hypertensive kidney disease), and respiratory (worsened asthma and asthma-like issues). Chronic inflammation related to obesity may also increase the risk of certain cancer development.

We've learned that obesity can affect medical care—not only by increasing the severity of infections and risk for postoperative complications but also by the ability to seek medical care may be impaired for obese individuals, as well as the interest of providers in providing care. Obesity may lead to discrimination, which may affect health care delivery; this in turn may lead to aggravation of the chronic illnesses associated with obesity and may also exacerbate obesity's effect on acute illnesses, including COVID-19 and other viruses. Obesity can be a stigma. It can affect relationships; childbearing and child rearing; job interviews, performance, and satisfaction; as well as overall quality of life. On the other hand, as being obese has also become more accepted in society, at least in some circles (eg, "About that Bass" by Meghan Trainor), where it is no longer a stigma, but that may lead to the opposite problem—acceptance of obesity and decreased drive and willingness to do something about it.

Furthermore, obesity is no longer just an adult problem, but increasingly it is recognized in childhood and in adolescents. Management is complex and involves a combination of behavioral, pharmacologic, endoscopic, and surgical care, all with lifelong follow-up to ensure compliance. The optimal therapy or combination of therapies has been elusive. Combating obesity requires a multifaceted approach. As we understand more about weight regulation, lifestyle alternations can become more effective for the prevention as well as for the treatment of obesity. In addition to lifestyle modifications, medications can be used to enhance appetite as well as weight regulation. Bariatric surgery has advanced, but less-invasive endoscopic approaches are becoming more refined. That's not the end of the problem, however. Once weight has been lost, maintenance of that weight loss requires a re-setting of energy balance—something medical science is now just beginning to understand; therapeutic approaches and maintenance of remission from obesity may require differing approaches.

Dr Kaplan has assembled a cadre of leading physicians and investigators in the first part of a two-part series wherein obesity is defined, the scope of the epidemic is described, and the complex interactions of obesity with society, medical care, and various important health issues are explained. This should help the gastroenterologist understand the effects of obesity not only on the gastrointestinal system but also in life in general from childhood to adulthood, and the role of the gastroenterologist in the recognition, treatment, and maintenance of therapy for the obese patient.

Alan L. Buchman, MD, MSPH
Intestinal Rehabilitation and Transplant Center
Department of Surgery/
UI Health University of Illinois at Chicago
840 South Wood Street
Suite 402 (MC958)
Chicago, IL 60612, USA

E-mail address:
buchman@uic.edu

# What is Obesity?
## Definition as a Disease, with Implications for Care

Jonathan Q. Purnell, MD, FTOS

## KEYWORDS

• Obesity • Chronic disease • Obesity treatment • Prognosis

## KEY POINTS

- Chronic diseases, including obesity, share similarities in how they are defined, conveyance of risk for adverse health outcomes, therapeutic approaches, need for lifelong treatment, and variable responsiveness to interventions.
- Obesity in unique amongst common chronic diseases in that pathophysiologic mechanisms include biologically driven alterations in behaviors (food intake, activity).
- Increased risk for the development of obesity complications can occur through an excess increase in total body fat, expansion of region fat depots, and accumulation of intra-organ (ectopic) fat, alone or in combination.
- Currently accepted clinical adiposity measures (body mass index, waist circumference) fail to capture the full spectrum of these distributions and subsequent risks, but remain mainstays of clinical care due to cost and ease-of-use.
- Obesity bias and stigma, including reluctance to consider medical and surgical weight management options, are common and need to be recognized and overcome in order to provide optimal patient management.

## INTRODUCTION

Normal health, reproduction, and survival are dependent on the availability of lipids. Lipids function as structural elements of cell membranes and lipoproteins, "sensing" molecules during nutrient absorption, key mediators of inflammation, immediate energy sources for skeletal and cardiac muscle, and long-term energy reserves in adipose tissue. Excessive lipid accumulation in the form of obesity or adiposity, however, has become the most common chronic disease in developed countries and is a primary driver in recent worldwide increases in noncommunicable diseases and health care costs.

Knight Cardiovascular Institute and Division of Endocrinology, Diabetes, and Clinical Nutrition, Oregon Health & Science University, Mailcode: HRC5N, 3181 Southwest Sam Jackson Park Road, Portland, OR 97239, USA
*E-mail address:* purnellj@ohsu.edu

Gastroenterol Clin N Am 52 (2023) 261–275
https://doi.org/10.1016/j.gtc.2023.03.001
0889-8553/23/© 2023 Elsevier Inc. All rights reserved.

gastro.theclinics.com

Obesity is clearly not a new phenomenon. Female figurines with obesity date back tens of thousands of years.[1] Yet, despite major scientific advances during the past 30 years in our understanding of the physiology of body weight regulation and the pathophysiology that leads to unwanted weight gain, obesity is often regarded as a modern lifestyle choice. A condition for which the patient bears sole responsibility and can turn around if they chose to do so. This chapter explores how obesity is like other chronic diseases commonly managed in the clinic and the implications of acknowledging this for patient care as well as the consequences of inaction.

## DEFINING A CHRONIC DISEASE

Historically, what constitutes a disease included a clinical manifestation in the form of a symptom, physical exam finding, or a laboratory abnormality. Coinciding with advances in public health measures, the development of effective antiinfectious agents, and increasing economic wealth, the leading causes of morbidity and mortality worldwide have shifted from "communicable" to "non-communicable diseases."[2]

However, most noncommunicable diseases, including diabetes and cardiovascular diseases, start off asymptomatic, may involve an alteration in only a single laboratory or vital sign, and may not exhibit organ damage for years. And while prevention is a common goal for both communicable and noncommunicable diseases, once manifested, treatment expectations for noncommunicable diseases do not automatically assume complete cure or disease resolution as expected for communicable diseases. Instead, noncommunicable diseases typically require lifelong commitments to combined lifestyle and pharmacologic interventions to which any individual may experience variable degrees of effectiveness and during which the underlying condition may progress or worsen despite the continuation of therapies.

Much has been written about operationalizing a definition for chronic disease,[3] including obesity.[4] For the most common chronic diseases, including hypertension, diabetes, and hypercholesterolemia, three essential elements can be identified (Table 1). First, these diseases arise from a normal physiology that typically regulates a vital life process. This could be blood pressure regulation, glucose and lipid metabolism, or oxygenation capacity. Second, this physiology changes, typically permanently, to become a pathophysiology involving a new, regulated set point that maintains a process outside of what is considered normal limits. For example, blood pressures shift toward higher levels (hypertension) or blood glucose levels increase (diabetes). Finally, as a result of this pathophysiologic shift in regulated levels, some impairment in health ensues, such as diabetic retinopathy, hypertensive renal disease, heart attack, or stroke. This health impairment need not occur immediately nor in all affected subjects to be labeled a chronic disease. From a public health perspective and in clinical care, identification of increase risk for an adverse health outcome is all that is needed. In this regard, chronic diseases can be risk factors for other chronic diseases. For example, diabetes risk is strongly linked with increasing body mass index (BMI), even extending down into overweight and normal ranges for both men and women,[5] and diabetes is a strong risk factor for cardiovascular diseases.[6] Understanding these relationships helps to focus preventive and treatment strategies on "upstream" conditions that reduce the incidence of "downstream" adverse outcomes.

It is well established that chronic diseases arise from interactions between environmental influences (typically lifestyle) and genetic predisposition,[7] that the earlier the disease onset the stronger the genetic influence,[8] that disease onset is variable by age and between sexes, that once set in motion they are often progressive in severity,[9] and that because of this, early intervention is key to reducing morbidly and mortality.

**Table 1**
Important features characterizing common chronic, non-communicable diseases

| | Type 2 Diabetes | Hyperlipidemia | Hypertension | Obesity |
|---|---|---|---|---|
| Normal physiology | Glucose regulation by insulin, glucagon. | Production and clearance of lipoprotein particles | Baroreceptor, renin-angiotensin-aldosterone system, and osmoreceptors governing blood pressure. | Gut-brain and adipocyte interactions sensing food intake, energy expenditure, and body weight. |
| Pathophysiology | Impaired insulin receptor signaling and insulin secretion. | Enhanced lipoprotein production, reduced clearance, or both. | Increased arteriole tone, abnormal salt handling. | Leptin resistance, absence or excess accumulation of regional and ectopic fat stores. |
| Impaired health | Microvascular and macrovascular complications. | Heart disease, peripheral vascular disease, chylomicronemia syndrome. | Hypertensive cardiomyopathy, stroke, chronic kidney disease. | Type 2 diabetes, cardiopulmonary impairment, hypertension, gastroesophageal reflux, dyslipidemia, obstructive sleep apnea, menstrual irregularity and male hypogonadism, osteoarthritis, fatty liver, and more. |

For example, patients with diabetes and hypertension pass through clinical phases now referred to a prediabetes[10] and prehypertension.[11] At these stages, lifestyle still holds promise to halt their progression and avoid damaging consequences.[12,13] However, the directionality of the pathophysiologic change is typically one-way. Meaning that most individuals may experience a small improvement or stabilization in their condition in response to lifestyle alone and, rarely, be able to restore normal physiologic ("set point") conditions. Even so, lifelong continuation of the lifestyle improvement is required for sustained benefit. If the intervention is stopped, then disease progression will again resume. Often, disease progression occurs despite the continuation of lifestyle therapy,[14] necessitating the addition of medical therapy or procedural intervention.

## Obesity as a Chronic Disease

### The physiology of normal weight regulation

Much of our current understanding of weight regulation emerged following the discovery of the adipocyte hormone leptin 30 years ago.[15] It is now known that body weight is governed through interactions between the brain and brainstem, gastrointestinal system, and fat depots to maintain weight levels within a narrow range over time despite wide variations in food availability and activity levels.[16] Gut hormonal signals released or inhibited during nutrient absorption carry signals to the brain reflecting the number of calories ingested and govern eating behaviors such as fullness (satiety) leading to meal cessation and feelings of hunger that trigger food seeking behaviors.[17] Leptin is released in proportion to the amount of fat storage (fat cell size and number) and signals the amount of available adipose stores to the brain. Alterations in calorie intake, energy expenditure, and fat mass are thus "sensed" by an interconnected network of brain centers that, in turn, integrates these signals and determines if adjustments in food intake and energy expenditure are necessary to maintain weight. These systems operate without conscious control and can, for a period of time, be willfully overridden, but will elicit continuous counter-regulatory forces until gut hormone and leptin levels (and body weight) are restored to their previous (preintervention) levels. Understandably, given the importance of maintaining adequate lipid stores for survival and reproduction, weight regulatory systems are complex and potent in their capacity for defending a weight set point.[18]

### Pathophysiologic alterations in leptin signaling lead to unwanted weight gain and hyperleptinemia

Although the exact molecular mechanisms are unknown, the fundamental, albeit oversimplified, pathophysiologic change that leads to positive energy balance and unwanted weight gain is the emergence of leptin resistance. Analogous to insulin resistance resulting in compensatory hyperinsulinemia, expression of leptin resistance[19] leads to increased food intake without adequate compensatory changes in energy expenditure, facilitating fat store expansion and leptin level increases until central neural leptin signaling is again restored at a new, higher, body weight set-point. In this way, expression of unwanted weight gain and obesity can be understood as a failure of the normal weight regulatory system to adequately "counter-regulate" in the face of rising adipose stores, and not the result of a patient simply making poor food choices, failing to exercise enough, or "overeating." This higher fat mass and accompanying leptin levels are then "defended" by these central nervous system centers against efforts to limit calories and increase energy expenditure, just as it was at the previous, lower weight set-point.[20–23] This can be misinterpreted to be a manifestation of a "remitting-relapsing" process analogous to auto-immune diseases or multiple-sclerosis, when in fact a true remission was never achieved. A better description is that the condition of obesity was being managed by the intervention, not cured. The set point was not permanently altered but instead remained elevated and continues to be the force behind the failure to maintain the lost weight.

It is worth noting that unique amongst chronic diseases, key mediators of the expression and maintenance of obesity include observable behaviors involving eating and activity. Although strong cultural and habitual influences govern these behaviors, motivation for food,[24] food-seeking behaviors including hunger,[25] satiety,[26,27] and spontaneous activity levels[28] all have underlying biologic bases and can be manipulated by pharmacologic and surgical weight loss interventions.[29,30] An analogous behavioral physiologic response is the activation of thirst mechanism during dehydration or hypernatremia in the regulation of blood pressure.[31] Because osmostat control of thirst is well accepted, however, even though a reduction in plasma volume through voluntary restriction of water ingestion can lower blood pressure, this is not an acceptable treatment for hypertension. Before these biologic bases governing eating and activity behaviors were understood, treatments for overweight and obesity focused exclusively on behavior modification techniques that inevitably failed to lead to sustained weight loss of more than a few percentage points.[32] Patients are often relieved to know that these behaviors are, in fact, controlling them rather than the other way around.

The natural history of unwanted weight gain and life course of obesity follows similar patterns as other chronic diseases. In order to develop obesity, patients experiencing unwanted weight gain transition from a healthy weight through a "pre-obese" state currently referred to as overweight. It is useful to think of overweight as a state of pre-obesity in the same way that we now recognize prediabetes and prehypertension as similar transitional states toward their respective disease states. Even though not all individuals within these categories progress to obesity, type 2 diabetes, or hypertension, respectively, they are recognized as being at high-risk to do so and therefore represent important opportunities for the prevention of disease progression through enhanced lifestyle intervention and, increasingly, pharmacologic therapies.

Although expression of overweight and obesity can occur at any age, obesity prevalence peaks in the fifth and sixth decades in both men and women.[33] Women are vulnerable to expressing unwanted weight gain during three hormonal transition stages: puberty, pregnancy, and menopause.[34] Genetics have a strong (up to 70%) influence on the determination of adult weight[35–37] with several studies show gene-dosing effects on both expression of,[38] and protection from,[39] obesity. The earlier the onset of excessive weight gain, the stronger the genetic influence.[8] Lifestyle can restrain or exacerbate the severity of weight gain, but in most cases has a limited capacity to alter one's body weight set point once obesity is expressed.[12,32,40] Because peak body weight may not be realized until later in life, a person with obesity who manages their weight through lifestyle, pharmacologic, or surgical interventions may experience weight regain despite continuing therapy. This can be understood as a progression of the underlying disease pathophysiology, in the same way that type 2 diabetes often progresses despite ongoing lifestyle or medical management as a result of a continued decline in beta-cell function.[9] Establishing a lifetime maximum weight (excluding pregnancy) during history taking is therefore important since many patients seek help after voluntary weight loss through some combination of a low-calorie diet and exercise, including during the preparatory period before metabolic-bariatric surgery. A life-time maximum body weight represents the best estimate for the weight set point that their brains consider normal and allows either reassurance of medical or surgical efficacy for these patients even though the best that is achieved is weight stability or prevention of weight regain.

Finally, in line with the management of other chronic diseases, it is predictable that weight loss responses will vary between patients regardless of the intervention.[41,42] No single lifestyle approach, antiobesity medication, or metabolic-bariatric procedure would be expected to be effective in all patients. For many patients, and those more severely affected, combinations of lifestyle, drug therapy, and procedures involving complementary and synergistic pathways will be necessary.[43,44]

### Impaired health consequences of overweight and obesity (adiposity)

Obesity is the level of fat mass accumulation that impairs health. Most commonly, this includes increased risk for, or worsening of, type 2 diabetes, hypertension, hyperlipidemia, obstructive sleep apnea, osteoarthritis, nonalcoholic fatty liver disease, structural and vascular heart disease and stroke, cancer, and many more adverse health conditions (**Fig. 1**).[45] Adverse health complications can result not only from excess total fat accumulation, but also increases in regional fat depots and ectopic lipid deposition, especially in liver and muscle. Although total, regional, and ectopic fat accumulation often occurs together, obesity complications also manifest from excess regional and ectopic lipid accumulation even when total fat stores are normal. For example, disproportionate enlargement visceral depots (abdominal, epicardial, and perirenal) are strongly associated with type 2 diabetes and heart disease.[46–49] In cases of extreme loss of subcutaneous fat, either partial or total lipodystrophies, accumulation of visceral fat and ectopic lipids can lead to severe metabolic disorders, including insulin-dependent diabetes, chylomicronemia syndrome, and heart disease.[50–52] Lipedema, the abnormal accumulation of subcutaneous fat of the lower abdomen, thighs, and lower extremities can be associated with chronic pain and joint dysfunction.[53] Excess lipid deposition in liver, muscle, and pancreas have been suggested to primary mediators of type 2 diabetes and, in the liver, are a precursor to nonalcoholic steatohepatitis and cirrhosis.[49,54]

Current clinical guidelines define overweight (that level of fat mass conferring intermediate risk for adverse health outcomes between normal weight and obesity) and obesity using indirect estimates of total and regional fat accumulation (body mass index or BMI, and waist circumference) that have been shown to convey increased risks

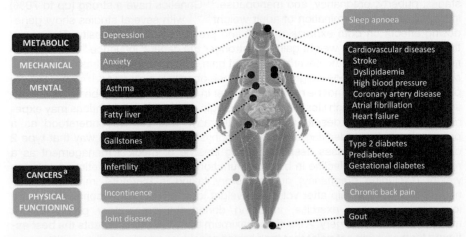

**Fig. 1.** Obesity-related complications. [a]Including breast, colorectal, endometrial, esophageal, kidney, ovarian, pancreatic and prostate. (*Courtesy of* Rachel Batterham, OBE, PhD, FRCP, London, UK.)

for obesity complications and mortality (**Table 2**).[55] These thresholds are lower in people of South and Southeast Asian origin,[56] where rates of obesity-related complications have been steadily increasing in conjunction with population-based weight gain.[57] Excess liver fat (nonalcoholic fatty liver disease) can often be detected by imaging techniques including abdominal ultrasound, computed tomography, and magnetic resonance imaging, or presumed when liver enzymes are elevated in the absence of other causes of hepatitis.[58]

In clinic and epidemiological studies, obesity has become synonymous with an increased BMI. However, because excess fat that leads to impaired health can occur with increased regional and ectopic lipids, a more inclusive term for levels to designate fat accumulation that impairs health would be adiposity. Ideally, the practitioner would have a means of estimating adiposity in the clinic that, in conjunction with a laboratory test indicating concurrent organ function or risk for future disease, would allow for the determination of prognosis and guide intervention based on outcomes studies using similar measurements. Practically, however, this would require a screening and monitoring tool that is low cost, easy to access, and available in the clinic, and allow for simultaneous estimation of all excess fat stores. The best current candidate for this would be whole-body magnetic resonance imaging.[59] However, cost, availability, and body size limitations currently preclude widespread use of this imaging modality in the clinic and as part of large outcomes studies.

Therefore, despite their limitations, BMI and waist circumferences remain the primary clinical measures in determining the presence of overweight and obesity in patients. As first-level screening tools, these measurements allow the identification of at-risk individuals in the same way that cholesterol levels are used in the management of cardiovascular risk, fasting blood glucose and hemoglobin A1c for diabetes risk and complications, and liver enzymes for liver disease screening. Each is highly standardized, widely available, and cost-affordable. However, it is acknowledged

**Table 2**
**Classification of overweight and obesity by BMI, waist circumference, and associated disease rihsks**

|  | BMI (kg/m²) | Obesity Class | Disease Risk[a] Relative to Normal Weight and Waist Circumference[c] | |
|---|---|---|---|---|
|  |  |  | Men 102 cm (40 in) or Less Women 88 cm (35 in) or Less | Men > 102 cm (40 in) Women > 88 cm (35 in) |
| Underweight | < 18.5 |  | - | - |
| Normal | 18.5–24.9 |  | - | - |
| Overweight | 25.0–29.9 |  | Increased | High |
| Obesity | 30.0–34.9 | I | High | Very High |
|  | 35.0–39.9 | II | Very High | Very High |
| Extreme Obesity | 40.0[b] | III | Extremely High | Extremely High |

[a] Disease risk for type 2 diabetes, hypertension, and CVD.
[b] Increased waist circumference also can be a marker for increased risk, even in persons of normal weight.
[c] For men of South and Southeast Asian origin, a waist circumference greater than 35.4 in and women from these groups, above 31.5 in are at high risk.

*Modified from* National Institute of Health - National Heart, Lung, and Blood Institute (NHLBI – NIH). Losing Weight, Body Mass Index. Available at https://www.nhlbi.nih.gov/health/educational/lose_wt/BMI/bmi_dis.htm.

that not all individuals with elevations in these measures progress to diabetes, end-stage liver disease, or experience a stroke or heart attack in their lifetime. Yet, they remain well-accepted screening tools in chronic disease management. As each of these tools undergoes refinement, thresholds that convey risk and guide the initiation of therapy will change. In the management of obesity, immediate refinement needs are in updating thresholds of BMI, WC, and ectopic fat measures for assigning risk for complications and initiating therapy. For example, the metabolic improvements from sleeve gastrectomy and gastric bypass extend below a BMI of 35 kg/m², [60] yet this has received only limited acceptance in current guidelines and by insurance providers. [61,62] And a BMI of 25 kg/m² may represent a current threshold for healthy weight status, but as obesity therapeutics advance and lower weight levels can be safely achieved, determining what is a healthy weight for an individual will likely include some combination of BMI, measurement of regional and ectopic fat, and status of an obesity-related complication. For example, management of weight in a patient with type 2 diabetes may allow for lowering weight below currently accepted thresholds for healthy BMI (<25 kg/m²) for further cardiometabolic improvement, especially in patients of Asian ancestry.

### Implications for Care of Those with Obesity (Adiposity)

Management of chronic diseases follows a standardized approach. Based on screening tests, lifestyle measures are initiated during preclinical phases. In those who progress to disease development, lifestyle is continued, and medical therapy begun. Although obesity has been recognized to be a chronic disease, it continues to be the only such condition in which medical or surgical approaches may be considered optional or "adjuncts" to lifestyle rather than essential next steps by many guidelines and practitioners. Doing so, however, limits those who would benefit from access to safe and effective therapies.

Side-stepping pharmacologic and surgical options for weight management even though they are available, effectively not treating obesity as a disease, is likely the result of a convergence of several factors: poor or misunderstanding of how body weight is regulated, limited office visit time, poor insurance reimbursement for obesity management, and often failure of insurance to cover costs for antiobesity medications or surgical procedures. [63,64] Even these factors, however, cannot fully explain reports that as little as 1% to 3% of eligible patients with overweight and obesity are appropriately being prescribed antiobesity medications [63] or referred for metabolic-bariatric surgery. [65]

An additional factor that is endemic in society, and by extension often into the medical community, is obesity stigma or bias—the assignment of blame to the patient for their condition and subsequent judgment of their behavior as inadequate or self-destructive. [66] Practitioners often enter their medical training having to "unlearn" these biases. In addition, pharmacologic and surgical treatment options are often perceived as "too extreme" or lack adequate safety profiles, despite evidence that these modalities result in meaningful and sustained improvements in weight, obesity complications, and reductions in total and disease-specific mortalities. [67–69] This obesity medical-surgical treatment hesitancy leads to an over reliance on lifestyle treatments alone and reinforces negative perceptions of people with obesity when, inevitably, target weight goals go unmet, and weight regain occurs.

Such societal bias and treatment hesitancy can change, however, as has happened with other stigmatized conditions, including HIV, mental illness, and substance abuse. Through better understanding of the integrated physiology of weight regulation with glucometabolic control, obesity can then become a primary target in the treatment of many other common chronic diseases, rather than a "modifiable" risk factor. For example, dyslipidemia, prediabetes, type 2 diabetes, nonalcoholic fatty liver disease, gastro-esophageal reflux, arthritis, sleep apnea, and heart failure can be prevented, significantly improved, or put into full remission with medical-surgical weight management,[70–75] especially when treatment is initiated early. In fact, these obesity complications often occur simultaneously, and targeting obesity can have a multiplicative effect to reduce overall drug burden and improve outcomes. It is important, however, that patients and providers understand obesity therapies are long-term and, if stopped, any benefits will be lost as patients regain their lost weight. Unfortunately, stopping an antiobesity medication after successful weight loss is still common. Subsequent weight regain is then labeled as "medication failure" or blamed on the patient, but this would be akin to successfully treating hypertension with an angiotensin-converting enzyme and then stopping it 3 months later and instructing the patient that "now you can manage it on your own."

As discussed above, weight loss in response to lifestyle, medical, or surgical interventions is variable. This is similar to other chronic diseases and, accordingly, treatment guidelines typically recommend combination therapies to achieve target goals. For example, once a hemoglobin A1c level crosses the 6.5% threshold, the American Diabetes Association recommends initially instituting metformin and lifestyle simultaneously (not waiting for the demonstration of the failure of lifestyle).[76] If target hemoglobin A1 is subsequent not met, or again rises after an initial response, metformin is continue and a decision algorithm guides the addition of other medications depending on patient characteristics.[76] It is now common to have patients with diabetes taking up to four different medications before initiating insulin. In weight management, this need for combination therapy has already been acknowledged by the fact that several currently approved antiobesity medications consist of two separate medications (Qysmia: phentermine and topiramate; and Contrave: bupropion and naltrexone). It is anticipated that as new evidence emerges, future obesity treatment guidelines will include not only additional medication combinations but also recommendations for medication treatment to accompany the pre- and postmetabolic-bariatric procedures to ensure optimal weight loss maintenance and health outcomes.

Failure to consider obesity as a disease also underlies the current debate about whether to offer weight loss treatment to those with "metabolically-healthy" obesity typically defined as those with obesity with normal blood pressure, lipid, and glucose levels. However, preclinical phases of diabetes and hypertension (prediabetes and prehypertension, respectively) are no longer considered benign conditions but, in fact, do convey risk for adverse outcomes including disease progression, microvascular damage, and increased macrovascular events.[77–80] Similar evidence exists for patients with metabolically healthy obesity, the vast majority of whom will convert over time to metabolically unhealthy status and have elevated risks for heart disease and strokes.[81,82] Delaying therapy also results in "pound-year" exposure and residual risk such that when therapy is finally begun, it will not be possible to reestablish normal status for many obesity complications, including osteoarthritis and heart disease.

Failure to acknowledge obesity as a disease has consequences for patient care when patients are excluded from coverage and, in many cases, life-saving therapies. This also becomes an equity issue since obesity disproportionately affects people living in lower socio-economic strata and who come from communities of color. Additional consequences include continued ballooning of health care expenditures in response to the rising incidences of obesity rates and complications,[83,84] delays in assigning research priorities into pathophysiologic mechanisms that could lead to novel new therapies, and failure to enact health care policy that could regulate environmental drivers of obesity pathophysiology,[85] which is vital for arresting and reversing the current worldwide trends in increasing obesity prevalence.

## SUMMARY

Body weight is regulated by a complex physiology involving multiple organ systems. Unwanted weight gain, abnormal distribution of fat, and accumulation of ectopic lipids represent pathophysiologic alterations to the physiologic weight set point that puts patients at risk for obesity complications. Unique to chronic diseases is the discovery of underlying biological signals and central neurocircuitry mediating behaviors (eating, spontaneous activity) that are drivers of the expression of obesity. These research breakthroughs provide the framework for the pharmacological and surgical management of patients with obesity. Advances in imaging, genetics, and biological markers will allow for further refinement of high-risk phenotypes than currently allowed by BMI and waist circumference.

In the chronic disease model, both prevention and treatment are important for patient management, and one should not be withheld or prioritized to the exclusion of the other. Preventive lifestyle strategies are vital to reversing the year-after-year increases in obesity prevalence now occurring in populations around the world and should be continued in those who progress to obesity. Implementation of antiobesity medications and metabolic-bariatric surgery to reduce patient and population-level obesity complications and mortality should be viewed as necessary, not optional, next steps when lifestyle alone is insufficient. Overcoming personal, cultural, and professional obesity stigma and communicating respectfully and empathetically with patients who are overweight and with obesity will be key to successful outcomes. As new evidence emerges, concepts of earlier initiation and combination medical and medical surgical therapies will no doubt become as standard as they are for the management of type 2 diabetes, hypertension, and heart disease.

## CLINICS CARE POINTS

- Manage obesity like other chronic diseases, starting with lifestyle in the overweight stage (preobesity), and then progressing to antiobesity medications and metabolic-bariatric procedures as indicated.

- Important for patient care are acknowledging obesity stigma and optimizing provider-patient communication using appropriate person-first language.

- A weight history will help identify medical and lifestyle contributors to obesity. Establishing lifetime maximal body weight can help determine treatment effectiveness.

- Body mass index and waist circumference are imperfect metrics but currently remain the best estimates of body adiposity and risk in the clinic setting.

- Once started, effective treatments are continued long-term, including antiobesity medications.

- Weight loss response will be variable to any individual treatment and unwanted weight gain may progress following an initial response. Therefore, combination therapy (drug-drug, drug-surgery) will be necessary for many patients to achieve optimal improvements in weight and obesity complications.

- Obesity management can be an initial treatment approach for many other chronic diseases, such as prediabetes, diabetes, dyslipidemia, fatty liver, and osteoarthritis.

## DISCLOSURE

J.Q. Purnell is a global advisory board member for Novo Nordisk and Boehringer Ingelheim. He is a scientific advisory board member for Luciole Pharmaceuticals.

## REFERENCES

1. Conard NJ. A female figurine from the basal Aurignacian of Hohle Fels Cave in southwestern Germany. Nature 2009;459(7244):248–52.
2. WHO. Noncommunicable diseases. Available at: https://www.who.int/health-topics/noncommunicable-diseases#tab=tab_1. Accessed August 1, 2022.
3. Goodman RA, Posner SF, Huang ES, et al. Defining and Measuring Chronic Conditions: Imperatives for Research, Policy, Program, and Practice. Preventing Chronic Dis 2013;10:E66.
4. Allison DB, Downey M, Atkinson RL, et al. Obesity as a disease: a white paper on evidence and arguments commissioned by the Council of the Obesity Society. Obesity (Silver Spring) 2008;16(6):1161–77.
5. Willett WC, Dietz WH, Colditz GA. Guidelines for healthy weight. N Engl J Med 1999;341(6):427–34.
6. Shah AD, Langenberg C, Rapsomaniki E, et al. Type 2 diabetes and incidence of cardiovascular diseases: a cohort study in 1.9 million people. Lancet Diabetes Endocrinol 2015;3(2):105–13.
7. Prentice AM. Obesity–the inevitable penalty of civilisation? Br Med Bull 1997; 53(2):229–37.
8. Loos RJF, Yeo GSH. The genetics of obesity: from discovery to biology. Nat Rev Genet 2022;23(2):120–33.
9. U.K. Progressive Diabetes Study Group. U.K. prospective diabetes study 16. Overview of 6 years' therapy of type II diabetes: a progressive disease. U.K. Prospective Diabetes Study Group. Diabetes 1995;44(11):1249–58.
10. Ackermann RT, Cheng YJ, Williamson DF, et al. Identifying adults at high risk for diabetes and cardiovascular disease using hemoglobin A1c National Health and Nutrition Examination Survey 2005-2006. Am J Prev Med 2011;40(1):11–7.
11. Chobanian AV, Bakris GL, Black HR, et al. The Seventh Report of the Joint National Committee on Prevention, Detection, Evaluation, and Treatment of High Blood Pressure: the JNC 7 report. JAMA 2003;289(19):2560–72.
12. Knowler WC, Barrett-Connor E, Fowler SE, et al. Reduction in the incidence of type 2 diabetes with lifestyle intervention or metformin. N Engl J Med 2002; 346(6):393–403.
13. Sacks FM, Svetkey LP, Vollmer WM, et al. Effects on blood pressure of reduced dietary sodium and the Dietary Approaches to Stop Hypertension (DASH) diet. DASH-Sodium Collaborative Research Group. N Engl J Med 2001;344(1):3–10.
14. United Kingdom Prospective Diabetes Study (UKPDS). 13: Relative efficacy of randomly allocated diet, sulphonylurea, insulin, or metformin in patients with newly diagnosed non-insulin dependent diabetes followed for three years. BMJ 1995;310(6972):83–8.
15. Zhang Y, Proenca R, Maffei M, et al. Positional cloning of the mouse obese gene and its human homologue. Nature 1994;372(6505):425–32.
16. Affinati A.H. and Myers M.G., Jr., Neuroendocrine control of body energy homeostasis, In: Feingold K.R., Anawalt B., Boyce A., et al., Endotext, 2000, MDText.com, Inc; South Dartmouth (MA), Copyright © 2000-2022, MDText.com, Inc., 1-38.

17. Pucci A. and Batterham R.L., Endocrinology of the gut and the regulation of body weight and metabolism, In: Feingold K.R., Anawalt B., Boyce A., et al., Endotext. South Dartmouth, 2000, MDText: Portland, Oregon, 1-29.
18. Schwartz MW, Seeley RJ, Zeltser LM, et al. Obesity Pathogenesis: An Endocrine Society Scientific Statement. Endocr Rev 2017;38(4):267–96.
19. Frederich RC, Hamann A, Anderson S, et al. Leptin levels reflect body lipid content in mice: evidence for diet-induced resistance to leptin action. Nat Med 1995; 1(12):1311–4.
20. Weigle DS, Brunzell JD. Assessment of energy expenditure in ambulatory reduced-obese subjects by the techniques of weight stabilization and exogenous weight replacement. Int J Obes 1990;14(Suppl 1):69–77, discussion 77-81.
21. Leibel RL, Rosenbaum M, Hirsch J. Changes in energy expenditure resulting from altered body weight. N Engl J Med 1995;332(10):621–8.
22. Sumithran P, Prendergast LA, Delbridge E, et al. Long-term persistence of hormonal adaptations to weight loss. N Engl J Med 2011;365(17):1597–604.
23. Fothergill E, Guo J, Howard L, et al. Persistent metabolic adaptation 6 years after "The Biggest Loser" competition. Obesity (Silver Spring) 2016;24(8):1612–9.
24. Wang GJ, Volkow ND, Fowler JS. The role of dopamine in motivation for food in humans: implications for obesity. Expert Opin Ther Targets 2002;6(5):601–9.
25. Wren AM, Seal LJ, Cohen MA, et al. Ghrelin enhances appetite and increases food intake in humans. J Clin Endocrinol Metab 2001;86(12):5992.
26. Batterham RL, Cowley MA, Small CJ, et al. Gut hormone PYY(3-36) physiologically inhibits food intake. Nature 2002;418(6898):650–4.
27. Naslund E, Barkeling B, King N, et al. Energy intake and appetite are suppressed by glucagon-like peptide-1 (GLP-1) in obese men. Int J Obes Relat Metab Disord 1999;23(3):304–11.
28. Teske JA, Billington CJ, Kotz CM. Neuropeptidergic mediators of spontaneous physical activity and non-exercise activity thermogenesis. Neuroendocrinology 2008;87(2):71–90.
29. Zink AN, Bunney PE, Holm AA, et al. Neuromodulation of orexin neurons reduces diet-induced adiposity. Int J Obes (Lond) 2018;42(4):737–45.
30. Bray GA, Heisel WE, Afshin A, et al. The Science of Obesity Management: An Endocrine Society Scientific Statement. Endocr Rev 2018;39(2):79–132.
31. Gizowski C, Bourque CW. Neurons that drive and quench thirst. Science 2017; 357(6356):1092–3.
32. Tsai AG, Wadden TA. Systematic review: an evaluation of major commercial weight loss programs in the United States. Ann Intern Med 2005;142(1):56–66.
33. Afshin A, Forouzanfar MH, Reitsma MB, et al. Health Effects of Overweight and Obesity in 195 Countries over 25 Years. N Engl J Med 2017;377(1):13–27.
34. Srivastava G., Kushner R.F., Apovian C.M., Use of the historial weight trajectory to guide an obesity-focused patient encounter. In: Feingold K.R., Anawalt B., Boyce A., et al., editors. Endotext. South Dartmouth (MA): 2000. MDText: Portland, Oregon, 1-18.
35. Stunkard AJHJ, Pedersen NL, McClearn GE. The body-mass index of twins who have been reared apart. N Engl J Med 1990;322:1483–7.
36. Stunkard AJ, Sorensen TI, Hanis C, et al. An adoption study of human obesity. N Engl J Med 1986;314(4):193–8.
37. Maes HH, Neale MC, Eaves LJ. Genetic and environmental factors in relative body weight and human adiposity. Behav Genet 1997;27(4):325–51.

38. Speliotes EK, Willer CJ, Berndt SI, et al. Association analyses of 249,796 individuals reveal 18 new loci associated with body mass index. Nat Genet 2010;42(11): 937–48.

39. Akbari P., Gilani A., Sosina O., et al., Sequencing of 640,000 exomes identifies GPR75 variants associated with protection from obesity, *Science*, 373 (6550), 2021, 1-11.

40. Levin BE, Keesey RE. Defense of differing body weight set points in diet-induced obese and resistant rats. Am J Physiol 1998;274(2):R412–9.

41. Gilis-Januszewska A, Barengo NC, Lindström J, et al. Predictors of long term weight loss maintenance in patients at high risk of type 2 diabetes participating in a lifestyle intervention program in primary health care: The DE-PLAN study. PloS one 2018;13(3):e0194589.

42. Kelly AS, Auerbach P, Barrientos-Perez M, et al. A Randomized, Controlled Trial of Liraglutide for Adolescents with Obesity. N Engl J Med 2020;382(22):2117–28.

43. Billes SK, Sinnayah P, Cowley MA. Naltrexone/bupropion for obesity: an investigational combination pharmacotherapy for weight loss. Pharmacol Res 2014; 84:1–11.

44. Miras AD, Perez-Pevida B, Aldhwayan M, et al. Adjunctive liraglutide treatment in patients with persistent or recurrent type 2 diabetes after metabolic surgery (GRAVITAS): a randomised, double-blind, placebo-controlled trial. Lancet Diabetes Endocrinol 2019;7(7):549–59.

45. Kyrou I., Randeva H.S., Tsigos C., et al., Clinical problems caused by obesity. In: Feingold K.R., Anawalt B., Boyce A., et al., editors. Endotext. South Dartmouth (MA): 2000. MDText: Portland, Oregon, 1-76.

46. Bray GA, Jablonski KA, Fujimoto WY, et al. Relation of central adiposity and body mass index to the development of diabetes in the Diabetes Prevention Program. Am J Clin Nutr 2008;87(5):1212–8.

47. Huang G, Wang D, Zeb I, et al. Intra-thoracic fat, cardiometabolic risk factors, and subclinical cardiovascular disease in healthy, recently menopausal women screened for the Kronos Early Estrogen Prevention Study (KEEPS). Atherosclerosis 2012;221(1):198–205.

48. Lu MT, Park J, Ghemigian K, et al. Epicardial and paracardial adipose tissue volume and attenuation - Association with high-risk coronary plaque on computed tomographic angiography in the ROMICAT II trial. Atherosclerosis 2016;251: 47–54.

49. Neeland IJ, Ross R, Després JP, et al. Visceral and ectopic fat, atherosclerosis, and cardiometabolic disease: a position statement. The Lancet Diabetes Endocrinol 2019;7(9):715–25.

50. Robbins DC, Horton ES, Tulp O, et al. Familial partial lipodystrophy: complications of obesity in the non-obese? Metabolism 1982;31(5):445–52.

51. Oral EA, Simha V, Ruiz E, et al. Leptin-replacement therapy for lipodystrophy. N Engl J Med 2002;346(8):570–8.

52. Akinci B., Sahinoz M., Oral E., Lipodystrophy syndromes: presentation and treatment. In: Feingold K.R., Anawalt B., Boyce A., et al., editors. Endotext. South Dartmouth (MA): 2000. MDText: Portland, Oregon, 1-35.

53. Herbst K.L., Subcutaneous adipose tissue diseases: dercum disease, lipedema, familial multiple lipomatosis, and madelung disease. In: Feingold K.R., Anawalt B., Boyce A., et al., editors. Endotext. South Dartmouth (MA): 2000. MDText: Portland, Oregon, 1-46.

54. Duell PB, Welty FK, Miller M, et al. Nonalcoholic Fatty Liver Disease and Cardiovascular Risk: A Scientific Statement From the American Heart Association. Arterioscler Thromb Vasc Biol 2022;42(6):e168–85.

55. Clinical Guidelines on the Identification, Evaluation, and Treatment of Overweight and Obesity in Adults–The Evidence Report. National Institutes of Health. Obes Res 1998;6(Suppl 2):51S–209S.

56. Appropriate body-mass index for Asian populations and its implications for policy and intervention strategies. Lancet 2004;363(9403):157–63.

57. Pan XF, Wang L, Pan A. Epidemiology and determinants of obesity in China. The Lancet Diabetes Endocrinol 2021;9(6):373–92.

58. Kanwal F, Shubrook JH, Younossi Z, et al. Preparing for the NASH epidemic: A call to action. Obesity (Silver Spring) 2021;29(9):1401–12.

59. Tejani S, McCoy C, Ayers CR, et al. Cardiometabolic Health Outcomes Associated With Discordant Visceral and Liver Fat Phenotypes: Insights From the Dallas Heart Study and UK Biobank. Mayo Clin Proc 2022;97(2):225–37.

60. Rubino F, Nathan DM, Eckel RH, et al. Metabolic Surgery in the Treatment Algorithm for Type 2 Diabetes: A Joint Statement by International Diabetes Organizations. Diabetes Care 2016;39(6):861–77.

61. Di Lorenzo N, Antoniou SA, Batterham RL, et al. Clinical practice guidelines of the European Association for Endoscopic Surgery (EAES) on bariatric surgery: update 2020 endorsed by IFSO-EC, EASO and ESPCOP. Surg Endosc 2020; 34(6):2332–58.

62. Mechanick JI, Apovian C, Brethauer S, et al. Clinical Practice Guidelines for the Perioperative Nutrition, Metabolic, and Nonsurgical Support of Patients Undergoing Bariatric Procedures - 2019 Update: Cosponsored by American Association of Clinical Endocrinologists/American College of Endocrinology, The Obesity Society, American Society for Metabolic and Bariatric Surgery. Obesity (Silver Spring) 2020;28(4):O1–58.

63. Thomas CE, Mauer EA, Shukla AP, et al. Low adoption of weight loss medications: A comparison of prescribing patterns of antiobesity pharmacotherapies and SGLT2s. Obesity (Silver Spring) 2016;24(9):1955–61.

64. Kaplan LM, Golden A, Jinnett K, et al. Perceptions of Barriers to Effective Obesity Care: Results from the National ACTION Study. Obesity (Silver Spring) 2018; 26(1):61–9.

65. Campos GM, Khoraki J, Browning MG, et al. Changes in Utilization of Bariatric Surgery in the United States From 1993 to 2016. Ann Surg 2020;271(2):201–9.

66. Rubino F, Puhl RM, Cummings DE, et al. Joint international consensus statement for ending stigma of obesity. Nat Med 2020;26(4):485–97.

67. Wilding JPH, Batterham RL, Calanna S, et al. Once-Weekly Semaglutide in Adults with Overweight or Obesity. N Engl J Med 2021;384(11):989–1002.

68. Marso SP, Bain SC, Consoli A, et al. Semaglutide and Cardiovascular Outcomes in Patients with Type 2 Diabetes. N Engl J Med 2016;375(19):1834–44.

69. Syn NL, Cummings DE, Wang LZ, et al. Association of metabolic-bariatric surgery with long-term survival in adults with and without diabetes: a one-stage meta-analysis of matched cohort and prospective controlled studies with 174 772 participants. Lancet 2021;397(10287):1830–41.

70. Courcoulas AP, King WC, Belle SH, et al. Seven-Year Weight Trajectories and Health Outcomes in the Longitudinal Assessment of Bariatric Surgery (LABS) Study. JAMA Surg 2018;153(5):427–34.

71. le Roux CW, Astrup A, Fujioka K, et al. 3 years of liraglutide versus placebo for type 2 diabetes risk reduction and weight management in individuals with prediabetes: a randomised, double-blind trial. Lancet 2017;389(10077):1399–409.
72. Blackman A, Foster GD, Zammit G, et al. Effect of liraglutide 3.0 mg in individuals with obesity and moderate or severe obstructive sleep apnea: the SCALE Sleep Apnea randomized clinical trial. Int J Obes (Lond) 2016;40(8):1310–9.
73. Armstrong MJ, Gaunt P, Aithal GP, et al. Liraglutide safety and efficacy in patients with non-alcoholic steatohepatitis (LEAN): a multicentre, double-blind, randomised, placebo-controlled phase 2 study. Lancet 2016;387(10019):679–90.
74. Purnell JQ, Dewey EN, Laferrere B, et al. Diabetes Remission Status During Seven-year Follow-up of the Longitudinal Assessment of Bariatric Surgery Study. J Clin Endocrinol Metab 2021;106(3):774–88.
75. Aminian A, Zajichek A, Arterburn DE, et al. Association of Metabolic Surgery With Major Adverse Cardiovascular Outcomes in Patients With Type 2 Diabetes and Obesity. JAMA 2019;322(13):1271–82.
76. ADAPP Committee. 9. Pharmacologic Approaches to Glycemic Treatment: Standards of Medical Care in Diabetes—2022. Diabetes Care 2021; 45(Supplement_1):S125–43.
77. Pan Y, Chen W, Wang Y. Prediabetes and Outcome of Ischemic Stroke or Transient Ischemic Attack: A Systematic Review and Meta-analysis. J Stroke Cerebrovasc Dis 2019;28(3):683–92.
78. Cai X, Zhang Y, Li M, et al. Association between prediabetes and risk of all cause mortality and cardiovascular disease: updated meta-analysis. BMJ 2020;370: m2297.
79. Carlsson LMS, Sjöholm K, Karlsson C, et al. Long-term incidence of microvascular disease after bariatric surgery or usual care in patients with obesity, stratified by baseline glycaemic status: a post-hoc analysis of participants from the Swedish Obese Subjects study. Lancet Diabetes Endocrinol 2017;5(4):271–9.
80. Huang Y, Wang S, Cai X, et al. Prehypertension and incidence of cardiovascular disease: a meta-analysis. BMC Med 2013;11:177.
81. Echouffo-Tcheugui JB, Short MI, Xanthakis V, et al. Natural History of Obesity Subphenotypes: Dynamic Changes Over Two Decades and Prognosis in the Framingham Heart Study. J Clin Endocrinol Metab 2019;104(3):738–52.
82. Eckel N, Li Y, Kuxhaus O, et al. Transition from metabolic healthy to unhealthy phenotypes and association with cardiovascular disease risk across BMI categories in 90 257 women (the Nurses' Health Study): 30 year follow-up from a prospective cohort study. The Lancet Diabetes Endocrinol 2018;6(9):714–24.
83. Ward ZJ, Bleich SN, Long MW, et al. Association of body mass index with health care expenditures in the United States by age and sex. PloS one 2021;16(3): e0247307.
84. Cawley J, Biener A, Meyerhoefer C, et al. Direct medical costs of obesity in the United States and the most populous states. J Manag Care Spec Pharm 2021; 27(3):354–66.
85. Wang Y, Zhao L, Gao L, et al. Health policy and public health implications of obesity in China. Lancet Diabetes Endocrinol 2021;9(7):446–61.

# Global Impact of Obesity

Nasreen Alfaris, MD, MPH[a],*, Ali Mohammed Alqahtani, MBBS[b],
Naji Alamuddin, MD, MTR, Diplomate ABOM[c], Georgia Rigas, MBBS FRACG[d]

## KEYWORDS

- Obesity • Epidemiology • Impact • Burden • Cost

## KEY POINTS

- The prevalence of obesity is rising globally.
- The review describes the global epidemiology of obesity including the alarming rise in childhood obesity and its consequences.
- The review also delves into the burden of the disease of obesity and explores the impact of obesity on health, quality of life, and economy.

## INTRODUCTION

The World health organization (WHO) defines obesity as an abnormal or excessive accumulation of fat that presents a risk to health. The WHO categorizes preobesity and obesity based on body mass index (BMI) categories (**Table 1**).[1] Despite the wide use of BMI for obesity, the standard obesity cut-off point ($\geq$30 kg/m$^2$) may not be suitable for non-Europids because of differing body (muscle: fat) compositions. Therefore, waist circumference may also be used to define obesity. Waist circumferences for different ethnic groups are outlined in **Table 2**.

Additionally, multiple epidemiologic studies have identified preobesity and obesity as predisposing factors to a number of noncommunicable diseases (NCD) including type 2 diabetes (T2DM), cardiovascular disease (CVD), and cancer. Obesity is also a major contributor to 120 million disability-adjusted life-years (DALYs).[2]

Unfortunately, despite unanimous commitment to halt the rise in preobesity and obesity, the prevalence of preobesity and obesity is rising globally (**Figs. 1** and **2**).[2]

In this review, we discuss the epidemiology of obesity in both children and adults in different regions of the world. We also explore the impact of obesity as a disease not only on physical and mental health but also its economic impact.

---

[a] King Fahad Medical City, 3895 Susah, Alwurud, Riyadh 12252-7111, Saudi Arabia; [b] King Fahad Medical City, PO Box 6855, Riyadh 13781, Saudi Arabia; [c] RCSI Bahrain, King Hamad University Hospital, Alsayh, Sheikh Eisa Bin Salman Bridge, 7J62+X92, Bahrain; [d] St George Private Hospital, 1 South Street, Kogarah, New South Wales 2217, Australia
* Corresponding author.
*E-mail address:* nasreen.alfaris@gmail.com

Gastroenterol Clin N Am 52 (2023) 277–293
https://doi.org/10.1016/j.gtc.2023.03.002
0889-8553/23/© 2023 Elsevier Inc. All rights reserved.

**gastro.theclinics.com**

**Table 1**
**Obesity classification by BMI for Europid individuals**

| Classification | BMI Cut-Off-Points (kg/m²⁾ |
|---|---|
| Healthy weight | 18.5–24.99 |
| Preobesity | 25–29.99 |
| Class I obesity | 30–34.99 |
| Class II obesity | 35–39.99 |
| Class III obesity | ≥40 |

## EPIDEMIOLOGY OF OBESITY
### Epidemiology in North America

Prevalence rates of adult obesity in North America have increased at an alarming rate in the last 50 years, making it currently the most common chronic disease (see **Fig. 1**).[3] According to the recent 2017 to 2018 National Health and Nutrition Examination Survey (NHANES), 31.1% of the US population have preobesity, 42.4% have obesity, and 9.0% have severe obesity.[4] While, the prevalence of preobesity has been stable since the 1960s, a disproportionate increase has been observed in those with severe obesity, being higher in women (11.5% vs 6.9%), and adults aged 40 to 59.[4] (see **Figs. 1** and **2**).

In Canada, no differences in obesity prevalence rates were observed between genders (26.9% men vs 27% women) however, preobesity disproportionately affects men (38.4% vs 28.5%).[5]

The prevalence of obesity varies based on several factors, including race, and ethnicity, gender, and level of educational attainment. In the US, obesity disproportionately affects African Americans and Hispanic adults (49.6% and 44.8% respectively). A higher proportion of non-Hispanic Black vs non-Hispanic White adults were found to have severe obesity (13.8% vs 9.3%). These higher prevalence ethnic groups were also noted to have higher rates of socioeconomic disadvantage and were less likely to have a college degree.[4]

When reviewing the prevalence rates in different racial groups across both genders, a divergence was observed among women, where the prevalence of obesity was highest for non-Hispanic Black women at 56.9%.[4]

**Table 2**
**International Diabetes Federation criteria for ethnic or country-specific values for waist circumference cut-off**

| Country and Ethnic Group | Sex | Waist Circumference (cm) |
|---|---|---|
| Europid | Men | >94 |
| | Women | >80 |
| South Asian | Men | >90 |
| | Women | >80 |
| Chinese | Men | >90 |
| | Women | >80 |
| Japanese | Men | >90 |
| | Women | >80 |

*Adapted from* Alberti KG, Zimmet P, Shaw J. Metabolic syndrome–a new world-wide definition. A Consensus Statement from the International Diabetes Federation. Diabet Med. 2006;23(5):469-480. https://doi.org/10.1111/j.1464-5491.2006.01858.x; with permission.

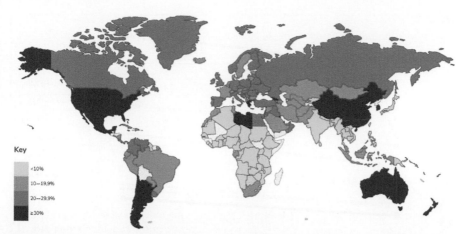

**Fig. 1.** Men living with obesity. (*Adapted from* World Obesity Federation, World Obesity Atlas 2022, Available at https://data.worldobesity.org/publications/World-Obesity-Atlas-2022.pdf; with permission.)

Geographical variations in obesity prevalence have also been observed, with the highest obesity rates seen in the southeast of the US. Obesity Prevalence ranged from 24.2% in Colorado to 39.7% in Mississippi.[6]

In Canada, there has been a 1.8% annual increase in adult obesity since 2010, and the prevalence is expected to be 38.5% of the adult population in 2030.[5] (**Figs. 3** and **4**)

### Epidemiology in Europe

In Europe, the prevalence of preobesity and obesity is estimated at 34% to 50% and 16% respectively, with wide country-to-country variations-particularly higher rates in Northern compared to Western/Southern European countries.[7] The highest prevalence of obesity in Europe occurred in Malta (28.7%) and the lowest in Romania (10.9%).[8]

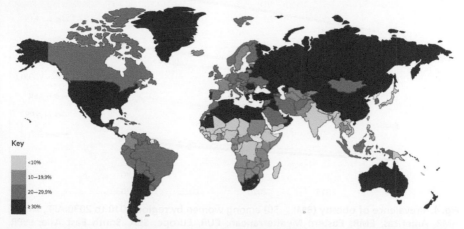

**Fig. 2.** Women living with obesity. (*Adapted from* World Obesity Federation, World Obesity Atlas 2022, Available at https://data.worldobesity.org/publications/World-Obesity-Atlas-2022.pdf; with permission.)

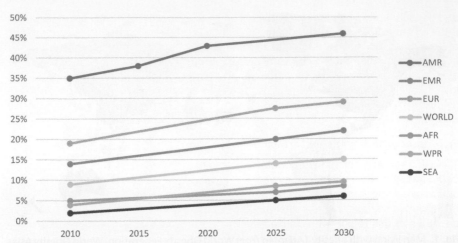

**Fig. 3.** Prevalence of obesity (BMI ≥ 30) among men by region 2010–2030. AFR, Africa; AMR, Americas; EMR, Eastern Mediterranean; EUR, Europe; SEA, South East Asia; WPR, Western Pacific Region. (*Adapted from* World Obesity Federation, World Obesity Atlas 2022, Available at https://data.worldobesity.org/publications/World-Obesity-Atlas-2022.pdf; with permission.)

These regional variations may be attributed to Europe's diversity, including considerable differences in geographical features, climate, language, history, economics, cultural traditions, territorial boundaries, social values and habits, food availability and norms about eating, physical features, physiology, and genetic predisposition.[9]

The European population is unique given the observed increased adult life expectancy and reduced birth rates compared to other regions. This demographic of aging population results in a rise in obesity prevalence rates well into the sixth decade of life,

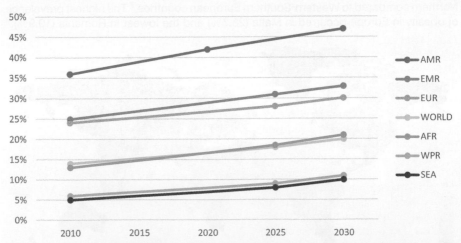

**Fig. 4.** Prevalence of obesity (BMI ≥ 30) among women by region 2010 to 2030. AFR, Africa; AMR, Americas; EMR, Eastern Mediterranean; EUR, Europe; SEA, South East Asia; WPR, Western Pacific Region. (*Adapted from* World Obesity Federation, World Obesity Atlas 2022, Available at https://data.worldobesity.org/publications/World-Obesity-Atlas-2022.pdf; with permission.)

and consequently a higher prevalence of sarcopenic obesity, currently estimated to be 20.2%.[10] Individuals with sarcopenic obesity tend to have higher rates of morbidity and mortality, possibly attributed to a reduction in anabolic metabolism and increased catabolism in older adults.[11] Several studies have projected that the European prevalence rates of obesity will be highest in the UK (37%) and Ireland (36%), with the lowest levels expected for men in The Netherlands (28%) and for women in Denmark (24%).[12,13] Obesity rates continue to increase in the European continent (see **Figs. 3** and **4**)

## Epidemiology in the Middle East and North Africa

The MENA region constituent countries share a variety of cultural and environmental characteristics. Nonetheless, they vary greatly in terms of their gross domestic product, socio-demographic profiles, and health care systems.[14] Obesity is considered a major public health concern in the MENA region as recent data demonstrated that six countries of this region were ranked among the top 20 countries globally in obesity prevalence particularly upper-middle-income countries in the region, with a higher predilection for women (**Table 3**).[15–17]

The rate of increase is also concerning as seen in Oman and Morocco where obesity rates among men increased from 2% to 23% and 10% to 33% in women respectively in four decades.[18] Furthermore, the gender gap in BMI has narrowed or reversed in some countries as men gain more weight than women. Obesity prevalence rates appear to increase significantly at the age of 40.[19]

Factors contributing to the MENA region's obesity epidemic include sedentary eating habits, physical inactivity, cultural, social, and economic changes, and urbanization.[15,20]

Obesity prevalence in the MENA region is predicted to continue to increase; it is estimated that by 2030, 21.7% of men and 33.2% of women will have obesity.[20] Obesity rates continue to increase in the MENA region (see **Figs. 3** and **4**); It is estimated that by 2030, 21.7% men and 33.2% women will have obesity.[20]

## Epidemiology in Sub-saharan Africa

The United Nations Development Program identifies 46 of Africa's 54 countries as "sub-Saharan."[21]

SSA has the fastest population growth rate of any major region, and the total population is expected to double by 2050.[22] This area of the world is considered to have the extremes of malnutrition, namely the coexistence of both undernutrition and overnutrition.[23]

Male obesity prevalence rates ranged from 16% in South Africa to 1.9% in Uganda, the latter being the lowest worldwide. Conversely, female obesity prevalence rates ranged from 41% in South Africa to 7.3% in Ethiopia.[20]

The literature on the impact of socioeconomic status on obesity within SSA is modest and conflicting.[24,25] However, it has been reported that women living in urban areas are more prone to obesity and BMI increases than those in rural settings.[25,26] Consequently, this has led to the highest urban excess BMI worldwide. This finding could be explained by the persistence of manual farming activities (particularly among women) and a lack of transportation in rural areas due to poor infrastructure. In contrast, employment in offices, the use of modern transportation methods, and the substitution of healthy food with processed food were the primary drivers of this disproportionate BMI increase.[27]

The overall prevalence of obesity among women and men in SSA is predicted to reach 20% of the population by 2030 (see **Figs. 3** and **4**). Furthermore, some SSA

**Table 3**
Countries with the highest obesity prevalence adapted from World Obesity Federation (WOF) Rankings

| Ranking | % Obesity (Men) | % Obesity (Women) | % Obesity (Children) |
|---|---|---|---|
| 1 | Nauru (59.85%) | American Samoa (65.32%) | Cook Islands (33.30%) |
| 2 | American Samoa (58.75%) | Nauru (64.81%) | Nauru (33.14%) |
| 3 | Cook Islands (53.97%) | Cook Islands (60.85%) | Palau (31.92%) |
| 4 | Palau (53.15%) | Palau (60.48%) | Niue (30.87%) |
| 5 | Marshall Islands (49.85%) | Marshall Islands (59.02%) | American Samoa (30.58%) |
| 6 | Tahiti (French Polynesia) (48.89%) | Tuvalu (57.85%) | Tahiti (French Polynesia) (29.09%) |
| 7 | Tuvalu (48.47%) | Tahiti (French Polynesia) (56.90%) | Marshall Islands (25.79%) |
| 8 | Niue (46.17%) | Niue (56.77%) | Tuvalu (25.60%) |
| 9 | Kiribati (42.87%) | Samoa (56.62%) | Kuwait (25.35%) |
| 10 | Tonga (42.72%) | Tonga (56.06%) | Tokelau (24.15%) |
| 11 | Federated States of Micronesia (41.48%) | Federated States of Micronesia (53.17%) | Tonga (23.76%) |
| 12 | Tokelau (41.40%) | Tokelau (52.18%) | United States (23.29%) |
| 13 | Samoa (41.28%) | Kiribati (51.96%) | Kiribati (22.47%) |
| 14 | United States (36.47%) | Kuwait (47.08%) | Qatar (22.14%) |
| 15 | Kuwait (34.28%) | Qatar (44.60%) | Bermuda (21.94%) |
| 16 | Qatar (33.46%) | Jordan (44.60%) | Argentina (20.76%) |
| 17 | Saudi Arabia (31.73%) | Saudi Arabia (43.74%) | Puerto Rico (20.55%) |
| 18 | New Zealand (31.07%) | Bermuda (43.17%) | Samoa (19.85%) |
| 19 | Australia (30.57%) | Egypt (42.48%) | Federated States of Micronesia (19.72%) |
| 20 | Canada (30.47%) | United Arab Emirates (42.46%) | Saudi Arabia (19.69%) |

*Adapted from* World Obesity Federation, World Obesity Atlas 2022, Available at https://data.worldobesity.org/publications/World-Obesity-Atlas-2022.pdf; with permission.

countries with a strong pace of urbanization are predicted to attain greater rates, with South Africa expected to reach 50% of the female population.[28]

### Epidemiology in Southeast Asia

The WHO SEA region represents over a quarter of the world's population, and obesity prevalence estimates are greatly distorted by India, whose population accounts for the majority of the SEA's population.[29] Countries in the SEA are in a state of nutrition transition, with the growing paradox of under-nutrition and obesity in the same population, being driven by the flourishing economic development and urbanization which have led to lifestyle changes.

Obesity prevalence in SEA shows great variability however with a predilection for women; the Maldives (19.7% women, 12.9% men) having the highest to Nepal (9.2% women, 5.1% men) having the lowest.[28]

Whilst SEA has some of the lowest prevalence of preobesity and obesity globally, the region is seeing an alarming trend in the rates of increase in the last 10 to 15 year.[30,31] In particular, Thailand and Indonesia prevalence rates are rapidly growing and anticipated to reach 20% and 14% in women, and 11% and 8% men respectively by 2030.[28]

Obesity prevalence in individual SEA countries varies from rural to urban and statewise due to various factors including heterogenelty in customs, dietary pattern, lifestyle, geographical condition, and economic development. For example, NCD risk factor surveillance reported that the prevalence of obesity was highest in South India (27.2%) followed by North India (23.8%) and lowest in West India (15%).[32]

Obesity Prevalence is projected to continue to increase, with a predicted 1 in 20 men and 1 in 11 women to be living with obesity by 2030 (see **Figs. 3** and **4**).

### Epidemiology in the Western Pacific Region

The WHO WPR comprises of 37 constituents who vary in their population density, such as China (1.4 billion) and Niue (1,000). Like other areas of the world, Some of the WPR countries are in a state of nutrition transition.[33]

Obesity prevalence in WPR shows great variability from American Samoa (80.1% women, 69.3% men) having the highest to Viet Nam Viet Nam (5% women, 3.9% men) having the lowest.[34]

It should be noted that the WPR prevalence estimates are greatly distorted by China, whose population accounts for the majority of the WPR's population.[29]

The socioeconomic context is believed to promote increased consumption of highly processed foods of low nutritional value, in addition to decreased opportunities for safe physical activity and active transportation.

Furthermore, in some cultures, traditional gender norms may confer differing expectations, roles/opportunities between genders for example, may preclude women from participating in physical activities, or privilege men with unrestricted access to foods considered as rewards.[33]

An obvious gender demarcation in obesity prevalence exists in Pacific Islander Territories, with a predilection toward women. In these territories different sociocultural factors might affect the gender disparities; for example, larger female body size is perceived to represent greater fertility.[33]

The prevalence of adult preobesity and obesity tends to be higher among women than men in most low- and middle-income countries (LMIC) in the WPR. However, the reverse is observed in high-income countries (HIC) including Australia, Hong Kong, Japan, and New Zealand.[35]

In the WPR the prevalence of preobesity and obesity in urban vs rural areas varies significantly and shows large disparities across different geographical areas within countries but do not show a clear pattern of how these disparities might be explained.

However, a 2021 study in China showed that the prevalence of adult preobesity/obesity was significantly higher in the rural population (25.4%), compared to populations in urban areas (21.2%). The differences were particularly observed among women, ethnic minorities, and among people in the lowest socioeconomic status. Furthermore, the mean BMI was persistently lower in women with higher levels of education compared with women with lower levels of education, but the inverse was true among men.[36,37]

Across the WPR around 1 in 10 men and 1 in 8 women are predicted to have obesity by 2030 (see **Figs. 3** and **4**).[28]

## IMPACT OF OBESITY
### Childhood Obesity

The WHO definition of child and adolescent preobesity and obesity is a BMI greater than 1 or 2 standard deviations above the median respectively, utilizing BMI for age and gender percentiles.[35,38]

Childhood obesity prevalence has doubled in more than 70 countries since 1980 and is predicted to affect 254 million children by 2030 (**Fig. 5**).[39] women are at a high risk of developing obesity secondary to their hormonal status.[40]

Many prenatal/early life experiences have been identified as contributing to the development of obesity.[41,42]

Children with preobesity or obesity are more likely to experience negative metabolic, mental health, and social sequelae (**Fig. 6**) These complications are often detected as early as in childhood, with more than half having ≥ 1 and one-quarter having ≥2 biochemical or clinical cardiovascular risk factors.[43] Large prospective cohort studies show that the duration of obesity is independently associated with an increased risk of developing T2DM.[44]

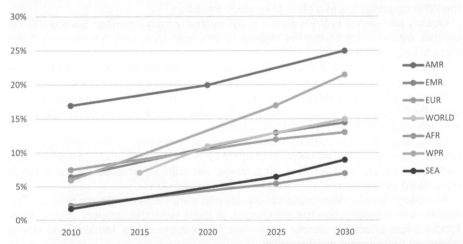

**Fig. 5.** Prevalence of obesity (BMI≥30 kg/m2) among children (5–19) globally in 2010 to 2030.AFR, Africa; AMR, Americas; EMR, Eastern Mediterranean; EUR, Europe; SEA, South East Asia; WPR, Western Pacific Region. (*Adapted from* World Obesity Federation, World Obesity Atlas 2022, Available at https://data.worldobesity.org/publications/World-Obesity-Atlas-2022.pdf; with permission.)

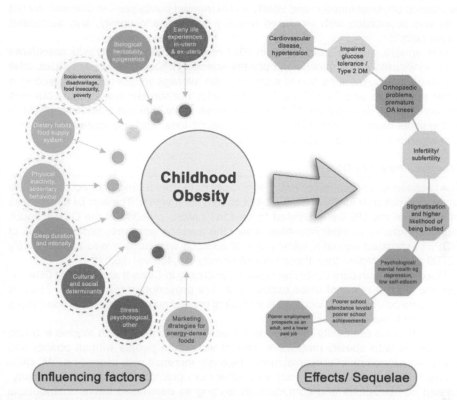

Influencing factors    Effects/ Sequelae

**Fig. 6.** Childhood obesity controllable influencing factors and selected effects on health. (*From* Weihrauch-Blüher S, Wiegand S. Risk Factors and Implications of Childhood Obesity. Curr Obes Rep. 2018;7(4):254-259; with permission.)

Many adolescents living with obesity continue to do so into adulthood, with increased morbidity and mortality due to cardiovascular, metabolic, or oncological disorders.[45–47]

In most LMIC, children from lower-income households are less likely to be living with preobesity/obesity; the opposite being true in HIC. The prevalence of childhood pre-obesity/obesity within individual countries shows heterogeneity among different ethnic groups and between geographical areas due to differences in customs, dietary patterns, lifestyle, geographical condition, and economic development.

## Impact on Health-Related Quality of Life

Health-related quality of life (HRQoL) is a multidimensional measure, encompassing emotional, mental health, physical, general health, social functioning, bodily pain, and subjective feelings of well-being which reflect an individual's subjective evaluation and reaction to health or illness.[48] One of the main reasons for seeking treatment of obesity is self-perceived reduction in quality of life.[49]

The impact of obesity on HRQoL is well documented in several studies.[49] The largest one being the Nurses Health Study which found that higher BMI was associated with more impairment in HRQoL. When the questionnaire was administered to the same group 4 years later, they found that weight gain was associated with decreased physical function and vitality and increased bodily pain. In contrast, weight loss was associated with increased physical function and vitality, and decreased bodily pain.[50]

Furthermore, a systematic review in 2017 reported that (i) obesity was associated with significantly lower generic and obesity-specific HRQoL (ii) improve HRQoL after bariatric surgery, perhaps due to a greater than average weight loss compared with other treatments and (iii) HRQoL improved after nonsurgical weight loss, but was not consistently demonstrated.[49] Currently newer, more effective antiobesity pharmacotherapies have yielded more significant weight loss, and associated greater improvements in reported HRQoL measures.[51,52]

### Economic Impact of Obesity

The economic impact of obesity, including both direct and indirect costs, are significant-not only for the individual, but society as a whole. The annual direct costs of obesity in the US are estimated to be $147 billion, or 9.3% of the GDP,[53] much higher compared to other countries, where the average economic cost is ~1.8% of GDP.[54] Estimated annual medical costs of an adult with obesity was approximately $2700 per year higher than those without obesity ($4,458 vs1,763).[55]

The direct health care costs rise rapidly particularly in Class II and Class III Obesity, and the biggest driver of these excess costs are prescription medications.[56] Higher health care costs are also incurred as a result of greater number of hospital admissions and longer hospital stays.[57,58]

Indirect costs of obesity result from decreased productivity, with studies showing that people with obesity miss more days of work than people without obesity and are at increased risk of unemployment; the costs increase with ascending BMI categories.[59] People with obesity may also suffer from premature death due to obesity-related complications and comorbidities leading to decreased future contributions to economy.[60]

Despite better scientific understanding of obesity as a disease not a lack of willpower, the ensuing weight stigma has resulted in people living with obesity being less likely to participate in opportunistic health screening programs.[61] Consequently, they present with more advanced stages of disease at the time of diagnosis.[62,63] The indirect costs associated with weight stigma and bias whilst important, are difficult to quantify.

### Health Impact of Obesity

Obesity affects the health of individuals in different ways: (i) metabolic for example, T2DM, hypertension, cardiovascular disease, nonalcoholic fatty liver disease (NAFLD), infertility, and sexual dysfunction, (ii) mechanical for example, Obstructive sleep apnea (OSA), osteoarthritis, gastroesophageal reflux and/or (iii) mental health sequelae (depression, anxiety, and so forth). **Fig. 7** reports the relative risk of obesity for developing different health conditions.

### T2DM

The burden of disease because of concurrent obesity and T2DM is significant. Approximately 50% to 90% of people with T2DM have either preobesity or obesity, while people with a BMI of more than 35 kg/m$^2$ are 20 times more likely to develop T2DM than those with a healthy BMI.[64] Obesity is closely linked with poor metabolic control in patients with T2DM, putting them at a greater risk of developing various microvascular and macrovascular complications associated with T2DM, thereby further increasing their burden of disease.[65] Weight loss can lead to both regression

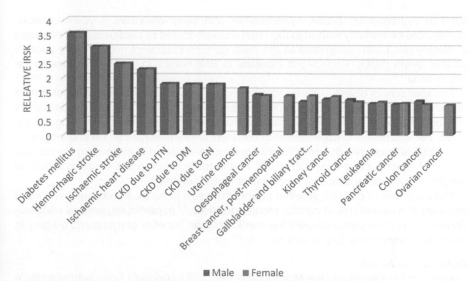

■ Male  ■ Female

**Fig. 7.** Relative risks of high body mass index (BMI) for different conditions.CKD, Chronic Kidney Disease; DM, Diabetes Mellitus; GN, Glomerulonephritis. (*Data from* GBD 2015 Obesity Collaborators, Afshin A, Forouzanfar MH, et al. Health Effects of Overweight and Obesity in 195 Countries over 25 Years. N Engl J Med 2017;377(1):13-27. doi:10.1056/NEJMoa1614362.)

of prediabetes to normoglycemia that is, diabetes prevention, and in some circumstances T2DM remission.[66,67]

### Nonalcoholic fatty liver disease /nonalcoholic steatohepatitis

NAFLD affects 20% to 25% of the adult population globally.[68] The rising prevalence and severity of NAFLD are closely associated with the rising obesity epidemic.[69] Approximately 60% to 90% of adults with obesity have evidence of NAFLD.[70,71] The spectrum of this disease ranges from simple steatosis to advanced disease such as NASH, cirrhosis associated with NASH, and hepatocellular cancer.

In recent years, NASH has been identified as the most common reason for liver transplant in the US and other countries with high prevalence rates of obesity.[72,73] In addition to increasing overall mortality, obesity appears to worsen liver-specific morbidity and mortality in people with NAFLD.[69]

### Obesity and cancer

A causal relationship has been established between high BMI and the development of several types of cancer, including those of the uterus, breast, esophagus, gallbladder and biliary tract, kidney, ovary, pancreas, thyroid, and colon cancers.[2,74,75] High BMI has been linked to approximately 90,000 cancer deaths in the United States each year, which could be averted if obesity was treated appropriately.[76]

The prevalence of different cancers in people living with obesity also varies between the genders, with uterine cancer being most prevalent in women and esophageal cancer most prevalent in men.[2]

### Cardiovascular diseases

The presence of obesity increases a person's risk of developing cardiovascular disease; the risk increases when combined with other obesity-related complications such as dyslipidemia, T2DM, hypertension, and sleep disorders.[77] While approximately 70% of mortality related to high BMI were attributed to cardiovascular diseases 2, obesity has been recognized as the most common cause of nonischemic sudden cardiac death (SCD). Each 5-unit increase in BMI results in a 16% increase in the risk of SCD.[78]

The spectrum of obesity-related cardiovascular diseases includes, but is not limited to, atherosclerosis, heart failure, and cardiac arrhythmia.[76] Additionally, obesity not only contributes to cardiovascular disease but also creates barriers to making a diagnosis. For example, the assessment of coronary artery disease can be challenging in individuals with obesity due to ECG changes that are related to increasing the cardiac workload among other mechanisms.[79] Furthermore, there are the practicalities of weight or body dimension limits for various investigations.

The treatment of obesity, whether pharmacological or surgical, has been shown to decrease the overall risk of cardiovascular diseases.[77] In particular, several observational studies have demonstrated the cardiovascular benefits of metabolic surgery in adults with concurrent T2DM and obesity.[80]

### Reproductive health

Obesity profoundly affects the reproductive health of individuals living with obesity. A cohort study estimated the risk of infertility in women living with obesity of childbearing age to be approximately 78% when compared to those with a healthy BMI.[81] It has been reported that for every one-unit increase in BMI, a women's pregnancy rates fall by around 4%.[82] Furthermore, obesity can lower the response rate of assisted reproductive technologies and increases the risk of miscarriage. If a viable pregnancy does occur, the presence of maternal obesity increased the risk of maternal and fetal complications during the pregnancy and during delivery.[83]

Given that obesity affects the hypothalamic–pituitary–gonadal axis, it follows that it will also impact male fertility and subsequent reproductive capacity. Moreover, obesity from either parent can contribute to epigenetic changes which can be transferred to the future generations.[84]

### Musculoskeletal health

Obesity is linked with significant mobility impairment and a variety of musculoskeletal symptoms, which can result in disability and a reduction in HRQoL.[85] Musculoskeletal disorders associated with high BMI are considered the second leading cause of global disability (after T2DM), accounting for 5.7 million years lived with disability globally.[2] Osteoarthritis, low back pain, gait disturbance, osteoporosis, and soft tissue problems are just some of the musculoskeletal conditions associated with obesity.[86] It is estimated that one-fourth of all osteoarthritis surgeries could be avoided by addressing obesity alone.[87]

A randomized controlled trial showed that a 10% reduction in weight led to an improvement in symptoms and physical functioning by 28% which is clinically meaningful.[88]

### SUMMARY

This review describes the global high prevalence of obesity and explores the impact that preobesity and obesity have on the health of people living with the disease. This review illustrates how the burden of obesity as a disease is rising globally which highlights the need for action to have accessible interventions to treat obesity in order to help reduce the prevalence of the disease and in turn decrease the global burden of obesity.

## CLINICS CARE POINTS

- The prevalence of pre obesity and obesity is rising globally.
- Pre- obesity and obesity predispose to a number of non-communicable diseases including T2DM, cardiovascular disease, and cancer.
- Childhood obesity prevelance has doubled in more than 70 countries since 1980 and is associated with negative metabolic, mental health and social sequelae.
- The economic impact of obesity includes both direct and indirect costs and rises rapidly in class II and class III obesity.

## REFERENCES

1. Available at: https://www.who.int/health-topics/obesity#tab=tab_1. Accessed June 11, 2022.
2. Afshin A, Forouzanfar MH, Reitsma MB, et al. Health Effects of Overweight and Obesity in 195 Countries over 25 Years. N Engl J Med 2017;377(1):13–27.
3. Flegal KM, Carroll MD, Ogden CL, et al. Prevalence and trends in obesity among US adults, 1999-2008. JAMA 2010;303(3):235–41.
4. Hales CM, Carroll MD, Fryar CD, et al. Prevalence of Obesity and Severe Obesity Among Adults: United States, 2017-2018. NCHS Data Brief 2020;360:1–8.
5. Canadian Health Measures Survey (CHMS) 2017. Available at: https://www150. statcan.gc.ca/t1/tbl1/en/tv.action?pid=1310037301&pickMembers%5B0%5D=3.3. Accessed May 17, 2022.
6. Centers for Disease Control and Prevention NCfCDPaHP, Division of Population Health. BRFSS Prevalence & Trends Data [online]. 2015. Available at: https:// www.cdc.gov/brfss/brfssprevalence/. Accessed May 17, 2022.
7. Gallus S, Lugo A, Murisic B, et al. Overweight and obesity in 16 European countries. Eur J Nutr 2015;54(5):679–89.
8. Available at: https://data.worldobesity.org/tables/prevalence-of-adult-overweight-obesity-2. Accessed April 6,2022.
9. Blundell JE, Baker JL, Boyland E, et al. Variations in the Prevalence of Obesity Among European Countries, and a Consideration of Possible Causes. Obesity Facts 2017;10(1):25–37.
10. Ethgen O, Beaudart C, Buckinx F, et al. The Future Prevalence of Sarcopenia in Europe: A Claim for Public Health Action. Calcif Tissue Int 2017;100(3):229–34.
11. Ahima RS. Metabolic syndrome: a comprehensive textbook. USA: Springer; 2016.
12. Pineda E, Sanchez-Romero LM, Brown M, et al. Forecasting Future Trends in Obesity across Europe: The Value of Improving Surveillance. Obesity Facts 2018;11(5):360–71.
13. Janssen F, Bardoutsos A, Vidra N. Obesity Prevalence in the Long-Term Future in 18 European Countries and in the USA. Obesity Facts 2020;13(5):514–27.
14. Burden of obesity in the Eastern Mediterranean Region: findings from the Global Burden of Disease 2015 study. Int J Public Health 2018;63(Suppl 1):165–76.
15. Al-Daghri NM, Al-Attas OS, Alokail MS, et al. Diabetes mellitus type 2 and other chronic non-communicable diseases in the central region, Saudi Arabia (Riyadh cohort 2): a decade of an epidemic. BMC Med 20 2011;9:76.
16. Musaiger AO. Overweight and obesity in eastern mediterranean region: prevalence and possible causes. J Obes 2011;2011:407237.

17. Trends in adult body-mass index in 200 countries from 1975 to 2014: a pooled analysis of 1698 population-based measurement studies with 19·2 million participants. Lancet 2016;387(10026):1377–96.
18. Al-Lawati JA, Jousilahti PJ. Prevalence and 10-year secular trend of obesity in Oman. Saudi Med J 2004;25(3):346–51.
19. Okati-Aliabad H, Ansari-Moghaddam A, Kargar S, et al. Prevalence of Obesity and Overweight among Adults in the Middle East Countries from 2000 to 2020: A Systematic Review and Meta-Analysis. J Obes 2022;2022:8074837.
20. Worldwide trends in body-mass index, underweight, overweight, and obesity from 1975 to 2016: a pooled analysis of 2416 population-based measurement studies in 128·9 million children, adolescents, and adults. Lancet 2017; 390(10113):2627–42.
21. website. hwauocrehrhTUNDPo. Available at: https://www.africa.undp.org/content/rba/en/home/regioninfo.html. The United Nations Development Program official website. Accessed May 2022, 2022.
22. United Nations DoEaSA-PD. United Nations, Department of Economic and Social Affairs- Population Dynamics 2022. Available at: https://www.un.org/development/desa/pd/. Accessed May 2022.
23. Wojcicki JM. The double burden household in sub-Saharan Africa: maternal overweight and obesity and childhood undernutrition from the year 2000: results from World Health Organization Data (WHO) and Demographic Health Surveys (DHS). BMC Publ Health 2014;14:1124.
24. Bhurosy T, Jeewon R. Overweight and obesity epidemic in developing countries: a problem with diet, physical activity, or socioeconomic status? Sci World J 2014; 2014:964236.
25. Ziraba AK, Fotso JC, Ochako R. Overweight and obesity in urban·Africa: A problem of the rich or the poor? BMC Publ Health 2009;9:465.
26. Mařincová L, Šafaříková S, Cahlíková R. Analysis of main risk factors contributing to obesity in the region of East Africa: meta-analysis. Afr Health Sci 2020;20(1): 248–56.
27. Rising rural body-mass index is the main driver of the global obesity epidemic in adults. Nature 2019;569(7755):260–4.
28. World Obesity Federation, World obesity Atlas 2022, Available at: https://data.worldobesity.org/publications/World-Obesity-Atlas-2022.pdf. Accessed June 11, 2022.
29. https://www.statista.com/statistics/632565/asia-pacific-total-population-by-country/. Accessed June16,2022.
30. https://www.who.int/southeastasia/health-topics/obesity. Accessed June 15,2022.
31. Biswas T, Townsend N, Magalhaes RJS, et al. Current Progress and Future Directions in the Double Burden of Malnutrition among Women in South and Southeast Asian Countries. Curr Dev Nutr 2019;3(7):nzz026.
32. Ahirwar R, Mondal PR. Prevalence of obesity in India: A systematic review. Diabetes Metab Syndr 2019;13(1):318–21.
33. . https://www.who.int/publications/i/item/9789290618133.
34. Kessaram T, McKenzie J, Girin N, et al. Noncommunicable diseases and risk factors in adult populations of several Pacific Islands: results from the WHO STEPwise approach to surveillance. Aust N Z J Public Health 2015;39(4):336–43.
35. Kliegman RMBR, Jenson HB, Stanton. Nelson's textbook of peadiatrics. Sheila gahagan chapter 47 Overweight and obesity. 20th edition 2016. p. 307–316 2016.
36. Tian X, Zhao G, Li Y, et al. Overweight and obesity difference of Chinese population between different urbanization levels. J Rural Health. Winter 2014;30(1): 101–12.

37. Wang L, Zhou B, Zhao Z, et al. Body-mass index and obesity in urban and rural China: findings from consecutive nationally representative surveys during 2004-18. Lancet 2021;398(10294):53–63.

38. https://www.who.int/news-room/fact-sheets/detail/obesity-and-overweight. Accessed June 23,2022

39. Feigin VL, Roth GA, Naghavi M, et al. Global burden of stroke and risk factors in 188 countries, during 1990-2013: a systematic analysis for the Global Burden of Disease Study 2013. Lancet Neurol 2016;15(9):913–24.

40. Weng SF, Redsell SA, Swift JA, et al. Systematic review and meta-analyses of risk factors for childhood overweight identifiable during infancy. Arch Dis Child 2012; 97(12):1019–26.

41. Bouhours-Nouet N, Dufresne S, de Casson FB, et al. High birth weight and early postnatal weight gain protect obese children and adolescents from truncal adiposity and insulin resistance: metabolically healthy but obese subjects? Diabetes Care 2008;31(5):1031–6.

42. Ortega-García JA, Kloosterman N, Alvarez L, et al. Full Breastfeeding and Obesity in Children: A Prospective Study from Birth to 6 Years. Child Obes 2018;14(5):327–37.

43. Maximova K, Kuhle S, Davidson Z, et al. Cardiovascular risk-factor profiles of normal and overweight children and adolescents: insights from the Canadian Health Measures Survey. Can J Cardiol 2013;29(8):976–82.

44. Hu Y, Bhupathiraju SN, de Koning L, et al. Duration of obesity and overweight and risk of type 2 diabetes among US women. Obesity 2014;22(10):2267–73.

45. Berenson GS. Health consequences of obesity. Pediatr Blood Cancer 2012;58(1): 117–21.

46. Tirosh A, Shai I, Afek A, et al. Adolescent BMI trajectory and risk of diabetes versus coronary disease. N Engl J Med 2011;364(14):1315–25.

47. Weihrauch-Blüher S, Wiegand S. Risk Factors and Implications of Childhood Obesity. Curr Obes Rep 2018;7(4):254–9.

48. Fontaine K, Barofsky I. Obesity and health-related quality of life. Obes Rev 2001; 2(3):173–82.

49. Kolotkin RL, Andersen JR. A systematic review of reviews: exploring the relationship between obesity, weight loss and health-related quality of life. Clin Obes 2017;7(5):273–89.

50. Fine JT, Colditz GA, Coakley EH, et al. A prospective study of weight change and health-related quality of life in women. JAMA 1999;282(22):2136–42.

51. Wilding JPH, Batterham RL, Calanna S, et al. Once-Weekly Semaglutide in Adults with Overweight or Obesity. N Engl J Med 2021;384(11):989–1002.

52. Jastreboff AM, Aronne LJ, Ahmad NN, et al. Tirzepatide Once Weekly for the Treatment of Obesity. N Engl J Med 2022. https://doi.org/10.1056/NEJMoa2206038.

53. Finkelstein EA, Trogdon JG, Cohen JW, et al. Annual medical spending attributable to obesity: payer-and service-specific estimates. Health Aff 2009;28(5): w822–31.

54. Okunogbe A, Nugent R, Spencer G, et al. Economic impacts of overweight and obesity: current and future estimates for eight countries. BMJ Glob Health 2021; 6(10). https://doi.org/10.1136/bmjgh-2021-006351.

55. Cawley J, Meyerhoefer C. The medical care costs of obesity: an instrumental variables approach. J Health Econ 2012;31(1):219–30.

56. Cawley J, Meyerhoefer C, Biener A, et al. Savings in Medical Expenditures Associated with Reductions in Body Mass Index Among US Adults with Obesity, by Diabetes Status. Pharmacoeconomics 2015;33(7):707–22.

57. Cecchini M. Use of healthcare services and expenditure in the US in 2025: The effect of obesity and morbid obesity. PLoS One 2018;13(11):e0206703.

58. Zizza C, Herring AH, Stevens J, et al. Length of hospital stays among obese individuals. Am J Public Health 2004;94(9):1587–91.

59. Kleinman N, Abouzaid S, Andersen L, et al. Cohort analysis assessing medical and nonmedical cost associated with obesity in the workplace. J Occup Environ Med 2014;56(2):161–70.

60. Biener A, Cawley J, Meyerhoefer C. The impact of obesity on medical care costs and labor market outcomes in the US. Clinical chemistry 2018;64(1):108–17.

61. Graham Y, Hayes C, Cox J, et al. A systematic review of obesity as a barrier to accessing cancer screening services. Obesity Science & Practice 2022;8(6): 715–27.

62. Bray GA. A guide to obesity and the metabolic syndrome. Florida: CRC; 2011.

63. Kværner AS, Hang D, Giovannucci EL, et al. Trajectories of body fatness from age 5 to 60 y and plasma biomarker concentrations of the insulin-insulin-like growth factor system. Am J Clin Nutr 2018;108(2):388–97.

64. Kyrou I, Randeva HS, Tsigos C, et al. Clinical problems caused by obesity, 2018, Endotext [Internet]. Oregon, USA.

65. Sonmez A, Yumuk V, Haymana C, et al. Impact of Obesity on the Metabolic Control of Type 2 Diabetes: Results of the Turkish Nationwide Survey of Glycemic and Other Metabolic Parameters of Patients with Diabetes Mellitus (TEMD Obesity Study). Obes Facts 2019;12(2):167–78.

66. Group DPPR. The Diabetes Prevention Program (DPP) description of lifestyle intervention. Diabetes Care 2002;25(12):2165–71.

67. Garvey WT, Ryan DH, Henry R, et al. Prevention of type 2 diabetes in subjects with prediabetes and metabolic syndrome treated with phentermine and topiramate extended release. Diabetes Care 2014;37(4):912–21.

68. Younossi ZM, Koenig AB, Abdelatif D, et al. Global epidemiology of nonalcoholic fatty liver disease-Meta-analytic assessment of prevalence, incidence, and outcomes. Hepatology 2016;64(1):73–84.

69. Polyzos SA, Kountouras J, Mantzoros CS. Obesity and nonalcoholic fatty liver disease: From pathophysiology to therapeutics. Metabolism 2019;92:82–97.

70. Amarapurkar DN, Hashimoto E, Lesmana LA, et al. How common is non-alcoholic fatty liver disease in the Asia-Pacific region and are there local differences? J Gastroenterol Hepatol 2007;22(6):788–93.

71. Williams CD, Stengel J, Asike MI, et al. Prevalence of nonalcoholic fatty liver disease and nonalcoholic steatohepatitis among a largely middle-aged population utilizing ultrasound and liver biopsy: a prospective study. Gastroenterology 2011;140(1):124–31.

72. Alqahtani SA, Broering DC, Alghamdi SA, et al. Changing trends in liver transplantation indications in Saudi Arabia: from hepatitis C virus infection to nonalcoholic fatty liver disease. BMC Gastroenterol 2021;21(1):245.

73. Younossi ZM, Stepanova M, Ong J, et al. Nonalcoholic Steatohepatitis Is the Most Rapidly Increasing Indication for Liver Transplantation in the United States. Clin Gastroenterol Hepatol 2021;19(3):580–9.e5.

74. Lauby-Secretan B, Scoccianti C, Loomis D, et al. Body Fatness and Cancer–Viewpoint of the IARC Working Group. N Engl J Med 2016;375(8):794–8.

75. Friedenreich CM, Ryder-Burbidge C, McNeil J. Physical activity, obesity and sedentary behavior in cancer etiology: epidemiologic evidence and biologic mechanisms. Mol Oncol 2021;15(3):790–800.
76. Calle EE, Rodriguez C, Walker-Thurmond K, et al. Overweight, obesity, and mortality from cancer in a prospectively studied cohort of U.S. adults. N Engl J Med 2003;348(17):1625–38.
77. Powell-Wiley TM, Poirier P, Burke LE, et al. Obesity and Cardiovascular Disease: A Scientific Statement From the American Heart Association. Circulation 2021; 143(21):e984–1010.
78. Aune D, Schlesinger S, Norat T, et al. Body mass index, abdominal fatness, and the risk of sudden cardiac death: a systematic review and dose-response meta-analysis of prospective studies. Eur J Epidemiol 2018;33(8):711–22.
79. Poirier P, Giles TD, Bray GA, et al. Obesity and cardiovascular disease: pathophysiology, evaluation, and effect of weight loss: an update of the 1997 American Heart Association Scientific Statement on Obesity and Heart Disease from the Obesity Committee of the Council on Nutrition, Physical Activity, and Metabolism. Circulation 2006;113(6):898–918.
80. Doumouras AG, Wong JA, Paterson JM, et al. Bariatric Surgery and Cardiovascular Outcomes in Patients With Obesity and Cardiovascular Disease:: A Population-Based Retrospective Cohort Study. Circulation 2021;143(15): 1468–80.
81. Ramlau-Hansen CH, Thulstrup AM, Nohr EA, et al. Subfecundity in overweight and obese couples. Hum Reprod 2007;22(6):1634–7.
82. van der Steeg JW, Steures P, Eijkemans MJ, et al. Obesity affects spontaneous pregnancy chances in subfertile, ovulatory women. Hum Reprod 2008;23(2): 324–8.
83. Mahutte N, Kamga-Ngande C, Sharma A, et al. Obesity and Reproduction. J Obstet Gynaecol Can 2018;40(7):950–66.
84. Houfflyn S, Matthys C, Soubry A. Male Obesity: Epigenetic Origin and Effects in Sperm and Offspring. Curr Mol Biol Rep 2017;3(4):288–96.
85. Hergenroeder AL, Wert DM, Hile ES, et al. Association of body mass index with self-report and performance-based measures of balance and mobility. Phys Ther 2011;91(8):1223–34.
86. Anandacoomarasamy A, Caterson I, Sambrook P, et al. The impact of obesity on the musculoskeletal system. Int J Obes (Lond) 2008;32(2):211–22.
87. Coggon D, Reading I, Croft P, et al. Knee osteoarthritis and obesity. Int J Obes Relat Metab Disord 2001;25(5):622–7.
88. Christensen R, Astrup A, Bliddal H. Weight loss: the treatment of choice for knee osteoarthritis? A randomized trial. Osteoarthritis Cartilage 2005;13(1):20–7.

# The Physiological Regulation of Body Fat Mass

Priya Sumithran, MBBS, PhD, Associate Professor[a,b,*]

## KEYWORDS

- Body weight • Body fat • Weight regulation • Obesity

## KEY POINTS

- Experimental data support the presence of a system that senses a reduction in body weight below a desired range, and effects changes in energy intake and expenditure to promote restoration of energy balance.
- The adipocyte hormone leptin is the key afferent signal in this negative feedback loop that opposes depletion of fat mass. The equivalent signal that elicits a response to counteract weight gain has not been identified.
- Identifying ways to durably modify these physiological responses is likely to improve the long-term success of obesity treatments.

## INTRODUCTION

Obesity is increasingly recognized as a complex, chronic condition with physiologic roots.[1] Central to this recognition is the understanding that our body weight is not entirely within our voluntary control. For most people, weight loss achieved through intentional changes in behavior alone (such as caloric restriction and increased physical activity) is difficult to sustain over the long term, and weight is usually partially or completely regained over time.[2]

A potential explanation for this is that body weight, or one of its components, is physiologically regulated, meaning that a deviation in weight beyond a desired range is "sensed," triggering adjustments in appetite and energy expenditure that promote restoration of energy balance. This review examines this concept and its implications for the treatment of obesity.

[a] Department of Medicine (St Vincent's), University of Melbourne, St Vincent's Hospital, Clinical Science Building Level 4, 29 Regent Street, Fitzroy, Victoria 3065, Australia; [b] Department of Endocrinology, Austin Health
* Department of Medicine, University of Melbourne, St Vincent's Hospital, Clinical Sciences Building Level 4, 29 Regent Street, Fitzroy, Victoria 3065, Australia.
*E-mail address:* priyas@unimelb.edu.au

Gastroenterol Clin N Am 52 (2023) 295–310
https://doi.org/10.1016/j.gtc.2023.03.003
0889-8553/23/© 2023 Elsevier Inc. All rights reserved.

## DISCUSSION
### Stability of Body Weight

Most individuals maintain a fairly stable body weight for prolonged periods during adulthood. A mean weight gain of ~2 kg over 5 years is observed in population-based cohorts.[3–5] This indicates that even if food intake and physical activity vary from day to day, energy intake and expenditure are matched with precision of ~0.2% over the longer term.

Moreover, short-term changes in weight brought about through periods of imposed calorie deficit or excess are usually followed by return to the preintervention body weight when ad libitum food intake is resumed. In humans, this is most commonly illustrated by weight loss attempts by people with obesity. Restriction of energy intake and increased physical activity initially result in weight loss, which is followed by weight regain in the majority after discontinuation of the intervention.[2] The converse is observed with extended overfeeding.[6] Although in humans, behaviors aimed at maintaining a particular body weight are influenced by a range of external factors, including social pressures, restoration of previous body weight (or weight trajectory) after cessation of food restriction or excess is seen also in animal models[7] in which these influences are not expected to be significant.

Because an adequate amount of body fat is essential for normal physical functions, including reproduction, it is likely that if body weight is regulated, fat is an important component of this process. Several studies in animals have examined how the body responds to alteration of adipocyte mass through surgical removal or addition of fat. In many species, particularly those with large seasonal variations in body fat content, removal of regional fat pads leads to expansion of other fat depots so that total body fat returns to prelipectomy levels within weeks to months (reviewed in Ref.[8]). This is not uniformly observed across species and is variable depending on the fat pad excised,[8] but overall, data from lipectomy studies point toward defense of a minimum level of body fat. In humans, prospective, controlled trials of small-volume liposuction also support this idea, as removal of fat from abdominal ± gluteofemoral regions is followed by accumulation of predominantly abdominal fat within 6 to 12 months.[9,10] In contrast, surgical addition of fat does not appear to prompt a reduction in native fat depots in animals,[11] although limits to the amount of fat that can be viably added, and the variable extent to which vascular and nerve supply are reestablished, may affect the ability of transplanted fat to be detected and responded to.

"Regulation" of body fat implies the existence of a mechanism that senses adipose mass and engages the responses necessary to maintain it within a desired range. It was proposed 70 years ago that a hypothalamic satiety center adjusts food intake in response to changes in circulating levels of one or more metabolites to maintain stability of body fat stores.[12] This "lipostatic" theory is supported by studies in humans and animals demonstrating alterations in appetite, food intake, and energy expenditure in apparent opposition to imposed changes in weight.

### Compensatory Responses in Appetite and Energy Expenditure Oppose Weight Loss

In humans, weight loss induced by dietary restriction leads to a sustained increase in appetite. In a study of adults with obesity who lost 14% body weight over 10 weeks, self-reported ratings of hunger, desire to eat, and prospective food consumption (how much food participants thought they could eat) were higher at 10 weeks compared with pre–weight loss ratings and remained elevated after 12 months of attempted maintenance of weight loss, during which weight was partially regained[13] (**Fig. 1**).

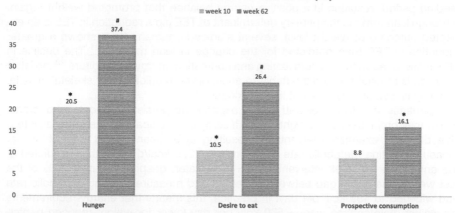

**Fig. 1.** Median changes (%) from baseline (week 0) in area under the curve values for visual analogue scale ratings of hunger, desire to eat, and prospective food consumption after diet-induced weight loss. P values from Wilcoxon Signed Rank tests for paired comparisons between each of weeks 10 and 62 (*P<.05; #P≤.001) compared with baseline (week 0). (*Data from* Sumithran P, Prendergast LA, Delbridge E, et al. Long-term persistence of hormonal adaptations to weight loss. The New England Journal of Medicine. Oct 2011;365(17):1597-604. https://doi.org/10.1056/NEJMoa1105816.)

Establishing that an increase in appetite leads to increased food intake is difficult in humans, as natural eating habits are likely to be modified under laboratory observation, whereas obtaining accurate self-reports of food intake is challenging in free-living participants. Valuable insight comes from the seminal Minnesota Experiment and reanalysis of its data. For 12 men in continuous residence for 24 weeks of semi-starvation, 12 weeks of restricted refeeding, and 8 weeks of unrestricted refeeding, hyperphagia of ~50% above prestarvation intake was observed during the first 4 weeks of unrestricted refeeding.[14] The magnitude of hyperphagia was most strongly related to the degree of body fat depletion and was also independently related to depletion of fat-free mass, indicating that the drive to overeat is the outcome of regulatory control aiming to restore both fat and lean mass. Animals similarly exhibit an increased drive to eat in response to weight loss.[15,16] In diet-induced obese (DIO) rats that have been food-restricted to induce weight loss and then allowed to eat ad libitum, caloric intake was 20% higher on the first day of ad libitum feeding compared with pre–weight loss consumption and remained elevated until weight had been fully regained.[15]

Weight loss of 10% induced by caloric restriction in people with obesity also leads to altered neural activity (detected by functional MRI) in response to palatable food cues in several regions involved in the regulatory, emotional, and cognitive control of food intake, including the hypothalamus, amygdala, hippocampus, prefrontal cortex, and limbic system.[17,18] Although small sample sizes and lack of correlation with eating behavior prevent drawing conclusions about clinical outcomes, these findings provide an objective indication of changes in the salience of food cues after weight loss.

Changes in energy expenditure that favor weight regain are also observed after caloric restriction. In the abovementioned study of DIO rats that exhibited hyperphagia after a period of food restriction,[15] total energy expenditure (TEE) decreased during the weight loss period and remained below baseline values during the ad libitum feeding period, resulting in a positive energy balance that promoted weight regain. Although lean mass is the primary determinant of TEE (so a reduction in TEE is an expected outcome of weight loss), several studies in humans have shown a greater reduction in TEE than predicted for the change in lean mass.[19–21] The decline in TEE involves reductions in both resting and nonresting energy expenditure,[22] the latter of which is at least partly attributable to an increase in efficiency of skeletal muscle, resulting in less energy spent at low workloads.[23,24]

Importantly, a below-expected energy expenditure persists in people who remain below their preintervention weight.[25,26] In a study of participants undergoing an intensive diet and exercise intervention[25] resulting in a mean weight loss of 58 kg, measured resting metabolic rate was a mean of 275 kcal/d lower than predicted at the end of the 30-week intervention. Six years later, despite regain of 70% of the lost weight, the mean gap between expected and measured resting metabolic rate had widened to 499 kcal per day. In practice, this means that energy requirements for weight maintenance were ~500 kcal per day lower for weight-reduced participants than expected for people of a similar age and body composition who had not lost weight (**Fig. 2**).

Changes in metabolism are also seen in response to weight loss. In DIO rats that have been food restricted, return to ad libitum feeding results not only in hyperphagia but also in increased feed efficiency (a measure of weight gained per kilocalorie of energy consumed),[16] suppressed oxidation of dietary fat, and greater accumulation of ingested fat in adipose tissue[27] during weight regain, compared with obese rats that were not food restricted. Studies in humans maintaining a reduced weight have also demonstrated lower fasting or 24-hour rates of fat oxidation and impaired ability to increase fat oxidation appropriately in response to a high-fat diet,[28–30] compared with pre–weight loss or body mass index (BMI) -matched control participants.

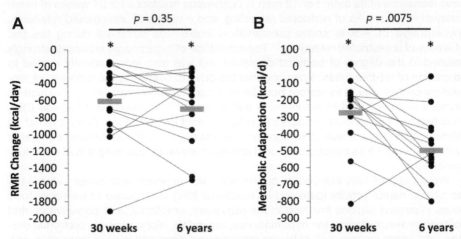

**Fig. 2.** Individual (*circles*) and mean (*rectangles*) changes in (*A*) resting metabolic rate and (*B*) metabolic adaptation at the end of "The Biggest Loser" 30-week weight loss competition and after 6 years. Horizontal bars and corresponding $P$ values indicate comparisons between 30 weeks and 6 years. *$P<.001$ compared with baseline. RMR, resting metabolic rate. (*From* Fothergill E, Guo JE, Howard L, et al. Persistent Metabolic Adaptation 6 Years After "The Biggest Loser" Competition. Obesity. Aug 2016;24(8):1612-1619. https://doi.org/10.1002/oby.21538; with permission.)

Considered together, these data support the presence of a system that senses a reduction in body weight below a desired range, and effects changes in energy intake and expenditure that promote restoration of energy balance, regardless of the time since weight loss occurred.

### Peripheral Hormonal Responses to Weight Loss

The key afferent signal in this negative feedback loop that opposes the depletion of fat mass is the adipocyte hormone leptin. In conditions of energy balance at usual body weight, leptin is secreted in proportion to fat mass.[31] The binding of leptin to its receptor in the arcuate nucleus of the hypothalamus activates neurons expressing proopiomelanocortin (the precursor of a number of peptides including the anorectic α-melanocyte stimulating hormone) and inhibits those expressing the orexigenic neuropeptide Y and agouti-related peptide. Both sets of neurons project to second-order neurons expressing the melanocortin 4 receptor (MC4R) and interact with other centers within and beyond the hypothalamus to modulate appetite and efferent signals regulating energy expenditure and sympathetic nervous system activity.[32]

When circulating leptin is low or absent, a range of physiologic responses results in lowering of energy expenditure and stimulation of appetite. These responses are clearly demonstrated in people with rare monogenic syndromes caused by deficiency of leptin, who have severe obesity and excess adiposity, markedly increased hunger and impaired satiety, and exhibit food-seeking behavior for all types of foods,[33] as well as abnormalities in immune function, and gonadal and thyroid hormone secretion. Replacement of leptin reverses this phenotype, leading to preferential fat loss, profound effects on hunger and satiety, and restoration of the ability to discriminate between rewarding and less-palatable foods.[33] In contrast to the important role of leptin in thermogenesis in rodents, leptin replacement in leptin-deficient humans does not result in a discernible increase in energy expenditure, although it does appear to blunt the reduction in energy expenditure resulting from weight loss.[33]

Dietary energy restriction also induces a rapid, marked reduction in circulating leptin (before the depletion of fat stores), which is sustained, although less severe, during maintenance of weight loss.[13,34] Whether this is primarily related to a reduction in adipocyte size, number, or total body fat content is not clear. The overlap between some features of the weight-reduced state and characteristics of congenital leptin deficiency supports the idea that leptin plays a critical role in the physiologic response to a negative energy balance. Furthermore, in participants maintaining a diet-induced weight loss, leptin "replacement" to pre–weight loss levels reduces appetite and reverses many of the post–weight loss alterations in thyroid hormones, sympathetic nervous system tone, norepinephrine and epinephrine secretion, skeletal muscle energy efficiency, and regional brain activation in response to food cues.[17,35] These findings indicate that the leptin reduction associated with diet-induced weight loss brings about a state of relative leptin deficiency.

Appetite is also influenced by several hormones originating from the gut and pancreas, which convey information about nutrient intake to brain regions, including the hypothalamus and hindbrain (reviewed elsewhere[36]). These meal-related hormones include ghrelin, which promotes hunger and food reward, as well as numerous peptides released in response to nutrient intake: cholecystokinin (CCK), glucagon-like peptide-1 (GLP-1), peptide YY (PYY), and gastric inhibitory polypeptide (GIP) from enteroendocrine cells, and amylin, insulin, and pancreatic polypeptide (PP) from the endocrine pancreas. Most promote satiety and reduce gut motility, in addition to having a number of other roles (**Table 1**).

**Table 1**
**Selected appetite-related gut hormones and effect of caloric restriction**

| Gut Peptide | Source[a] | Major Actions | Change After Caloric Restriction |
|---|---|---|---|
| Ghrelin | P/D$_1$ (X/A-like) cells, stomach | ↑ Hunger; ↑ gut motility | ↑ |
| GLP-1 | L cells; predominantly distal to terminal ileum | ↑ Satiety<br>↓ Gastric emptying, gut motility<br>↓ β-cell apoptosis<br>↑ Glucose-stimulated insulin secretion | ↔/↓/↑ |
| PYY | L cells; predominantly distal to terminal ileum | ↑ Satiety<br>↓ Gastric emptying, gut motility | ↓ |
| GIP | K cells; proximal small intestine | ↑ Satiety<br>↓ Gastric emptying<br>↓ β-cell apoptosis<br>↑ Glucose-stimulated insulin secretion<br>↑ Adipose tissue uptake of glucose and fatty acids | ↑ |
| CCK | I cells; proximal small intestine | ↑ Satiety<br>↓ Gut motility<br>↑ Gallbladder contraction<br>↑ Pancreatic enzyme secretion | ↓ |
| Amylin | β cells; endocrine pancreas | ↑ Satiety<br>↓ Gastric emptying | ↓ |
| PP | PP cells; endocrine pancreas | ↓ Appetite<br>↓ Gastric emptying<br>↓ Pancreatic secretions | ↑ |

*Abbreviations:* ↓, decreased; ↔, unchanged; ↑, increased.
[a] Enteroendocrine cells are heterogeneous, and subsets coexpress several peptides, but the traditional classification is used here for simplicity.

The release of many of these hormones is altered after diet-induced weight loss. Consistently reported changes include increases in circulating ghrelin, GIP, and PP and reductions in PYY, CCK, insulin, and amylin.[13,37–39] Variable changes in circulating GLP-1 following weight loss[40,41] are likely due to differences in the methods used to measure it, and the hormonal fraction measured.[42] Based on the role of these hormones in hunger, satiety, and food reward, many of these changes are expected to favor regain of lost weight by increasing the drive to eat and reducing satiety. Importantly, these responses are not only transiently seen during the period of negative energy balance. One year after completion of a weight loss intervention, circulating levels of leptin, PYY, CCK, ghrelin, GIP, and PP remain altered compared with pre–weight loss values,[13] and fasting ghrelin remains elevated compared with pre–weight loss levels 3 years after completion of a weight loss intervention, despite regain of three-quarters of the lost weight.[43]

Although there is a lack of data demonstrating associations between weight loss–induced peripheral hormone changes and weight regain,[44] many issues make detection and interpretation of these relationships challenging. First, circulating hormone levels may not reflect central sensitivity to their actions. Furthermore, there is clearly some redundancy, with several hormones having overlapping effects. The relative contribution of gut hormones to appetitive drive is likely to differ according to meal composition and perhaps also between individuals. In addition, how each component of the response to weight loss interacts with each individual's environmental and psychosocial context to affect their propensity to weight regain is something that we do not currently have the means to measure.

However, relevance of a reduction in satiety hormones to increased appetite after weight loss is suggested by the sustained weight loss and appetite control achieved with obesity treatments that augment levels or actions of satiety hormones alone or in combination.[45,46] In contrast to the hormone profile seen after diet-induced weight loss, increased postprandial secretion of the satiety hormones GLP-1 and PYY is seen after the bariatric procedures Roux-en-Y gastric bypass (RYGB) and sleeve gastrectomy.[47] The synergistic role of these hormones in the inhibition of food intake in weight-reduced patients after RYGB is indicated by the demonstration that blockade of the actions of either hormone resulted in increased secretion of the other and no change in food intake at a test meal, whereas combined blockade of the actions of GLP-1 and PYY led to a ~20% increase in food intake.[48]

Of note, a physiologic response to weight loss occurs regardless of the quantity of stored fat. Maintenance of a 10% reduction in body weight is associated with similar reductions in TEE in people with and without obesity,[21] and no relationship was found between baseline BMI and changes in appetite-related hormones after weight loss in people with varying degrees of excess weight (BMI, 26–51 kg/m$^2$).[49]

### Compensatory Responses to Overfeeding and Weight Gain

In contrast to the large body of data strongly indicating that a compensatory physiologic response initiated by a drop in leptin opposes reduction of body fat below a minimum level, studies examining whether an upper level of weight or fat is also counteracted are not as consistent, and the mechanisms by which this might occur are less clear.

Periods of enforced overfeeding, such as under experimental conditions or during cultural overfeeding practices, are usually followed by restoration of body weight and adiposity to preintervention levels over weeks to months.[6,50] For example, in a study of 12 pairs of male monozygotic twins, overfeeding by 6000 kcal per week for 100 days resulted in mean weight gain of 16% (8 kg), with return of weight and body fat close to baseline values by 4 months after cessation of the experiment.[6]

In rats and mice that are overfed to induce weight gain, voluntary food intake is profoundly reduced until their weight has returned to pre-overfeeding levels.[51,52] However, in humans, although a reduction in hunger and increase in satiety are observed within a few meals of introducing a hypercaloric diet,[53] short-term excess energy intake is associated with incomplete short-term compensation.[54,55] There is also considerable heterogeneity in the reported changes in appetite-related gut hormones in response to overfeeding (reviewed in Ref.[56]).

Although findings are mixed,[57] many studies have found that prolonged overfeeding leads to a greater increase in TEE than would be expected for the change in lean mass in both humans[21] and animals.[58] An increase in nonexercise activity thermogenesis (energy spent in physical activity other than volitional exercise, including activities of daily living, fidgeting, spontaneous muscle contraction, and maintaining posture) was correlated with resistance to fat gain in a study of supervised overfeeding for 8 weeks in 16 adults without obesity.[59] This appears not to be explained by a change in time spent in different postures (sitting, lying, standing) after overfeeding.[60]

Together, changes in appetite, food intake, and energy expenditure after overfeeding, along with an increase in the thyroid hormone triiodothyronine,[61] lend support to the idea that weight gain, like weight loss, is opposed by responses favoring restoration of weight stability. However, in contrast to the compensatory response to calorie restriction, leptin does not seem to play a significant role in this response.

During overfeeding, most (>60%) of the weight gained is adipose tissue,[56] and fat gain is accompanied by an increase in circulating leptin. Although leptin administration has powerful effects on appetite, food intake, and adiposity in people with low endogenous levels, it has little effect in weight-stable people with obesity,[62] who generally have high circulating leptin. Moreover, after a period of overfeeding in mice, hypophagia and a return to pre-overfeeding weight when allowed to feed ad libitum are seen even if circulating leptin levels are prevented from increasing.[51] Therefore, although a deficiency of leptin has profound obesity-promoting effects, elevated circulating leptin levels are not sufficient to counteract weight gain, and an increase in leptin is not required for the compensatory response to overfeeding. This suggests that leptin's primary role is to communicate an energy deficit to the brain to defend against fat loss, rather than to protect against fat gain.

The process by which weight gain is counteracted has not been identified. In mice and rats, implantation of metabolically inactive weights equivalent to ~10% to 15% body weight leads to a reduction in tissue mass that partially offsets the added weight.[63–65] A preferential loss of fat[63,64] and reduction in food intake[64,65] have been variably reported in response to implanted weight. It has been proposed that excess weight is sensed by osteocytes in weight-bearing bones.[64] A short-term proof-of-concept study in humans showed small reductions in weight (1.4%) and fat mass (4%) and no changes in self-reported food intake when weighted vests were worn for 3 weeks.[66] However, studies in mice and rats subjected to decreasing or increasing gravity,[67] and observations of weight loss in humans undergoing spaceflight,[68] are not consistent with a bone-based weight-sensing system being the primary means of defense against weight gain.

## UNRESOLVED QUESTIONS AND CONTROVERSIES

Much of our knowledge about body weight is seemingly contradictory. How do we reconcile our understanding that our weight is strongly influenced by genes[69] with the fact that the number of adults with obesity worldwide increased nearly sevenfold between 1975 and 2016?[70] How can the diverse range of biologic, psychosocial, environmental, and socioeconomic risk factors for obesity be incorporated into a cohesive model of weight regulation?

Undoubtedly, changes in the environment over the last 5 decades, such as an increase in portion sizes, availability, and marketing of inexpensive, energy-dense foods high in fat and/or sugar, as well as reduction in work-related physical activity,[71,72] have contributed to the increase in the population prevalence of obesity. However, there is clearly wide interindividual variability in the "defended" level of fat mass and in susceptibility to weight changes in response to energy imbalance. The fact that some people readily develop obesity under conducive environmental conditions, whereas others do not, is largely due to differences in genetic predisposition. Genome-wide association studies have identified hundreds of loci associated with BMI and obesity, most of which are predominantly expressed in the brain and central nervous system, in areas central to appetite (hypothalamus and pituitary gland), addiction and reward (insula and substantia nigra), cognition, emotion, and memory (hippocampus and limbic system).[73–75]

For example, heterozygous loss-of-function mutations in the MC4R gene are found in an estimated 0.3% of a UK birth cohort and are associated with an 18-kg greater body weight and 3.7 times increased risk of obesity at age 18 compared with noncarriers.[76] Conversely, approximately 6% of a UK cohort of European ancestry carries gain-of-function MC4R variants associated with 50% lower risk of obesity.[77] More often, inherited susceptibility to obesity is not the result of single gene mutations, but rather the cumulative effect of numerous common gene variants. A 13-kg difference in weight and 25-fold difference in risk of severe obesity were found between middle-aged adults in the highest versus lowest decile category for a polygenic risk score comprising 2.1 million gene variants.[78] Therefore, although a predisposition to develop, or not develop, obesity in a given environment is conferred by our genes, the increasingly obesogenic environment over recent decades has likely resulted in greater manifestation of inherited susceptibility among those most at risk.

An unresolved question is whether in people with an underlying genetic predisposition, the development of obesity is simply a natural response to the obesogenic environment, or if a specific factor (or factors) within the environment disrupts or overrides normal regulatory mechanisms to drive an increase in body weight. The latter is suggested by data from a short-term inpatient study showing that participants consumed ~500 kcal per day more, and ate more quickly, when offered an ultraprocessed diet for 2 weeks compared with an unprocessed diet matched for calories, energy density, macronutrients, sugar, sodium, and fiber that was rated as equally pleasant.[79] Whether dietary carbohydrates similarly promote overconsumption is a matter of active debate,[80,81] although similar long-term weight outcomes for low-carbohydrate and low-fat diets[82] indicate that reducing dietary carbohydrate consumption alone is insufficient to promote a sustained reduction in appetite and energy intake.

Several models of body weight control have been put forward to explain observations of weight stability over long periods and apparent compensatory responses to changes in energy balance, not all of which postulate that body fat is regulated. These are discussed in detail elsewhere[83,84] and presented briefly here. The lipostatic *"set point"*[12] proposes a negative feedback loop around a target level of body fat, mediated by central detection of a circulating signal from fat, with deviations from the target level triggering adjustments in energy intake or expenditure to restore body fat to the desired level. In contrast, in the *"settling point"* model, there is no active defense of weight or fat—an imbalance between energy intake and maintenance requirements leads to a change in body weight and composition, which, in turn, reduces the imbalance, leading to stabilization of weight at a new steady state.[85] The settling point model better accounts for the observed gradual weight gain during adulthood than the set point model, but does not explain compensatory adaptations to weight changes.

There are also hybrid models that combine elements of both set and settling point concepts. These include the *"dual intervention point"*[83] model, in which body weight/fat is maintained between independent lower and upper bounds. A counterregulatory physiologic response is enacted if weight deviates beyond either bound, whereas a settling point system operates between them. Another example is the *"general model of intake regulation,"*[86] which proposes that food intake is influenced by both uncompensated factors (primarily environmental, which affect but are not affected by food intake) and compensated factors (primarily physiologic, which are reciprocally linked with intake). These hybrid models attempt to account for interactions between environmental, genetic/biologic, and other factors in the determination of individual body weight.

Assuming that fat mass is defended, uncertainty remains about exactly how the defended level is determined and whether it can be modified. Evidence that the defended level of fat mass can be experimentally manipulated comes from studies of animals with ablative lesions in the lateral or ventromedial hypothalamus, which appear to defend body fat at lower and higher levels (respectively) than nonlesioned animals.[87,88] For example, compared with sham-lesioned animals, rats with lateral hypothalamic lesions maintain body weight around 15% lower, and defend this weight in the same manner, when subjected to food restriction or overfeeding[88] (**Fig. 3**). Along with the observation that their total daily resting expenditure is as expected for their size,[89] these results indicate that lateral hypothalamic lesions lower the defended fat mass, rather than representing a state of displacement from the higher fat mass level. Although experimental data are lacking, adjustments in defended fat mass appear to occur naturally in humans during various life stages, such as during and after pregnancy.

The ability to lower the defended level of fat mass would have tremendous implications for the treatment of obesity. As yet, apart from the example provided by lateral hypothalamic lesions, there is no clear evidence that this is achievable. Data from animal studies could raise the possibility that certain centrally acting obesity medications, and bariatric surgeries, act by reducing the defended level of fat mass. The anorectic effect of fenfluramine, semaglutide, and vertical sleeve gastrectomy (VSG) is temporary in rats and mice, although reduction in body weight is maintained.[90–92] This might simply represent their effect on appetite being offset by the increase in hunger expected with weight loss. On the other hand, if these treatments were reducing the level of defended fat mass, a temporary reduction in food intake until weight has

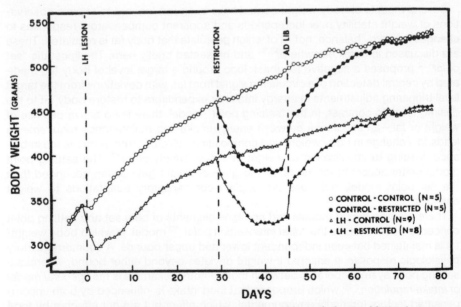

**Fig. 3.** Body weights of control rats and rats with lateral hypothalamic ablative lesions under restricted and ad libitum feeding conditions. LH, lateral hypothalamic lesion. (*From* Mitchel J.S. and Keesey R.E., Defense of a lowered weight maintenance level by lateral hypothalamically lesioned rats - evidence from a restriction-refeeding regimen, *Physiol Behav,* **18** (6), 1977, 1121–1125. with permission.)

reduced to the new regulated level is the expected result. Interestingly, imposed caloric restriction in rats that have undergone VSG is followed by hyperphagia and regain of weight back to the prerestriction (but not pre-VSG) weight, indicating "defense" of the post-VSG weight.[92] Regardless of whether these treatments reduce the level of defended fat mass, it is important to note that they act only while they are in use (in the case of medications) or functioning (in the case of bariatric surgery). Discontinuation of obesity medications, and reversal of bariatric surgery, results in rapid weight regain.

## SUMMARY

Disturbances in body weight and adiposity in both humans and animals are met by compensatory adjustments in energy intake and energy expenditure, strongly suggesting that body weight or fat is regulated. From a clinical viewpoint, this means that people with obesity who have lost weight through caloric restriction and are maintaining a body weight lower than their "defended" weight, are likely to have lower energy expenditure, greater hunger and hedonic drive to eat, and increased propensity to store fat, than they did before they lost weight. Strategies that address these physiological changes are likely to improve the long-term success of obesity treatments.

## CLINICS CARE POINTS

- The amount of body fat individuals carry is strongly influenced by interactions between genetic susceptibility to weight gain and environmental factors

- Physiological responses appear to oppose changes in fat mass and promote restoration of energy balance

- In the management of obesity, strategies to counteract these responses are associated with more successful maintenance of weight loss

## DISCLOSURE

P. Sumithran is supported by an Investigator Grant from the National Health and Medical Research Council, Australia (1178482) and has co-authored manuscripts assisted by medical writing provided by Novo Nordisk.

## REFERENCES

1. Bray GA, Kim KK, Wilding JPH, et al. Obesity: a chronic relapsing progressive disease process. A position statement of the World Obesity Federation. Obesity Reviews 2017;18(7):715–23.
2. Franz MJ, Vanwormer JJ, Crain AL, et al. Weight-loss outcomes: A systematic review and meta-analysis of weight-loss clinical trials with a minimum 1-year follow-up. J Am Diet Assoc 2007;107(10):1755–67.
3. Rosell M, Appleby P, Spencer E, et al. Weight gain over 5 years in 21,966 meat-eating, fish-eating, vegetarian, and vegan men and women in EPIC-Oxford. Int J Obes 2006;30(9):1389–96.
4. Ebrahimi-Mameghani M, Scott JA, Der G, et al. Changes in weight and waist circumference over 9 years in a Scottish population. Eur J Clin Nutr 2008; 62(10):1208–14.

5. Ball K, Crawford D, Ireland P, et al. Patterns and demographic predictors of 5-year weight change in a multi-ethnic cohort of men and women in Australia. Publ Health Nutr 2003;6(3):269–80.
6. Bouchard C, Tremblay A, Despres JP, et al. Overfeeding in identical twins: 5-year postoverfeeding results. Metabolism-Clinical and Experimental 1996;45(8): 1042–50.
7. Bernstein IL, Lotter EC, Kulkosky PJ, et al. Effect of force-feeding upon basal insulin levels of rats. PSEBM (Proc Soc Exp Biol Med) 1975;150(2):546–8.
8. Mauer MM, Harris RB, Bartness TJ. The regulation of total body fat: lessons learned from lipectomy studies. Neurosci Biobehav Rev 2001;25(1):15–28.
9. Hernandez TL, Kittelson JM, Law CK, et al. Fat Redistribution Following Suction Lipectomy: Defense of Body Fat and Patterns of Restoration. Obesity 2011; 19(7):1388–95.
10. Benatti F, Solis M, Artioli G, et al. Liposuction Induces a Compensatory Increase of Visceral Fat Which Is Effectively Counteracted by Physical Activity: A Randomized Trial. J Clin Endocrinol Metab 2012;97(7):2388–95.
11. Lacy EL, Bartness TJ. Autologous fat transplants influence compensatory white adipose tissue mass increases after lipectomy. Am J Physiol Regul Integr Comp Physiol 2004;286(1):R61–70.
12. Kennedy GC. The role of depot fat in the hypothalamic control of food intake in the rat. Proceedings of the Royal Society Series B-Biological Sciences 1953; 140(901):578–92.
13. Sumithran P, Prendergast LA, Delbridge E, et al. Long-term persistence of hormonal adaptations to weight loss. N Engl J Med 2011 2011;365(17):1597–604.
14. Dulloo AG, Jacquet J, Girardier L. Poststarvation hyperphagia and body fat overshooting in humans: A role for feedback signals from lean and fat tissues. Am J Clin Nutr 1997;65(3):717–23.
15. MacLean PS, Higgins JA, Jackman MR, et al. Peripheral metabolic responses to prolonged weight reduction that promote rapid, efficient regain in obesity-prone rats. Am J Physiol Regul Integr Comp Physiol 2006;290(6):R1577–88.
16. Levin BE, Keesey RE. Defense of differing body weight set points in diet-induced obese and resistant rats. Am J Physiol Regul Integr Comp Physiol 1998;274(2): R412–9.
17. Rosenbaum M, Sy M, Pavlovich K, et al. Leptin reverses weight loss-induced changes in regional neural activity responses to visual food stimuli. J Clin Invest 2008;118(7):2583–91.
18. Neseliler S, Hu W, Larcher K, et al. Neurocognitive and Hormonal Correlates of Voluntary Weight Loss in Humans. Cell Metabolism 2019;29(1):39–+.
19. Doucet E, St-Pierre S, Almeras N, et al. Evidence for the existence of adaptive thermogenesis during weight loss. Br J Nutr 2001;85(6):715–23.
20. Dulloo AG, Jacquet J. Adaptive reduction in basal metabolic rate in response to food deprivation in humans: a role for feedback signals from fat stores. Am J Clin Nutr 1998;68(3):599–606.
21. Leibel RL, Rosenbaum M, Hirsch J. Changes in energy-expenditure resulting from altered body-weight. N Engl J Med 1995;332(10):621–8.
22. Rosenbaum M, Leibel RL. Models of Energy Homeostasis in Response to Maintenance of Reduced Body Weight. Obesity 2016;24(8):1620–9.
23. Rosenbaum M, Vandenborne K, Goldsmith R, et al. Effects of experimental weight perturbation on skeletal muscle work efficiency in human subjects. Am J Physiol Regul Integr Comp Physiol 2003;285(1):R183–92.

24. Doucet E, Imbeault P, St-Pierre S, et al. Greater than predicted decrease in energy expenditure during exercise after body weight loss in obese men. Clinical Science 2003;105(1):89–95.

25. Fothergill E, Guo JE, Howard L, et al. Persistent Metabolic Adaptation 6 Years After "The Biggest Loser" Competition. Obesity 2016;24(8):1612–9.

26. Leibel RL, Hirsch J. Diminished energy-requirements in reduced-obese patients. Metabolism-Clinical and Experimental 1984;33(2):164–70.

27. Jackman MR, Steig A, Higgins JA, et al. Weight regain after sustained weight reduction is accompanied by suppressed oxidation of dietary fat and adipocyte hyperplasia. Am J Physiol Regul Integr Comp Physiol 2008;294(4):R1117–29.

28. Ballor DL, HarveyBerino JR, Ades PA, et al. Decrease in fat oxidation following a meal in weight-reduced individuals: A possible mechanism for weight recidivism. Metabolism-Clinical and Experimental 1996;45(2):174–8.

29. Astrup A, Buemann B, Christensen NJ, et al. Failure to increase lipid oxidation in response to increasing dietary-fat content in formerly obese women. Am J Physiol 1994;266(4):E592–9.

30. Filozof CM, Murua C, Sanchez MP, et al. Low plasma leptin concentration and low rates of fat oxidation in weight-stable post-obese subjects. Obes Res 2000;8(3):205–10.

31. Considine RV, Sinha MK, Heiman ML, et al. Serum immunoreactive leptin concentrations in normal-weight and obese humans. N Engl J Med 1996;334(5):292–5.

32. Friedman J. Leptin at 20: an overview. J Endocrinol 2014;223(1):T1–8.

33. Farooqi IS, O'Rahilly S. Leptin: a pivotal regulator of human energy homeostasis. Am J Clin Nutr 2009;89(3):980S–4S.

34. Keim NL, Stern JS, Havel PJ. Relation between circulating leptin concentrations and appetite during a prolonged, moderate energy deficit in women. Am J Clin Nutr 1998;68(4):794–801.

35. Rosenbaum M, Goldsmith R, Bloomfield D, et al. Low-dose leptin reverses skeletal muscle, autonomic, and neuroendocrine adaptations to maintenance of reduced weight. J Clin Invest 2005;115(12):3579–86.

36. Wren AM, Bloom SR. Gut hormones and appetite control. Gastroenterology 2007;132(6):2116–30.

37. Chearskul S, Delbridge E, Shulkes A, et al. Effect of weight loss and ketosis on postprandial cholecystokinin and free fatty acid concentrations. Am J Clin Nutr 2008;87(5):1238–46.

38. Pfluger PT, Kampe J, Castaneda TR, et al. Effect of human body weight changes on circulating levels of peptide YY and peptide YY3-36. J Clin Endocrinol Metab 2007;92(2):583–8.

39. Cummings DE, Weigle DS, Frayo RS, et al. Plasma ghrelin levels after diet-induced weight loss or gastric bypass surgery. N Engl J Med 2002;346(21):1623–30.

40. Verdich C, Toubro S, Buemann B, et al. The role of postprandial releases of insulin and incretin hormones in meal-induced satiety - effect of obesity and weight reduction. Int J Obes 2001;25(8):1206–14.

41. Adam TCM, Lejeune M, Westerterp-Plantenga MS. Nutrient-stimulated glucagon-like peptide 1 release after body-weight loss and weight maintenance in human subjects. Br J Nutr 2006;95(1):160–7.

42. Bak MJ, Albrechtsen NJW, Pedersen J, et al. Specificity and sensitivity of commercially available assays for glucagon-like peptide-1 (GLP-1): implications for GLP-1 measurements in clinical studies. Diabetes Obes Metab 2014;16(11):1155–64.

43. Purcell K, Sumithran P, Prendergast LA, et al. The effect of rate of weight loss on long-term weight management: a randomised controlled trial. Lancet Diabetes Endocrinol 2014;2(12):954–62.
44. Strohacker K, McCaffery JM, MacLean PS, et al. Adaptations of leptin, ghrelin or insulin during weight loss as predictors of weight regain: a review of current literature. Int J Obes 2014;38(3):388–96.
45. Jastreboff AM, Aronne LJ, Ahmad NN, et al. Tirzepatide Once Weekly for the Treatment of Obesity. N Engl J Med 2022;387(3):205–16.
46. Enebo LB, Berthelsen KK, Kankam M, et al. Safety, tolerability, pharmacokinetics, and pharmacodynamics of concomitant administration of multiple doses of cagrilintide with semaglutide 2.4 mg for weight management: a randomised, controlled, phase 1b trial. Lancet 2021;397(10286):1736–48.
47. Nielsen MS, Ritz C, Albrechtsen NJW, et al. Oxyntomodulin and Glicentin May Predict the Effect of Bariatric Surgery on Food Preferences and Weight Loss. J Clin Endocrinol Metab 2020;105(4):dgaa061.
48. Svane MS, Jorgensen NB, Bojsen-Moller KN, et al. Peptide YY and glucagon-like peptide-1 contribute to decreased food intake after Roux-en-Y gastric bypass surgery. Int J Obes 2016;40(11):1699–706.
49. Edwards KAL, Prendergast LA, Kalfas S, et al. Impact of starting BMI and degree of weight loss on changes in appetite-regulating hormones during diet-induced weight loss. Obesity 2022;30(4):911–9.
50. Pasquet P, Apfelbaum M. Recovery of initial body weight and composition after long-term massive overfeeding in men. Am J Clin Nutr 1994;60(6):861–3.
51. Ravussin Y, Edwin E, Gallop M, et al. Evidence for a Non-leptin System that Defends against Weight Gain in Overfeeding. Cell Metabolism 2018;28(2). https://doi.org/10.1016/j.cmet.2018.05.029.
52. Wilson BE, Meyer GE, Cleveland JC, et al. Identification of candidate genes for a factor regulating body-weight in primates. Am J Physiol 1990;259(6):R1148–55.
53. Thomas EA, Bechtell JL, Vestal BE, et al. Eating-related behaviors and appetite during energy imbalance in obese-prone and obese-resistant individuals. Appetite 2013;65:96–102.
54. Levitsky DA, Obarzanek E, Mrdjenovic G, et al. Imprecise control of energy intake: Absence of a reduction in food intake following overfeeding in young adults. Physiol Behav 2005;84(5):669–75.
55. He JY, Votruba S, Pomeroy J, et al. Measurement of Ad Libitum Food Intake, Physical Activity, and Sedentary Time in Response to Overfeeding. PLoS One 2012;7(5):e36225.
56. Bray GA, Bouchard C. The biology of human overfeeding: A systematic review. Obesity Reviews 2020;21(9). https://doi.org/10.1111/obr.13040.
57. Riumallo JA, Schoeller D, Barrera G, et al. Energy-expenditure in underweight free-living adults - impact of energy supplementation as determined by doubly labeled water and indirect calorimetry. Am J Clin Nutr 1989;49(2):239–46.
58. Jackman MR, MacLean PS, Bessesen DH. Energy expenditure in obesity-prone and obesity-resistant rats before and after the introduction of a high-fat diet. Am J Physiol Regul Integr Comp Physiol 2010;299(4):R1097–105.
59. Levine JA, Eberhardt NL, Jensen MD. Role of nonexercise activity thermogenesis in resistance to fat gain in humans. Science 1999;283(5399):212–4.
60. Levine JA, Lanningham-Foster LM, McCrady SK, et al. Interindividual variation in posture allocation: Possible rote in human obesity. Science 2005;307(5709):584–6.

61. Davidson MB, Chopra IJ. Effect of carbohydrate and non-carbohydrate sources of calories on plasma 3,5,3'-triiodothyronine concentrations in man. J Clin Endocrinol Metab 1979;48(4):577–81.

62. Heymsfield SB, Greenberg AS, Fujioka K, et al. Recombinant leptin for weight loss in obese and lean adults - A randomized, controlled, dose-escalation trial. JAMA 1999;282(16):1568–75.

63. Wiedmer P, Boschmann M, Klaus S. Gender dimorphism of body mass perception and regulation in mice. J Exp Biol 2004;207(16):2859–66.

64. Jansson JO, Palsdottir V, Hagg DA, et al. Body weight homeostat that regulates fat mass independently of leptin in rats and mice. Proceedings of the National Academy of Sciences of the United States of America 2018;115(2):427–32.

65. Adams CS, Korytko AI, Blank JL. A novel mechanism of body mass regulation. J Exp Biol 2001;204(10):1729–34.

66. Ohlsson C, Gidestrand E, Bellman J, et al. Increased weight loading reduces body weight and body fat in obese subjects - A proof of concept randomized clinical trial. Eclinicalmedicine 2020;22:100338.

67. Turner RT, Branscum AJ, Wong CP, et al. Studies in microgravity, simulated microgravity and gravity do not support a gravitostat. J Endocrinol 2020;247(3):273–82.

68. Matsumoto A, Storch KJ, Stolfi A, et al. Weight Loss in Humans in Space. Aviat Space Environ Med 2011;82(6):615–21.

69. Loos RJF, Yeo GSH. The genetics of obesity: from discovery to biology. Nat Rev Genet 2022;23(2):120–33.

70. Ezzati M, Bentham J, Di Cesare M, et al. Worldwide trends in body-mass index, underweight, overweight, and obesity from 1975 to 2016: a pooled analysis of 2416 population-based measurement studies in 128.9 million children, adolescents, and adults. Lancet 2017;390(10113):2627–42.

71. Swinburn B, Sacks G, Ravussin E. Increased food energy supply is more than sufficient to explain the US epidemic of obesity. Am J Clin Nutr 2009;90(6):1453–6.

72. Church TS, Thomas DM, Tudor-Locke C, et al. Trends over 5 Decades in US Occupation-Related Physical Activity and Their Associations with Obesity. PLoS One 2011;6(5):e19657.

73. Locke AE, Kahali B, Berndt SI, et al. Genetic studies of body mass index yield new insights for obesity biology. Nature 2015;518(7538):197–U401.

74. Finucane HK, Reshef YA, Anttila V, et al. Heritability enrichment of specifically expressed genes identifies disease-relevant tissues and cell types. Nature Genetics 2018;50(4):621.

75. Ndiaye FK, Huyvaert M, Ortalli A, et al. The expression of genes in top obesity-associated loci is enriched in insula and substantia nigra brain regions involved in addiction and reward. Int J Obes 2020;44(2):539–43.

76. Wade KH, Lam BYH, Melvin A, et al. Loss-of-function mutations in the melanocortin 4 receptor in a UK birth cohort. Nat Med 2021;27(6):1088.

77. Lotta LA, Mokrosinski J, de Oliveira EM, et al. Human Gain-of-Function MC4R Variants Show Signaling Bias and Protect against Obesity. Cell 2019;177(3):597.

78. Khera AV, Chaffin M, Wade KH, et al. Polygenic Prediction of Weight and Obesity Trajectories from Birth to Adulthood. Cell 2019;177(3):587–+.

79. Hall KD, Ayuketah A, Brychta R, et al. Ultra-Processed Diets Cause Excess Calorie Intake and Weight Gain: An Inpatient Randomized Controlled Trial of Ad Libitum Food Intake. Cell Metabol 2019;30(1):67–+.

80. Hall KD, Farooqi IS, Friedman JM, et al. The energy balance model of obesity: beyond calories in, calories out. Am J Clin Nutr 2022;115(5):1243–54.
81. Ludwig DS, Aronne LJ, Astrup A, et al. The carbohydrate-insulin model: a physiological perspective on the obesity pandemic. Am J Clin Nutr 2021;114(6): 1873–85.
82. Schwingshackl L, Hoffmann G. Long-term effects of low glycemic index/load vs. high glycemic index/load diets on parameters of obesity and obesity-associated risks: A systematic review and meta-analysis. Nutr Metabol Cardiovasc Dis 2013; 23(8):699–706.
83. Speakman JR, Levitsky DA, Allison DB, et al. Set points, settling points and some alternative models: theoretical options to understand how genes and environments combine to regulate body adiposity. Dis Model Mech 2011;4(6):733–45.
84. Berthoud HR, Morrison CD, Munzberg H. The obesity epidemic in the face of homeostatic body weight regulation: What went wrong and how can it be fixed? Physiol Behav 2020;222:112959.
85. Payne PR, Dugdale AE. A model for the prediction of energy balance and body weight. Ann Hum Biol 1977;4(6):525–35.
86. de Castro JM, Plunkett S. A general model of intake regulation. Neurosci Biobehav Rev 2002;26(5):581–95. Pii s0149-7634(02)00018-0.
87. Hoebel BG, Teitelbaum P. Weight regulation in normal and hypothalamic hyperphagic rats. J Comp Physiol Psychol 1966;61(2):189.
88. Mitchel JS, Keesey RE. Defense of a lowered weight maintenance level by lateral hypothalamically lesioned rats - evidence from a restriction-refeeding regimen. Physiol Behav 1977;18(6):1121–5.
89. Corbett SW, Wilterdink EJ, Keesey RE. Resting oxygen-consumption in overfed and underfed rats with lateral hypothalamic-lesions. Physiol Behav 1985;35(6): 971–7.
90. Levitsky DA, Strupp BJ, Lupoli J. Tolerance to anorectic drugs - pharmacological or artifactual. Pharmacol Biochem Behav 1981;14(5):661–7.
91. Gabery S, Salinas CG, Paulsen SJ, et al. Semaglutide lowers body weight in rodents via distributed neural pathways. Jci Insight 2020;5(6):e133429.
92. Stefater MA, Perez-Tilve D, Chambers AP, et al. Sleeve gastrectomy induces loss of weight and fat mass in obese rats, but does not affect leptin sensitivity. Gastroenterology 2010;138(7):2426–36. Research Support, N.I.H., Extramural.

# Appetite, Energy Expenditure, and the Regulation of Energy Balance

Michael Rosenbaum, MD[a,b,*]

## KEYWORDS

- Weight gain • Weight loss • Weight maintenance • Obesity • Treatment

## KEY POINTS

- Changes in energy balance (energy intake and output) oppose both the processes of achieving and the maintenance of weight changes from usual.
- The opposition to sustaining weight loss is mainly physiological rather than to a lack of willpower and is not limited to individuals with overweight or obesity.
- Correlates of achieving weight loss or weight gain are not the same as those predicting weight loss maintenance (avoidance of weight regain).
- Treatments to lose weight and sustain weight loss are likely to be different for most individuals.

## INTRODUCTION: RECAP OF THE FIRST LAW OF THERMODYNAMICS

This is a discussion of the regulation of energy balance, in particular as it applies to losing weight and keeping it off. This discussion is based on the First Law of Thermodynamics (conservation of energy) which was stated by Dr. Rudolf Clausius, and others, in about 1850[1] as:

$$\Delta H = Q - W$$

It states that any change in energy stores in a closed system ($\Delta H$) must reflect the difference between $Q$, the energy put into the system as "intake," and $W$, the energy "output" from the system as work (transfer of mechanical energy) or heat (transfer of chemical energy). Despite statements in scientific journals such as "It is not excess calories that cause obesity[2] and media quotations from researchers such as "It has

a Division of Molecular Genetics, Department of Pediatrics, Columbia University Irving Medical Center, 1150 St. Nicholas Avenue, 6th Floor, New York, NY 10032, USA; b Department of Medicine, Columbia University Irving Medical Center, 1150 St. Nicholas Avenue, 6th Floor, New York, NY 10032, USA
* Division of Molecular Genetics, Department of Pediatrics, Columbia University Irving Medical Center, 1150 St. Nicholas Avenue, 6th Floor, New York, NY 10032.
E-mail address: mr475@cumc.columbia.edu

Gastroenterol Clin N Am 52 (2023) 311–322
https://doi.org/10.1016/j.gtc.2023.03.004
0889-8553/23/© 2023 Elsevier Inc. All rights reserved.

nothing to do with the calories,"[3] the principles of energy balance and energy conservation as stated in the First Law remain intact.[4]

The human body can be viewed as a closed system except in certain circumstances which remove or increase anatomic energy stores (eg, liposuction or transplant) independent of changes in energy intake (diet) or output (work and heat) on the part of the patient. This law applies to energy stores in the human: fat (usually more than 85% of total energy stores), protein (usually <15% of total energy stores), and carbohydrate (usually <1% of total energy stores).

Dietary energy intake and $Q$ are not the same. Calories ingested are not all absorbed into the system and therefore $Q$ is affected by nutrient harvesting which is affected by the microbiome (discussed elsewhere in this issue) and food absorption which differs between individuals and may be affected by various disease states such as lactose intolerance and medications such as orlistat.

Changes in weight and changes in stored as energy ($\Delta H$) are not the same. The caloric density of fat mass (FM, about 9500 kcal/kg) is 6x that of fat-free mass (FFM)[5] so the energy imbalance required to "melt away fat" while preserving FFM (as claimed by numerous advertisements), is much greater than that required to lose some mixture of FM and FFM. The partitioning of weight change during dietary alteration is affected by adiposity such that individuals with higher percentages of body fat tend to lose or gain weight more slowly with the same degree of caloric increase or decrease because a higher fraction of that weight change is the more calorically dense fat mass.[5]

What is not covered by the first law of thermodynamics are the factors that influence energy intake and output ($Q$ and $W$) or how the differences between intake and output affect body composition ($\Delta H$). The topics of this review are the effects of changes in energy balance ($Q-W$, predominantly weight loss) and energy stores ($\Delta H$, predominantly fat and muscle) on energy intake, energy expenditure, neuroendocrine function, and autonomic function and the differences between factors opposing dynamic changes in energy stores and maintenance of an altered body weight.

## BACKGROUND: EVIDENCE THAT BODY ENERGY STORES ARE REGULATED

The remarkable constancy of human body weight and composition constitutes tacit evidence that body weight is regulated such that at "usual weight" energy intake and output (Q and W) are coupled and vary directly. Increases or decreases in energy expenditure are followed, not necessarily immediately, by compensatory changes in intake and vice-versa. This "coupling" is evident in the observation that despite ingesting an average of approximately 900,000 kcal/y, the average American gains only about 0.5 to 1.5 kg/y or about 4000 kcal of stored energy. If energy intake and output were not coupled then simply increasing or decreasing energy expenditure by 50 kcal/day (approximately the energy expended in a ½ mile walk at 2 MPH) without any change in energy intake would a weight loss of about 4.5 kg of body weight over 1 year.

Teleologically, increases in stored energy (particularly fat) would favor survival and maintenance of reproductive integrity (earlier onset of puberty, greater fertility, and greater likelihood of successful breastfeeding), especially in times of limited food availability. Based on the pressures of natural selection and predation in the environment in which humans evolved, the human genome should be enriched with alleles favoring energy intake and storage (when food is available) and conservation (when the diet is limited).

The strong heritability (the proportion of the variance in a given trait that is attributable to genes in individuals living in a specified environment) of body fatness, and multiple components of energy intake and output and responses to overfeeding and underfeeding involved in the regulation of body composition,[6–11] (**Table 1**), indicate the consequences of the natural selection pressures described above.

## DISCUSSION
### Measurement of Energy Intake and Expenditure

#### Overview

Adults attempting nonsurgical weight loss typically lose weight for approximately 6 months followed by a brief (3–6 month) weight plateau, and then inexorable weight regain.[12–14] If the "coupling" between energy intake and expenditure that occurs to "defend" was equipotent in defending reduced weight then sustained weight loss would be relatively easy. Energy homeostatic systems would work in concert to simply maintain energy balance. Unfortunately, the opposite is true and energy intake and expenditure vary indirectly during and after weight loss such that there are both a decline in energy expenditure and an increase in appetite. Energy homeostatic systems response to a complex interaction of short-term and longer-term signals reflecting nutritional status (both energy stores and balance) as well as hedonic preferences and learned behaviors (**Fig. 1**).

The processes of dynamic weight loss ($Q < W$) and attempts to sustain weight loss ($Q = W$) are associated with hypometabolism, hyperphagia, changes in neuroendocrine function (decreased circulating concentrations of bioactive thyroid hormones and leptin), and autonomic nervous system (ANS) function (decreased sympathetic nervous system tone and increased parasympathetic nervous system tone) which "conspire" to favor regain of lost weight.[14–18]

#### Energy Intake

Efforts to model weight regain indicate that the increase in appetite (approximately 100 kcal/day above baseline) is a more potent effector of weight regain than the

**Table 1**
**Heritability of body fatness, energy expenditure, energy intake, and weight gain during under- and over-feeding**

| Trait | Heritability |
| --- | --- |
| Body Fatness[7] | 35%–75% |
| Energy Expenditure: | |
|   Total | 40% |
|   Resting | 50% |
|   Diet-induced | 40% |
|   Physical Activity | 25%–40% |
| Energy Intake: | |
|   Meal Initiation (hunger)<br>  Macronutrient content<br>  Portion size<br>  Satiation | All 25%–40% |
| Weight gain during overfeeding<br>Weight loss during underfeeding | 50%–60% correlation within twin pairs<br>65%-90% correlation within twin pairs |

Heritability of body fatness, energy expenditure, energy intake, and weight gain during under- and over-feeding based on a literature review. Heritability refers to the portion of the variability in given trait that is attributable to genetics rather than absolute values. What is most likely heritable in the case of adiposity is the rank order of body fatness in a given population based on diet and lifestyle. The population in which that heritability is expressed interacts with genetics to affect absolute levels of fatness.
*Data from* Refs.[6–11]

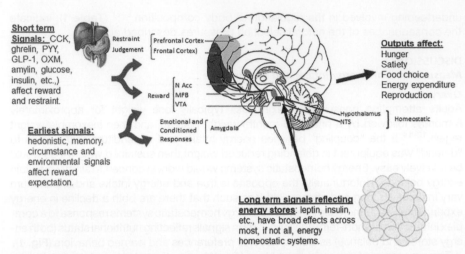

**Short term Signals:** CCK, ghrelin, PYY, GLP-1, OXM, amylin, glucose, insulin, etc.,) affect reward and restraint.

Restraint Judgement

Prefrontal Cortex / Frontal Cortex)

Reward

N Acc
MFB
VTA

Emotional and Conditioned Responses

Amygdala

**Earliest signals:** hedonistic, memory, circumstance and environmental signals affect reward expectation.

Hypothalamus
NTS

Homeostatic

**Outputs affect:** Hunger Satiety Food choice Energy expenditure Reproduction

**Long term signals reflecting energy stores:** leptin, insulin, etc., have broad effects across most, if not all, energy homeostatic systems.

**Fig. 1.** Simplified schematic of earliest, short-term, and long-term signals affecting central energy homeostatic systems. N Acc, nucleus accumbens; NTS, nucleus of the tractus solitarius; MFB, median forebrain bundle; VTA, ventral tegmental area.

disproportionate decline in energy expenditure[19–22] and a bigger contributor to the increasing prevalence of obesity than decreased physical activity.[23,24]

Functional magnetic resonance imaging (fMRI) studies of responses to visual food suggest that having obesity is associated with the dysregulation of functional connectivity of brain networks involved in reward, cognition, reward, self-referential processing, and emotional regulation.[25–27] All of these differences between those with and without obesity would favor weight gain. It should be noted that some of these studies do not control for whether or not participants are at their lifetime maximal weights or in the process of attempted weight loss at the time of testing raising questions of whether there are differences in energy balance between participants with and without obesity.

Between groups studies comparing those with and without obesity cannot differentiate whether differences in neuronal responses to food are a cause or a consequence of weight gain. In contrast, changes in neuronal signaling in participants studied before and after weight loss (within-group analyses) reflect the effects of dynamic weight loss (negative energy balance) and/or effects of reduced energy stores (weight stability and energy balance).

Weight maintenance after diet-induced weight reduction in humans is associated with region-specific changes in fMRI signaling in response to visual food cues (**Table 2**). Specifically, responsiveness is increased in brain areas related to reward (mainly the orbitofrontal cortex) and decreased in the hypothalamus and brain areas related to restraint (mainly the prefrontal cortex).[28–30] Early changes in these pathways during weight loss have been found to be premonitory of the success of weight loss and reduced weight maintenance.[29]

The increased food reward and decreased restraint following weight loss noted in these fMRI studies should translate, respectively, into increased hunger and delayed satiation. Numerous studies have shown increased hunger and delayed satiation both during weight loss and attempts to sustain weight loss with dietary intervention[31,32] and that these changes persist even years after successful weight loss.[33] These findings are not uniform and may be affected by the type of weight loss–for example,

**Table 2**
**Brain responses to visual food cues during weight stability before and after approximately 10% weight loss**

| Reduced Weight Greater than Initial Weight | | Initial Weight Greater than Reduced Weight. | |
|---|---|---|---|
| Trait | Neuronal Structures | Trait | Neuronal Structures |
| Emotional and cognitive responses to food (reward) | Globus Pallidus<br>Insula<br>Ventral Striatum<br>Habenula | Emotional and cognitive planning in response to food (control) | Cingulate gyrus<br>Fusiform gyrus<br>Precentral gyrus |
| Executive decision-making functions | Middle frontal gyrus<br>Lingual gyrus<br>Superior temporal gyrus | Knowledge representation | Inferior parietal lobule |
| | | Hypothalamic signaling directly or indirectly affects all aspects of energy homeostasis | Hypothalamus |

Changes in neuronal activity in response to food cues during weight stability in individuals before and after weight loss. Data indicate that following weight loss food, reward is higher and the decision to eat is processed faster. At usual weight, awareness of previous eating experiences and restraint around food is higher. *Data from* Refs.[28–30] somewhat diminished in surgical vs. nonsurgical,[34] or intermittent fasting vs. continuous caloric restriction,[35]induced weight loss. In large studies, such as the National Weight Control Registry,[36] Look AHEAD[36] and the Diabetes Prevention Trials (DPP)[37] dietary restraint has been positively associated with the degree of weight loss and negatively associated with the rate of weight regain during a supervised lifestyle intervention in adults with type 2 diabetes or prediabetes.

### Energy Expenditure

Homeostatic changes affecting energy expenditure reflect, at least in part, changes in skeletal muscle (increased work efficiency), neuroendocrine function (decreased circulating concentrations of bioactive thyroid hormones and leptin), and autonomic nervous system tone [increased parasympathetic (PNS) and decreased sympathetic (SNS) nervous system tone][15,38–42] but the relationship of these physiological changes to subsequent weight maintenance over time is undefined, beyond evidence that they are still active even years after successful weight loss[43–46] (see article by Sumithran in this issue). Circulating concentrations of leptin decline in proportion to, or slightly more than predicted by, loss of body fat during reduced weight maintenance and substantially more during active weight loss.[40]

Maintenance of a 10% or greater reduction in body weight by individuals with or without obesity is accompanied by an average decline in 24 hour energy expenditure (TEE) that is approximately 300 to 400 kcal/day below that predicted by the changes in weight and composition[15,46–48] and which persists in individuals successfully maintaining reduced weight for periods from 3 months to 6 years.[46] This finding is further supported by studies by outpatient studies, such as the National Weight Control Registry in which individuals who are successful at keeping weight off for periods of over 10 years still need to increase exercise and decrease caloric intake to compensate for a similar decrease in energy expenditure compared to those who are naturally the same weight.[44,49,50] The degree of adaptive thermogenesis (changes in energy expenditure beyond those predicted by changes in body weight and composition) following weight loss is quite variable (approximately +5% to −35% below predicted following a 10% or greater dietary weight loss), with most adaptive thermogenesis occurring in response to early (10%) weight loss.

TEE can be further compartmentalized into the resting energy expenditure (REE which is approximately 60% of TEE and consists of the predominantly biochemical work of maintaining transmembrane ion gradients and cardiorespiratory energy expended at rest), diet-induced thermogenesis (DIT which is approximately 5%–10% of TEE and consists of the work of digestion) and nonresting energy expenditure (NREE which is approximately 35% of TEE and consists of the predominantly mechanical work of physical activity). Even in sedentary individuals who do not alter their level of physical activity, reduction in NREE accounts for the majority ($\sim$150–250 kcal/day) of the disproportionate decline in energy expenditure; the remainder is accounted for by declines in REE.[15,51] The decline in REE is more pronounced during caloric restriction than during maintenance of the same reduced weight[15,51] and persists during the weight regain when individuals are below their usual weight.[52] Notably, additional weight loss (>10%) results in further declines (adjusted for metabolic mass) in NREE but to a lesser extent than occurred following a 10% reduction period without further reduction in REE.[53]

The decline in NREE is due mainly to an approximate 20% increase in skeletal muscle chemomechanical contractile efficiency during low levels of muscle work,[39,54–56] that is, levels of work commensurate with those of daily living rather than vigorous exercise. Increased relative expression in muscle of the more efficient myosin heavy chain (MHC) and sarcoplasmic endoplasmic reticulum $Ca^{2+}$-dependent ATPase (SERCA) isoforms (MHC I and SERCA2) during reduced weight maintenance are significantly correlated with the degree of increased muscle efficiency.[40] These responses are apparent consequences of the neuroendocrine and autonomic changes described later in discussion.

The simultaneous declines in expenditure and satiety, coupled with increased hunger and food reward, following weight loss are synergistic in creating create the optimal biological circumstances for weight regain. Of note, some, but not all, studies of subjects following bariatric surgery show a "blunting" of this disproportionate decline in energy expenditure resulting—in humans—from relative increases in REE or the thermic effect of feeding (TEF) as well as less effect on energy intake than seen following a lifestyle intervention.[57,58] In mice and rats, compensatory decreases in energy expenditure following weight loss caused by bariatric surgery are minimal, perhaps due to a lack of effect of surgical weight loss on sympathetic nervous system (SNS) tone and the importance of SNS tone in regulating brown adipose tissue (BAT) thermogenesis in rodents (see later in discussion).

## Mechanisms Affecting Energy Intake and Expenditure

### Overview
Homeostatic changes affecting energy expenditure are the result, at least in part, of changes in skeletal muscle (increased work efficiency), neuroendocrine function (decreased circulating concentrations of bioactive thyroid hormones and leptin), and autonomic nervous system tone (increased parasympathetic nervous system tone and decreased sympathetic nervous system tone).[16,40,59] Body composition measurements are necessary to compare changes in energy expenditure between individuals and before and after weight change or any intervention, and have also been reported as significant covariates of postweight loss weight trajectories with greater weight regain and increase in appetite associated with greater losses of weight as FFM rather than FM.[60] These pathways have been well described[15,38–42] and are still active even years after successful weight loss.[43–46] The individual variability in these responses to weight loss is substantial but it is clear that the coordinate actions of these systems creates the perfect storm for weight regain in most individuals.[40] The administration of exogenous leptin in physiological doses restores most of the energy and behavioral physiology to preweight loss status in weight-stable weight-reduced subjects with comparatively little effect when administered at usual weight or during weight loss.[31,38,40] Signals from adipose tissue including leptin, adiponectin, and various other cytokines clearly play key roles in regulating body weight[61] while increased skeletal muscle efficiency is the primary driving force of the decline in energy expenditure[38,40] during reduced weight maintenance.

### Neuroendocrine function
The primary neuroendocrine effect of weight loss and maintenance of a reduced body weight is the lower activity of the hypothalamic–pituitary–thyroid axis as a consequence of reduced circulating leptin.[33,40] After more extreme reductions in fat mass, hypothalamic–pituitary–gonadal (HPG) axis activity declines, as is seen in individuals with very low body fat content due to exercise or eating disorders. The leptin-responsive hypothalamic pro-opiomelanocortin (POMC)–melanocortin 4 receptor (MC4R) and neuropeptide Y (NPY)/agouti-related peptide (AgRP) pathways in the paraventricular nucleus (PVN) of the hypothalamus provide a nexus for the effects of relative hypoleptinemia, negative energy balance, and decreased energy stores on energy intake and expenditure. Decreased circulating (and CNS) concentrations of leptin

during and following weight loss result in decreased activity of the HPT axis (decreased thyroid-stimulating hormone [TSH], triiodothyronine [T3], and thyroxine [T4], and increased reverse T3 [rT3]) and, in cases of extreme weight loss or leptin deficiency, a decline in the activity of the HPG axis.[40] The decline in thyroid hormone decreases REE and also decreases the expression in muscle of the less chemomechanically efficient molecular isoforms: MHC II and SERCA1.[38,56]

Circulating concentrations of leptin decline in proportion to, or slightly more than predicted by, loss of body fat during reduced weight maintenance and substantially more during active weight loss.[40] The administration of exogenous leptin in physiological doses restores most of the energy and behavioral physiology to preweight loss status in weight-stable weight-reduced subjects with comparatively little effect when administered at usual weight or during weight loss.[28,31,40] Signals from adipose tissue including leptin, adiponectin, and various other cytokines clearly play key roles in regulating body weight[61] while increased skeletal muscle efficiency is the primary driving force of the decline in energy expenditure[38,40] during reduced weight maintenance.

### Autonomic nervous system

Parasympathetic (PNS) and sympathetic (SNSP) branches of the ANS provide major outflow tracts linking afferent biochemical signals regarding energy stores (eg, leptin) to efferent tracts regulating energy homeostasis via the CNS. Following weight loss, there is a significant reduction increase in PNS tone and in SNS tone which accounts for some of the disproportionate declines in both REE and NREE as well as suppression of the HPT axis.[41] ANS tone may modulate feeding behavior by effects on gut peptides via a "brain-gut" axis.[62–64]

More specifically, increased PNS output (as occurs in weight-reduced individuals) from the nucleus ambiguus in the dorsal motor nucleus of the vagus slows the heart rate and decreases REE.[42] Activation of the SNS (the opposite of what occurs as a result of weight loss) augments hypothalamic–pituitary–thyroid (HPT) axis activity centrally and production of epinephrine in the adrenal medulla peripherally and is associated with increased heart rate, decreased skeletal muscle work efficiency and, especially in rodents, increased lipolysis in white adipose tissue (WAT) and thermogenesis by brown adipose tissue BAT (due to the uncoupling of mitochondrial substrate oxidation from adenosine triphosphate (ATP) generation) with retrograde signaling to the CNS that affects energy homeostasis.[65] Recent advances in positron emission tomography (PET) scanning technology have allowed detailed imaging of human BAT, but the magnitude of its thermogenic role in adult humans remains unclear.

### Leptin

Signals from adipose tissue including leptin, adiponectin, and various other cytokines clearly play key roles in regulating body weight[61] through direct and indirect effects on appetitive behavior increased skeletal muscle efficiency[38,40] during reduced weight maintenance. The administration of exogenous leptin in physiological doses restores most of the energy and behavioral physiology to preweight loss status in weight-stable weight-reduced subjects. This is not surprising given the known inhibitory effects of leptin on hypothalamic expression the orexiant agouti-related peptide (AgRP) and stimulatory effects on the HPT axis and the SNS.[40] What is surprising is the lack of effect of exogenous leptin administration leptin on these systems when administered at usual weight or during weight loss (when circulating concentrations of leptin are lower than during weight maintenance).[28,31,40] The disparities in leptin responsiveness, coupled with the relatively brief period of weight loss (6–9 months) during pharmacotherapy for obesity, suggest that treatment to reduced weight versus maintaining reduced weight may need different physiological approaches. They also suggest that the major function of leptin is to signal inadequate energy stores to the CNS when circulating leptin concentrations are below a certain individualized threshold and that there is no difference in leptin sensitivity to higher leptin levels between individuals with and without obesity.

## SUMMARY

Conventional wisdom holds that "behavioral" issues related to the persistence of "bad habits" that provoke weight gain in the first place account for much or all of the virtually inexorable weight regain following dietary weight loss. However, the control of energy stores is achieved through coordinated regulation of energy intake and expenditure mediated by signals emanating from adipose, muscle, gastrointestinal, and other endocrine tissues, and integrated by the liver and by regulatory (hypothalamus, brainstem), hedonic–emotional (amygdala, ventral striatum, orbitofrontal cortex), and executive–restraint (cingulate, middle frontal, supramarginal, precentral, and fusiform gyri) elements of the central nervous system (CNS). Changes in these signals are not voluntary and are largely due to the reduction in circulating leptin that accompanies a reduction in fat mass and is largely relived by the administration of "replacement" doses of exogenous leptin, and constitute the physiological basis for the high recidivism to obesity of otherwise successfully treated patients. For individuals successfully sustaining weight loss, the "price" is a lifetime of conscious effort to decrease energy intake and increase expenditure beyond the respective levels required of individuals who are "naturally" at the same weight. Considerations of therapy should be tempered by the fact that these responses are highly heterogeneous and that a "one-size-fits-all" approach to behavioral, surgical, or pharmacotherapeutic interventions is not likely to be successful.

## DISCLOSURE

Dr M. Rosenbaum has no relevant disclosure statements. Dr M. Rosenbaum is supported, in part, by NIH UL1 TR00040.

## REFERENCES

1. Wolfram S. History of thermodynamics. In: A new kind of science. Champaign, IL USA: Wolfram Media; 2002. p. 1019.
2. Taubes G. Treat obesity as physiology, not physics. Nature 2012;492:155.
3. Taubes G. Is sugar toxic? The New York Times Magazine 2011.
4. Hall K, Farooqi I, Friedman J, et al. The energy balance model of obesity: beyond calories in, calories out. Amer J Clin Nutr 2022;115:1243–54.
5. Hall K. What is the required energy deficit per unit weight loss. Int J Obes 2008; 32:573–6.
6. Rankinen T, Bouchard C. Genetics of food intake and eating behavior phenotypes in humans. Annu Rev Nutr 2006;26:413–34.
7. Nan C, Guo B, Warner C, et al. Heritability of body mass index in pre-adolescence, young adulthood and late adulthood. Eur J Epidemiol 2012;27: 247–53.
8. Bouchard C, Tremblay A, Nadeau A, et al. Genetic effect in resting and exercise metabolic rates. Metabolism 1989;38:364–70.

9. Bouchard C. Heredity and the path to overweight and obesity. Med Sci Sports Exerc 1991;23:285–91.
10. Bray G, Bouchard C. The biology of human overfeeding. Obes Rev 2020;21: e13040.
11. Bouchard C, Tremblay A. Genetic influences on the response of body fat and fat distribution to positive and negative energy balances in human identical twins. J Nutr 1997;127:943S–7S.
12. Unick J, Beavers D, Jakicic J, et al. Effectiveness of lifestyle interventions for individuals with severe obesity and type 2 diabetes: results from the Look AHEAD trial. Diab Care 2011;34:2152–7.
13. Foster G, Wyatt H, Hill J, et al. Weight and metabolic outcomes after 2 years on a low-carbohydrate versus low-fat diet: a randomized trial. Ann Int Med 2010;153: 147–57.
14. Wadden T, Neiberg R, Wing R, et al. Four-year weight losses in the Look AHEAD study: factors associated with long-term success. Obesity 2011;19:1987–98.
15. Leibel R, Rosenbaum M, Hirsch J. Changes in energy expenditure resulting from altered body weight. N Eng J Med 1995;332:621–8.
16. Leibel R, Rosenbaum M. Metabolic response to weight perturbation. In: Clément K, editor. Novel insights into adipose cell functions, research and perspectives in endocrine interactions. Heidelberg: Springer-Verlag; 2010. p. 121–33.
17. Liu G, Liang L, Bray G, et al. Thyroid hormones and changes in body weight and metabolic parameters in response to weight loss diets: the POUNDS LOST trial. Int J Obes 2017;41:878–86.
18. Mai K, Brachs M, Leupelt V, et al. Effects of a combined dietary, exercise and behavioral intervention and sympathetic system on body weight maintenance after intended weight loss: Results of a randomized controlled trial. Metabolism 2018;83:60–7.
19. Hall K, Kahan S. Maintenance of lost weight and long-term management of obesity. Med Clin North Am 2018;102:183–97.
20. Polidori D, Sanghvi A, Seeley R, et al. How strongly does appetite counter weight loss? Quantification of the feedback control of human energy intake. Obes 2016; 24:2289–95.
21. Klem M, Wing R, McGuire M, et al. A descriptive study of individuals successful at long term maintenance of substantial weight loss. Am J Clin Nutr 1998;66: 239–46.
22. Guo J, Brager D, Hall K. Simulating long-term human weight-loss dynamics in response to caloric restriction. Am J Clin Nutr 2018;107:558–65.
23. Hall K, Sacks G, Chandramohan G, et al. Quantification of the effect of energy imbalance on bodyweight. Lancet 2011;378:826–37.
24. Swinburn B, Sacks G, Lo S, et al. Estimating the changes in energy flux that characterize the rise in obesity prevalence. Amer J Clin Nutr 2009;89:1723–8.
25. Rothemund Y, Preuschhof C, Bohner G, et al. Differential activation of the dorsal striatum by high-calorie visual food stimuli in obese individuals. Neuroimage 2007;37:410–21.
26. Devoto F, Zapparoli L, Bonandrini R, et al. Hungry brains: A meta-analytical review of brain activation imaging studies on food perception and appetite in obese individuals. Neurosci Biobehav Rev 2018;95:271–85.
27. Syan S, McIntyre-Wood C, Minuzzi L, et al. Dysregulated resting state functional connectivity and obesity: A systematic review. Neurosci Biobehav Rev 2021;131: 270–92.

28. Rosenbaum M, Sy M, Pavlovich K, et al. Leptin reverses weight loss–induced changes in regional neural activity responses to visual food stimuli. J Clin Invest 2008;118:2583–91.

29. Neseliler S, Hu W, Larcher K, et al. Neurocognitive and hormonal correlates of voluntary weight loss in humans. Cell Metab 2019;29:39–49.

30. Sweet L, Hassenstab J, McCaffery J, et al. Brain responses to food stimulation in obese, normal weight, and successful weight loss maintainers. Obesity 2012;20: 2220–5.

31. Kissileff H, Thornton J, Torres M, et al. Leptin reverses decline in satiation in weight-reduced obese individuals. Am J Clin Nutr 2012;95:309–17.

32. Hopkins M, Blundell J. Energy balance, body composition, sedentariness and appetite regulation: pathways to obesity. Clin Sci 2016;130:1615–28.

33. Sumithran P, Prendergast L, Delbridge E, et al. Long-term persistance of hormonal adaptations to weight loss. N Eng J Med 2011;365:1597–604.

34. Salem V, Demetriou L, Behary P, et al. Weight loss by low-calorie diet vesus gastric bypass surgery in people With diabetes results in divergent brain activation patterns: A functional MRI study. Diab Care 2021;44:1842–51.

35. Beaulier K, Casanova N, Oustric P, et al. Matched weight loss through intermittent or continuous energy restriction does not lead to compensatory increases in appetite and eating behavior in a randomized controlled trial in women with overweight and obesity. J Nutr 2020;150:623–33.

36. Thomas J, BOnd D, Phelan S, et al. Weight-loss maintenance for 10 years in the National Weight Control Registry. Am J Prev Med 2014;46:17–23.

37. Delahanty L, Peyrot M, Shrader P, et al. Pretreatment, Psychological, and behavioral predictors of weight outcomes among lifestyle intervention participants in the Diabetes Prevention Program (DPP). Diab Care 2013;36:34–40.

38. Rosenbaum M, Goldsmith R, Haddad F, et al. Triiodothyronine and leptin repletion in humans similarly reverse weight-loss induced changes in skeletal muscle. Am J Physiol Endocrinol Metab 2018;315:E771–9.

39. Rosenbaum M, Vandenborne K, Goldsmith R, et al. Effects of experimental weight perturbation on skeletal muscle work efficiency in human subjects. Am J Physiol Endocrinol Metab 2003;285:R183–92.

40. Rosenbaum M, Leibel R. 20 years of leptin: role of leptin in energy homeostasis in humans. J Endocrinol 2014;223:T83–96.

41. Rosenbaum M, Hirsch J, Murphy E, et al. The effects of changes in body weight on carbohydrate metabolism, catecholamine excretion, and thyroid function. Amer J Clin Nutr 2000;71:1421–32.

42. Aronne L, Mackintosh R, Rosenbaum M, et al. Autonomic nervous system activity in weight gain and weight loss. Am J Physiol 1995;38:R222–5.

43. McCaffery J, Haley A, Sweet L, et al. Differential functional magnetic resonance imaging response to food pictures in successful weight-loss maintainers relative to normal-weight and obese controls. Am J Clin Nutr 2009;90:928–34.

44. Wing R, Hill J. Successful weight loss maintenance. Annu Rev Nutr 2001;21: 323–41.

45. DelParigi A, Chen K, Salbe A, et al. Successful dieters have increased neural activity in cortical areas involved in the control of behavior. Int J Obes 2007;31: 440–8.

46. Rosenbaum M, Hirsch J, Gallagher D, et al. Long-term persistence of adaptive thermogenesis in subjects who have maintained a reduced body weight. Amer J Clin Nutr 2008;88:906–12.

47. Dulloo A, Jacquet J, Montani J, et al. Adaptive thermogenesis in human body weight regulation: more of a concept than a measurable entity. Obes Rev 2012;13(Suppl 2):105–21.
48. Rosenbaum M, Leibel R. Adaptive thermogenesis in humans. Int J Obes 2010;34: S47–55.
49. Shick S, Wing R, Klem M, et al. Persons successful at long-term weight loss and maintenance continue to consume a low-energy low-fat diet. J Am Diet Assoc 1998;98:408–13.
50. Phelan S, Wing R. Prevalance of successful weight loss. Arch Int Med 2005;165: 2430.
51. Muller M, Enderele J, Bosy-Westphal A. Changs in energy expenditure with weight gain and weight loss in humans. Curr Obes Rep 2016;5:413–23.
52. Fothergill J, Guo J, Howard L, et al. Persistent metabolic adaptation 6 years after "The Biggest Loser" competition. Obes 2016;24:1612–9.
53. Rosenbaum M, Leibel RL. Models of energy homeostasis in response to maintenance of reduced body weight. Obesity 2016;24:1620–9.
54. Simoneau J, Rosenbaum M, Segal K, et al. Changes in human skeletal muscle characteristics following maintenance of a 10% reduction in body weight. Can J Appl Physiol 1995;20(Suppl):46P.
55. Goldsmith R, Joanisse D, Gallagher D, et al. Effects of experimental weight perturbation on skeletal muscle work efficiency, fuel utilization, and biochemistry in human subjects. Am J Physiol 2010;298:R79–88.
56. Baldwin K, Joanisse D, Haddad F, et al. Effects of weight loss and leptin on skeletal muscle in human subjects. Am J Physiol Endocrinol Metab 2011;301: R1259–66.
57. Munzberg H, Laque A, Yu S, et al. Appetite and body weight regulation after bariatric surgery. Obes Rev 2015;16:77–90.
58. Das S, Roberts S, Mccrory M, et al. Long-term changes in energy expenditure and body composition after massive weight loss induced by gastric bypass surgery. Amer J Clin Nutr 2003;78:28–30.
59. Dulloo A, Schutz Y. Adaptive thermogenesis in resistance to obesity therapies: Issues in quantifying thrifty energy expenditure phenotypes in humans. Curr Obes Rep 2015;4:230–40.
60. Turicchi J, O'Driscoll R, Finlayson G, et al. Associations between the proportion of fat-free mass loss during weight loss, changes in appetite, and subsequent weight change: results from a randomized 2-stage dietary intervention trial. Amer J Clin Nutr 2020;111:536–44.
61. MacLean P, Wing R, Davidson T, et al. NIH working group report: Innovative research to improve maintenance of weight loss. Obes 2015;23:7–15.
62. Rupp S, Stenbel A. Interactions between nesfatin-1 and the autonomic nervous system-An overview. Peptides 2022;149:170719.
63. Browning K, Verheijden S, Boeckxxstaens G. The vagus nerve in appetite regulation, mood, and intestinal inflammation. Gastroenterol 2017;152:730–44.
64. Konturek S, Konturek J, Pawlik T, et al. Brain-gut axis and its role in the control of food intake. J Physiol Pharmacol 2004;55:137–54.
65. Blaszkiewica M, Willows J, Johnson C, et al. The importance of peripheral nerves in adipose tissue for the regulation of energy balance. Biology 2019;8(1):10.

# Genetic Contributors to Obesity

Ramya Sivasubramanian, MD[a], Sonali Malhotra, MD[b,c],*

## KEYWORDS

- Pediatric obesity • Syndromic obesity • Genetic obesity

## KEY POINTS

- More common single genetic defects and syndromes causing severe obesity are melanocortin 4 gene, leptin deficiency and leptin receptor mutations, proopiomelanocortin deficiency, and Prader–Willi syndrome.
- Genes play a crucial role in the physiology of appetite regulation and energy homeostasis.
- Extreme obesity before the age of 5 years is considered as early-onset obesity as per Endocrine Society clinical practice guidelines.
- Pediatricians are the first checkpoint in raising concerns about genetic obesity: cardinal signs of genetic obesity include early-onset severe obesity, severe hyperphagia, endocrinopathies, and developmental anomalies.
- Genetic testing enables timely and definitive diagnosis.

## INTRODUCTION: THE KNOWN PREVALENCE AND HIDDEN BURDEN OF GENETIC FORMS OF OBESITY IN THE GENERAL POPULATION

Genetic forms of obesity contribute to approximately 7% of severe obesity in children and adolescents. The exact global prevalence of monogenic and syndromic forms of obesity is not well established; this may be most likely due to missed or delayed diagnosis or perhaps the failure to recognition of obesity as a disease. The challenge in determining the prevalence can be attributed to the lack of consensus on identifying and evaluating symptoms suggestive of genetic defects in a timely manner and hence a vastly undertested patient population.[1] Of the young patients who have been identified with severe early-onset obesity, the most commonly identified genetic defect has been in the melanocortin 4 receptor gene (*MC4R*). The prevalence of MC4R variants ranges widely across different studies from 0.5% to 8.5%.[2] More than 200 variants have been identified to date, primarily heterozygous dominant missense

---

[a] Department of Pediatrics, SUNY Downstate Medical Center, Brooklyn, NY, USA; [b] MGH Weight Center, Massachusetts General Hospital and Harvard Medical School, 50 Staniford Street, Suite 430, Boston, MA 02114, USA; [c] Rhythm Pharmaceuticals, 222 Berkeley Street, 12th Floor, Boston, MA 02116, USA
* Corresponding author. MGH Weight Center, 50 Staniford Street, Suite 430, Boston, MA 02114.
*E-mail address:* smalhotra1@mgh.harvard.edu

Gastroenterol Clin N Am 52 (2023) 323–332
https://doi.org/10.1016/j.gtc.2023.03.005
0889-8553/23/© 2023 Elsevier Inc. All rights reserved.

variants.[3] Heterozygous variants have been noted in 2% to 5% of pediatric patients with extreme obesity.[4,5] It cannot be concluded however if the rarity of the disease is due to sporadic diagnosis or if it is the true prevalence or both.[1] About 3% of patients with severe obesity are noted to carry mutations in the leptin receptor gene (LEPR).[6] The trend of sporadicity in diagnosis and/or true prevalence is further emphasized in genetic defects involving proopiomelanocortin (POMC), PCSK, NTRK2, and SIM 1. These genetic defects have been diagnosed in lesser than 10 to 50 cases globally.[7] While focusing on syndromic forms of obesity, Prader–Willi syndrome (PWS) is the most commonly identified cause. The reported incidence of PWS is 1/10,000 to 1/30,000, with the United States, in particular, having approximately 10,000 to 20,000 living individuals with PWS.[8] To delve further into the specifics of genetic and syndromic obesities, this chapter will focus on its pathophysiology: the genetic interplay in hunger and satiety regulation, clinical presentation, diagnostic tools, and medical and surgical management of genetic forms of obesity.

## DISCUSSION
### The Genetic Interplay in the Physiology of Appetite Regulation

Energy homeostasis is facilitated by the balance of hunger and satiety; this is regulated through afferent and efferent signaling via neural circuits that maintain orexigenic and anorexigenic effects.

This homeostasis involves the following components:[9,10]

- Gut hormones
- Vagus nerve
- Neurons, namely neuropeptide Y/agouti related protein (NPY/AgRP) neurons and POMC neurons
- Neuropeptides, namely orexin and melanin-concentrating hormone (MCH), thyrotropin-releasing hormone (TRH), and corticotropin-releasing hormone (CRH)
- Insulin, leptin
- Key genes including proprotein convertase subtilisin/Kexin type 1 (PCSK1) and melanocortin 4 receptor (MC4R)
- Alpha-melanocyte-stimulating hormone (α-MSH)

### Orexigenic pathway (appetite stimulating)
In a state of fasting, fundal mucosa releases a gut hormone known as ghrelin.[9,10] This hormone binds to a receptor known as the growth hormone secretagogue receptor (GHS-R), which is found in several areas of the brain. Ghrelin specifically binds to the GHS-R in the NPY/AgRP neurons within the arcuate nucleus of the hypothalamus. This binding signals the release of neuropeptides that stimulate appetite (orexigenic neuropeptides) such as orexin- and melanin-concentrating hormone. This binding of ghrelin also promotes appetite by its antagonistic action on MC4R in the paraventricular nucleus (PVN) of the hypothalamus. On the other hand, stimulation of NPY/AgRP neurons inhibits the secretion of anorexigenic neuropeptides, TRH and CRH, in the PVN. All of these pathways induce the feeding behavior by stimulating the hunger.[9,10]

### Anorexigenic pathway (appetite inhibitor)
While ghrelin functions as the appetite-stimulating hormone, in a postfed state several gut hormones act to inhibit ghrelin. Such gut hormones are peptide YY3-36(PYY3–36), oxyntomodulin, insulin, and glucagon. Insulin and leptin cross the blood-brain-barrier and interact with the insulin and leptin receptors, respectively, on POMC neurons

(anorexigenic neurons) to stimulate it, hence inducing the release of alpha-MSH (α-MSH) that in turn stimulates the MC4-R to induce the feeling of satiety.[11] Stimulated POMC neurons also achieve satiety by anorexigenic neuropeptides, TRH, and CRH in PVN and simultaneous inhibition of orexigenic neurons, MCH and orexin.[9,10] Parallelly, leptin binds to leptin receptors on NPY/AgRP to inhibit it, thus preventing it from inducing feelings of hunger. Other stimuli such as stretch of the stomach and gut hormone signals that reach PVN through the vagus nerve will further promote satiety through the nucleus tractus solitarius. External factors such as cold exposure can stimulate the preoptic area, which sends signals to the dorsomedial hypothalamic nuclei, which in turn send signals to rostral raphe pallidus (rRPa). On receiving the stimuli, rRPa induces thermogenesis through brown adipose tissue, thereby promoting energy expenditure.[9,10]

### Importance of Diagnosing Genetic Obesity Early for Timely Intervention

General Pediatricians are the first checkpoints in screening for childhood obesity during well child visits. Extreme obesity with onset before the age of 5 years is considered early-onset obesity as per Endocrine Society clinical practice guidelines.[12] This is vital to acknowledge as early-onset severe obesity is one of the most tell-tale signs of genetic obesity. Other cardinal signs of genetic obesity include hyperphagia, endocrinopathies, and developmental anomalies.[12] The clinical picture can vary across monogenic obesity, that is, single-gene mutations, predominantly located in the leptin-melanocortin pathway, and syndromic obesity, that is, obesity occurring in the setting of multiple organ system involvements. Clinical presentations of both types of obesity are highlighted in the following section.

## CLINICAL FEATURES OF SINGLE-GENE DEFECTS/MONOGENIC OBESITY
### Leptin Deficiency

This disorder is inherited in an autosomal recessive manner and mostly associated with consanguinity. Lesser than 1000 cases have been identified worldwide. Apart from obesity, patients can have short stature, emotional lability, cognitive delays/disability, and hyperphagia. Hypogonadotropic hypogonadism, presenting with delayed puberty can also be seen in this condition.[6,13]

### Leptin Receptor Mutation

Three percent of individuals with severe-onset obesity may have LEPR mutation. Patients with LEPR mutations present with the onset of hyperphagia as early as the neonatal period, even within one week after birth. These patients can have alterations in immune function and frequent infections. Similar to the LEP gene defect, patients with LEPR mutations can also have delayed puberty due to hypogonadotropic hypogonadism.[13–15]

### Melanocortin 4 Receptor Mutation

This defect is noted to have codominance inheritance or is rarely homozygous (more severe presentation) and is the most common cause of genetic obesity. MC4R has been identified in 3% to 6% of children with severe early-onset obesity. These patients are observed to have increased lean mass and linear growth. Biochemical evaluation may reveal hyperinsulinemia.[16–19]

### Proopiomelanocortin Deficiency

Lesser than 10 individuals worldwide have been diagnosed with POMC deficiency.[20] These patients present with obesity as early as within the first few months of life along with associated hyperphagia.[20] Infants also are noted to have cholestatic jaundice or neonatal hypoglycemia.[20] POMC deficiency most importantly presents as a classic triad of obesity, adrenal insufficiency, and pale skin pigmentation with red hair.[21]

POMC gene codes the POMC polypeptide, which in healthy individuals gets cleaved into vital polypeptides: adrenocorticotropin hormone (ACTH), α-MSH, and β-MSH. When there is a gene defect involving the POMC gene, the lack of POMC cleavage into ACTH leads to hypocortisolism, hence neonatal hypoglycemia. Lack of β-MSH leads to deficient melanogenesis, leading to pale skin and red hair. Deficiency of α-MSH leads to lack of satiety and hence hyperphagia and severe obesity.[21]

### Proprotein Convertase Deficiency

Lesser than 20 cases have been identified worldwide. Key clinical findings include early-onset obesity, hyperphagia, postprandial hypoglycemia, and enteropathy, causing diarrhea.[22] Patients also have ACTH deficiency, causing secondary adrenal insufficiency, hypogonadotropic hypogonadism, and impaired glucose tolerance.[22]

### Other rare forms of genetic obesity

Defects in neurotrophic tyrosine kinase receptor has been diagnosed in lesser than 10 cases worldwide; however it presents with early-onset obesity, hyperphagia, developmental delay, short-term memory impairment, and nociception anomalies.[6,7] Similarly, patients with brain-derived neurotrophic factor gene variants, although its prevalence is unclear, are noted to have hyperphagia, severe obesity, cognitive impairment, and hyperactivity.[6,7] Single-minded homolog1 gene defects have been reported in lesser that 50 cases worldwide, with patients demonstrating severe obesity and neurobehavioral abnormalities, emotional lability, or autism-like presentation. Tubby bipartite transcription factor defect presents as early-onset obesity, and patients have characteristic vision deterioration.[6,7]

### TYPES AND CLINICAL FEATURES OF SYNDROMIC OBESITY
#### Prader–Willi Syndrome

PWS is the most common cause of syndromic obesity.[8] Interestingly, patients with PWS can present in neonates as low birth weight, feeding difficulties, and severe hypotonia. In early childhood, patients develop constant preoccupation with food and gradual onset of severe obesity.[23] These patients have characteristic facial features, strabismus, and scoliosis. They also present with delayed motor, social, and language developmental milestones with various degrees of behavioral concerns. Other manifestations include hypogonadism with genital hypoplasia, incomplete pubertal development, infertility, and short stature.[8]

### Rapid-Onset Obesity with Hypothalamic Dysregulation, Hypoventilation, and Autonomic Dysregulation Syndrome

This disorder is less prevalent, with only around 100 cases identified globally. It is defined by rapid early-onset obesity, hyperphagia, seizures, alveolar hypoventilation, central hypothyroidism, endocrinopathies, sodium and water dysregulation, autonomic dysfunction, and neuroendocrine tumor.[24]

### Alström Syndrome

This syndrome has been identified in approximately 700 cases globally. Patients are noted to have severe obesity and type 2 diabetes mellitus.[7] These patients can have hyperlipidemia with pancreatitis. Dilated cardiomyopathy or congestive heart failure is seen in 70% of patients by adolescence.[25] Visual defects are of significant concern in children with Alström syndrome, as they have an onset of retinitis pigmentosa by 15 months of age, retinal degeneration, and neurosensory deafness before 10 years of age.[7,25]

### Bardet–Biedl Syndrome

The prevalence of Bardet–Biedl syndrome (BBS) is lesser than 1: 100,000 in Europe and North America. Patients with BBS have a myriad of symptoms apart from severe obesity, including hyperphagia, several congenital anomalies such as polydactyly, renal defects, congenital heart disease, olfactory deficit, and dental defects.[7,26] Patients can be diagnosed with rod-cone retinal dystrophy and retinitis pigmentosa.[26]

### Pseudohypoparathyroidism Type 1a

This syndrome has an autosomal dominant inheritance, and patients present with obesity, short stature, round facies, brachydactyly, typically, short fourth metacarpal, and other skeletal anomalies with subcutaneous ossifications. Biochemical evaluation can show hypocalcemia and hyperphosphatemia.[27]

### Other rare syndromic obesities

Several syndromic obesities are notable for their unique presentations despite their rarity in general population; these include Wilms tumor aniridia-genitourinary anomalies mental retardation and obesity (WAGRO), Cohen, Smith-Magenis, Borjeson-Forssman-Lehmann, Carpenter, and Kabuki syndromes to name a few. Patients can present with Wilms tumor, aniridia, ambiguous genitalia, mental retardation, and obesity; this is termed WAGRO syndrome.[28] Cohen syndrome is an autosomal recessive disorder in which patients are noted with obesity, hypotonia, microcephaly, distinctive facial features, nonprogressive psychomotor retardation, and progressive myopia.[29] Smith-Magenis syndrome, on the other hand, constitutes of obesity, neurobehavioral disorder, sleep disturbance, and multiple developmental anomalies.[30] Although literature does not indicate the prevalence of Borjeson–Forssman–Lehmann[31] syndrome, patients with this syndrome are tend to present with obesity, microcephaly and severe mental disability, epilepsy, delayed puberty due to hypogonadism, and gynecomastia.[31] Carpenter syndrome (also referred to as acrocephalopolysyndactyly type II) presentation constitutes obesity, acrocephaly, preaxial polydactyly, soft tissue syndactyly, brachy- or agenesis mesophalangy of the hands and feet, congenital heart disease, umbilical Hernia, and cognitive deficits.[32] Kabuki syndrome is a rare syndrome that constitutes obesity, characteristic facial dysmorphism, intellectual deficits, visceral and skeletal malformations, growth deficiency, and several endocrinopathies.[33]

## AVAILABLE DIAGNOSTIC METHODS

Genetic testing enables timely and definitive diagnosis of genetic causes, thus providing patient and their families specific information on patients' underlying pathology, ways to mitigate the symptoms, and reducing self-blame for obesity and persistent weight gain.

Pediatric Endocrine Society guideline recommends genetic testing in children with extreme, early-onset obesity before 5 years of age with hyperphagia and/or a family history of extreme obesity.[12] Next-generation sequencing of the genes postulated to be involved in the clinical phenotype should be considered. Advantages of gene panels that makes them tier-1 tests are that they are of low costs, have a shorter turnaround time, and nonspecific tests are minimal.[34] Having stated the advantages, they are still less sensitive in comparison with whole exome sequencing (WES).[35,36] WES is favored as a first-line approach in evaluation of monogenic disorders due to the ability to identify greater number of genes compared with gene panels.[35,36] WES uses high-throughput DNA sequencing technology to determine subset of genome and sequences the exon DNA[35,36]; this helps establish specific defective genetic variants attributable to patient's altered protein sequences. WES holds promise for precision medicine in pediatric obesity.[36] However, shortfalls of WES include its sensitivity to sequence (GC) content as well as capturing design and enrichment[37]; this makes whole genome sequence (WGS) even more favorable than WES. WGS provides a more comprehensive coverage of the exome and other clinically relevant genomic sequences.[37] WGS offers a genome-wide read, which provides a more reliable detection of copy-number variations attributing to the ongoing disease.[37,38] The only disadvantages are that WGS is more expensive than WES and requires more time to produce results than WES.[37]

## AVAILABLE THERAPEUTICS FOR GENETIC FORMS OF OBESITY
### Pharmacologic Options

- Metreleptin (recombinant leptin analogue)

This drug currently has Food and Drug Administration (FDA) approval for treatment of congenital and acquired lipodystrophy. It has been considered among children with obesity caused by *LEP* gene defects.[39] Metreleptin reduces hunger and body weight among children and adults with congenital leptin deficiency.[39]

- Sibutramine (serotonin-norepinephrine reuptake inhibitor)

This drug has showed promise in patients with *MC4R* mutation in maintaining body weight, improving body composition, and reducing obesity-related metabolic abnormalities.[40] However, FDA discontinued this medication to its cardiovascular adverse effects.[41]

- Exenatide and liraglutide (glucagon-like peptide 1 [GLP-1] agonists)

GLP-1 agonists have shown promise in obesity management.[42–44] One-year use of GLP-1 agonists in female subjects with PWS led to lowered ghrelin levels, food consumption, and lowered body mass index (BMI). A single 10-μg exenatide injection when compared with a placebo also helped achieve satiety and decreased glucose levels.[45,46]

- Oxytocin

A recent study has reported the efficacy of investigational therapy involving an oxytocin analogue: carbetocin. When administered, intranasally carbetocin showed a reduction in hunger.[47]

Apart from appetite and weight control, syndromic obesity also requires management of multitude of associated symptoms such as serotonin reuptake inhibitors, N-acetylcysteine, or topiramate, which are used to control skin picking and repetitiveness.[48] Similarly, sex steroids are recommended in the pubertal years in these children to allow for development of secondary sexual characteristics and optimal bone health.[49,50]

### Surgical Management of Genetic Obesity

Bariatric surgery (BS) is considered to be the most effective intervention for severe obesity. Adjustable gastric banding helped maintain long-term weight loss in patients with homozygous null mutations in *LEPR*. Response to BS in patients with heterozygous

*MC4R* mutations has also been found of similar efficacy as in the general population with severe obesity.[51,52]

Adolescents with PWS undergoing one-anastomosis gastric bypass have demonstrated clinically significant weight loss, improved gait, better lung function, and higher quality of life.[53] Patients with PWS have had promising outcomes with laparoscopic sleeve gastrectomy.[54] Although short-term outcomes in PWS have been efficient with BS, longer-term follow-up did not support sustainable long-term weight loss or comorbidity resolution. Although modest weight loss was achieved at 2 years postoperatively, weight gain was seen at further follow-ups at 3, 5, 8, and 10 years.[55]

Patients with other causes of syndromic obesity such as BBS have shown good outcome with BS.[56] A patient demonstrated BMI drop from 52.28 to 34.85 kg/m$^2$ when followed-up for 3.5 years after laparoscopic Roux-en-Y gastric bypass accompanied by lowered blood pressure, hyperuricemia, and mobility.[56] However, longer term studies would be beneficial in all genetic and syndromic obesity disorders to asses its true efficacy over a prolonged term.

## CLINICS CARE POINTS

- Genetic obesity contributes to ~7% of severe obesity in children and adolescents.

- More common single genetic defects and syndromes causing severe obesity are melanocortin 4 gene (*MC4R*), leptin deficiency and leptin receptor mutations, proopiomelanocortin deficiency, MC4R gene variants, and PWS.

- Genes play a crucial role in the physiology of appetite regulation and energy homeostasis.

- Extreme obesity before the age of 5 years is considered early-onset obesity as per Endocrine Society clinical practice guidelines.

- Pediatricians are the first checkpoints in raising concerns about genetic obesity and thus earlier identification: cardinal signs of genetic obesity include early-onset severe obesity, severe hyperphagia, endocrinopathies, and developmental anomalies.

- Genetic testing enables timely and definitive diagnosis. Some key medications of interest in tackling genetic contributors of obesity include: recombinant leptin analogues, SNRIs, GLP-1 agonists.

- BS has been used in some forms of genetic obesity; however, because of the small sample size and lack of long-term follow-up, its efficacy has not been established in this unique form of obesity.

## DISCLOSURE

S. Malhotra is an employee of Rhythm Pharmaceuticals. R. Sivasubramanian has nothing to disclose.

## REFERENCES

1. Dayton K, Miller J. Finding treatable genetic obesity: strategies for success. Curr Opin Pediatr 2018;30:526–31.
2. Vaisse C, Clement K, Guy-Grand B, et al. A frameshift mutation in human MC4R is associated with a dominant form of obesity. Nat Genet 1998;20:113–4.
3. Kuhnen P, Krude H, Biebermann H. Melanocortin-4 Receptor Signalling: Importance for Weight Regulation and Obesity Treatment. Trends Mol Med 2019;25: 136–48.

4. Vaisse C, Clement K, Durand E, et al. Melanocortin-4 receptor mutations are a frequent and heterogeneous cause of morbid obesity. J Clin Invest 2000;106: 253–62.

5. Farooqi IS, Yeo GS, Keogh JM, et al. Dominant and recessive inheritance of morbid obesity associated with melanocortin 4 receptor deficiency. J Clin Invest 2000;106:271–9.

6. Huvenne H, Dubern B, Clement K, et al. Rare Genetic Forms of Obesity: Clinical Approach and Current Treatments in 2016. Obes Facts 2016;9:158–73.

7. Thaker VV. Genetic and Epigenetic Causes of Obesity. Adolesc Med State Art Rev 2017;28:379–405.

8. Bohonowych J, Miller J, McCandless SE, et al. The Global Prader-Willi Syndrome Registry: Development, Launch, and Early Demographics. Genes 2019;10.

9. Andermann ML, Lowell BB. Toward a Wiring Diagram Understanding of Appetite Control. Neuron 2017;95:757–78.

10. Roh E, Kim MS. Brain Regulation of Energy Metabolism. Endocrinol Metab (Seoul) 2016;31:519–24.

11. Eneli I, Xu J, Webster M, et al. Tracing the effect of the melanocortin-4 receptor pathway in obesity: study design and methodology of the TEMPO registry. Appl Clin Genet 2019;12:87–93.

12. Styne DM, Arslanian SA, Connor EL, et al. Pediatric Obesity-Assessment, Treatment, and Prevention: An Endocrine Society Clinical Practice Guideline. J Clin Endocrinol Metab 2017;102:709–57.

13. Heymsfield SB, Avena NM, Baier L, et al. Hyperphagia: current concepts and future directions proceedings of the 2nd international conference on hyperphagia. Obesity 2014;22(Suppl 1):S1–17.

14. Farooqi S. Insights from the genetics of severe childhood obesity. Horm Res 2007;68(Suppl 5):5–7.

15. Kleinendorst L, Abawi O, van der Kamp HJ, et al. Leptin receptor deficiency: a systematic literature review and prevalence estimation based on population genetics. Eur J Endocrinol 2020;182:47–56.

16. Vollbach H, Brandt S, Lahr G, et al. Prevalence and phenotypic characterization of MC4R variants in a large pediatric cohort. Int J Obes 2017;41:13–22.

17. Hinney A, Volckmar AL, Knoll N. Melanocortin-4 receptor in energy homeostasis and obesity pathogenesis. Prog Mol Biol Transl Sci 2013;114:147–91.

18. Farooqi IS, Keogh JM, Yeo GS, et al. Clinical spectrum of obesity and mutations in the melanocortin 4 receptor gene. N Engl J Med 2003;348:1085–95.

19. Hainerova IA, Lebl J. Treatment options for children with monogenic forms of obesity. World Rev Nutr Diet 2013;106:105–12.

20. Koves IH, Roth C. Genetic and Syndromic Causes of Obesity and its Management. Indian J Pediatr 2018;85:478–85.

21. Gregoric N, Groselj U, Bratina N, et al. Two Cases With an Early Presented Proopiomelanocortin Deficiency-A Long-Term Follow-Up and Systematic Literature Review. Front Endocrinol 2021;12:689387.

22. Stijnen P, Ramos-Molina B, O'Rahilly S, et al. PCSK1 Mutations and Human Endocrinopathies: From Obesity to Gastrointestinal Disorders. Endocr Rev 2016;37: 347–71.

23. Miller JL. Approach to the child with prader-willi syndrome. J Clin Endocrinol Metab 2012;97:3837–44.

24. Harvengt J, Gernay C, Mastouri M, et al. ROHHAD(NET) Syndrome: Systematic Review of the Clinical Timeline and Recommendations for Diagnosis and Prognosis. J Clin Endocrinol Metab 2020;105.

25. Yakubi M, Cicek D, Demir M, et al. Diagnosing Alstrom syndrome in a patient followed up with syndromic obesity for years. Intractable Rare Dis Res 2022;11:84–6.

26. Elawad O, Dafallah MA, Ahmed MMM, et al. Bardet-Biedl syndrome: a case series. J Med Case Rep 2022;16:169.

27. Kuzel AR, Lodhi MU, Rahim M. Classic and Non-Classic Features in Pseudohypoparathyroidism: Case Study and Brief Literature Review. Cureus 2017;9:e1878.

28. Ferreira MAT, Almeida Junior IG, Kuratani DK, et al. WAGRO syndrome: a rare genetic condition associated with aniridia and additional ophthalmologic abnormalities. Arq Bras Oftalmol 2019;82:336–8.

29. Pirgon O, Atabek ME, Sert A. Metabolic syndrome manifestations in Cohen syndrome: description of two new patients. J Child Neurol 2006;21:536–8.

30. Gandhi AA, Wilson TA, Sisley S, et al. Relationships between food-related behaviors, obesity, and medication use in individuals with Smith-Magenis syndrome. Res Dev Disabil 2022;127:104257.

31. Voss AK, Gamble R, Collin C, et al. Protein and gene expression analysis of Phf6, the gene mutated in the Borjeson-Forssman-Lehmann Syndrome of intellectual disability and obesity. Gene Expr Patterns 2007;7:858–71.

32. Hidestrand P, Vasconez H, Cottrill C. Carpenter syndrome. J Craniofac Surg 2009;20:254–6.

33. Wang YR, Xu NX, Wang J, et al. Kabuki syndrome: review of the clinical features, diagnosis and epigenetic mechanisms. World J Pediatr 2019;15:528–35.

34. Saudi Mendeliome G. Comprehensive gene panels provide advantages over clinical exome sequencing for Mendelian diseases. Genome Biol 2015;16:134.

35. LaDuca H, Farwell KD, Vuong H, et al. Exome sequencing covers >98% of mutations identified on targeted next generation sequencing panels. PLoS One 2017;12:e0170843.

36. Bamshad MJ, Ng SB, Bigham AW, et al. Exome sequencing as a tool for Mendelian disease gene discovery. Nat Rev Genet 2011;12:745–55.

37. Meienberg J, Bruggmann R, Oexle K, et al. Clinical sequencing: is WGS the better WES? Hum Genet 2016;135:359–62.

38. Girirajan S, Brkanac Z, Coe BP, et al. Relative burden of large CNVs on a range of neurodevelopmental phenotypes. PLoS Genet 2011;7:e1002334.

39. Paz-Filho G, Mastronardi CA, Licinio J. Leptin treatment: facts and expectations. Metabolism 2015;64:146–56.

40. Hainerova IA, Zamrazilova H, Sedlackova D, et al. Hypogonadotropic hypogonadism in a homozygous MC4R mutation carrier and the effect of sibutramine treatment on body weight and obesity-related health risks. Obes Facts 2011;4: 324–8.

41. James WP, Caterson ID, Coutinho W, et al. Effect of sibutramine on cardiovascular outcomes in overweight and obese subjects. N Engl J Med 2010;363:905–17.

42. Khera R, Murad MH, Chandar AK, et al. Association of pharmacological treatments for obesity with weight loss and adverse events: a systematic review and meta-analysis. JAMA 2016;315:2424–34.

43. Senda M, Ogawa S, Nako K, et al. The glucagon-like peptide-1 analog liraglutide suppresses ghrelin and controls diabetes in a patient with Prader-Willi syndrome. Endocr J 2012;59:889–94.

44. Kim YM, Lee YJ, Kim SY, et al. Successful rapid weight reduction and the use of liraglutide for morbid obesity in adolescent Prader-Willi syndrome. Ann Pediatr Endocrinol Metab 2020;25:52–6.

45. Sze L, Purtell L, Jenkins A, et al. Effects of a single dose of exenatide on appetite, gut hormones, and glucose homeostasis in adults with Prader-Willi syndrome. J Clin Endocrinol Metab 2011;96:E1314–9.
46. Lomenick JP, Buchowski MS, Shoemaker AH. A 52-week pilot study of the effects of exenatide on body weight in patients with hypothalamic obesity. Obesity 2016; 24:1222–5.
47. Dykens EM, Miller J, Angulo M, et al. Intranasal carbetocin reduces hyperphagia in individuals with Prader-Willi syndrome. JCI Insight 2018;3.
48. Jafferany M, Patel A. Skin-picking disorder: a guide to diagnosis and management. CNS Drugs 2019;33:337–46.
49. Butler MG. Management of obesity in Prader-Willi syndrome. Nat Clin Pract Endocrinol Metab 2006;2:592–3.
50. Nolan BJ, Proietto J, Sumithran P. Intensive management of obesity in people with Prader-Willi syndrome. Endocrine 2022;77(1):57–62.
51. Aslan IR, Ranadive SA, Ersoy BA, et al. Bariatric surgery in a patient with complete MC4R deficiency. Int J Obes 2011;35:457–61.
52. Valette M, Poitou C, Le Beyec J, et al. Melanocortin-4 receptor mutations and polymorphisms do not affect weight loss after bariatric surgery. PLoS One 2012;7:e48221.
53. Tripodi M, Casertano A, Peluso M, et al. Prader-Willi syndrome: role of bariatric surgery in two adolescents with obesity. Obes Surg 2020;30:4602–4.
54. Martinelli V, Chiappedi M, Pellegrino E, et al. Laparoscopic sleeve gastrectomy in an adolescent with Prader-Willi syndrome: psychosocial implications. Nutrition 2019;61:67–9.
55. Liu SY, Wong SK, Lam CC, et al. Bariatric surgery for Prader-Willi syndrome was ineffective in producing sustainable weight loss: Long term results for up to 10 years. Pediatr Obes 2020;15:e12575.
56. Daskalakis M, Till H, Kiess W, et al. Roux-en-Y gastric bypass in an adolescent patient with Bardet-Biedl syndrome, a monogenic obesity disorder. Obes Surg 2010;20:121–5.

# Developmental Contributions to Obesity
## Nutritional Exposures in the First Thousand Days

Allison J. Wu, MD, MPH[a],*, Emily Oken, MD, MPH[b]

## KEYWORDS

• Pregnancy • Infant • Nutrition • Diet • Breastfeeding • Sugar-sweetened beverages

## KEY POINTS

- Nutritional exposures in the prenatal and postnatal periods contribute to offspring's long-term obesity risk and related health outcomes. There are complex mechanisms involved in intergenerational obesity, including epigenetics, the microbiome, and inflammation.
- High-quality research suggests that maternal consumption of a low-inflammatory diet or Mediterranean diet during pregnancy may be beneficial to weight status and adiposity for both mother and offspring.
- Feeding during infancy, including the timing of and composition of complementary feeding, and avoidance of fruit juice and sugar-sweetened beverages, also influences obesity risk into later life.

## INTRODUCTION

As has been discussed elsewhere in this issue, obesity is prevalent worldwide and has risen over the past decades among all sectors of the population, including children. For example, obesity, defined in childhood as body mass index (BMI) at or above the 95th percentile for age and sex, was prevalent in 5% of children 2 to 5 year old in the United States (US) from 1971 to 1974 and increased to over 13% in 2017 to 2018.[1] Childhood obesity has been shown to track into adulthood,[2] increasing risks of type 2 diabetes, non-alcoholic fatty liver disease, and other chronic adult diseases.

Funding: Dr E. Oken receives funding from the National Institutes of Health, United States (grants R01 HD034568 and UH3 OD023286).
a Division of Gastroenterology, Hepatology and Nutrition, Boston Children's Hospital, Harvard Medical School, 300 Longwood Avenue, Hunnewell Ground, Boston, MA 02115, USA;
b Division of Chronic Disease Research Across the Lifecourse, Department of Population Medicine, Harvard Medical School and Harvard Pilgrim Health Care Institute, 401 Park Drive, Suite 401E, Boston, MA 02215, USA
* Corresponding author.
E-mail address: Allison.Wu@childrens.harvard.edu

Gastroenterol Clin N Am 52 (2023) 333–345
https://doi.org/10.1016/j.gtc.2023.02.001
0889-8553/23/© 2023 Elsevier Inc. All rights reserved.

Obesity-related co-morbidities are increasingly being diagnosed earlier in the life course, including during childhood. The incidence of type 2 diabetes among US children has grown at about 5% per year, with the largest increases in racial and ethnic minority groups.[3]

Because of the myriad challenges surrounding the treatment and management of obesity and its sequelae, prevention is critical. An important period associated with the risk of development of obesity in childhood, and consequently throughout life, is the "first thousand days," — the period spanning from conception to 24 months of age.[4] Here we focus on reviewing the most recent evidence on specific nutritional exposures during the prenatal and early childhood periods (**Fig. 1**), shown to have persistent influences on obesity risk. We will briefly discuss potential mechanisms by which early-life nutrition may influence long-term obesity risk, and finally, review important implications for gastroenterologists, primary care providers, and other clinicians.

Genetics and a wealth of environmental factors also contribute to obesity risk, as covered elsewhere in this issue. Other modifiable early-life exposures (eg, environmental chemical exposures,[4] maternal prenatal smoking,[5] and stress[6]) have additionally been shown to influence later obesity and cardiometabolic risk, but will not be covered in this selective review. This review will focus on diet for several reasons. First, there is already substantial existing literature about other early-life factors as predictors of offspring obesity. Well-described prenatal obesity risk factors include maternal obesity entering pregnancy, excess gestational weight gain, and diabetes during pregnancy.[7–9] Among infants, both larger size at birth and faster weight gain in infancy predict subsequent obesity risk.[10] However, these factors are likely downstream of exposures like diet, environment, and genetics. Also, the goal of prevention is to extrapolate from observation to interventions, and conditions including obesity, diabetes, and weight gain do not directly translate to targeted interventions. Dietary intake is an example of a risk factor for which there may be more apparent and feasible behavior change interventions.

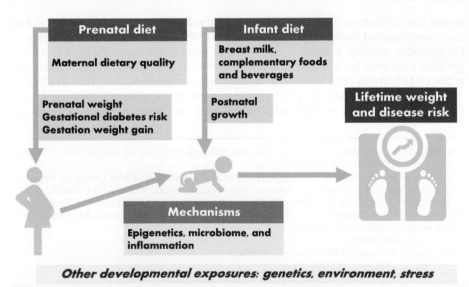

**Fig. 1.** Nutritional predictors of obesity in the first thousand days.

## DISCUSSION OF EVIDENCE
### Prenatal Nutrition and Offspring Obesity Risk

Prenatal nutritional exposures may influence not only fetal development but also subsequent lifelong health. Well-established examples include the importance of dietary folate to protect against neural tube defects,[11] and of dietary iron[12] and iodine[13] for the prevention of impaired neurodevelopment. Beyond individual essential nutrients, the quality of a pregnant woman's diet may have a persistent influence on complex chronic disease risk.

### Maternal dietary quality
Research over the past decade has increasingly focused on the quality of the overall diet, rather than the intake of individual nutrients or foods because foods are not consumed in isolation. Intakes of individual dietary components may be highly correlated, making it difficult or impossible to tease out the most important components; also, foods may interact with each other. Thus, many recent studies are focused on dietary patterns, which may be characterized as more or less healthful based on their associations with adverse health outcomes. Dietary patterns are defined as "the quantities, proportions, variety, or combination of different foods, drinks, and nutrients in diets, and the frequency with which they are habitually consumed,[14] whereas diet indices further represent a measure of "healthy" eating patterns."

- The Mediterranean diet

The main components of the Mediterranean diet include vegetables, fruits, nuts, legumes, whole grains, olive oil, and fish, as well as a low to moderate intake of dairy, and low intake of meat.[15] An extensive body of literature has shown the Mediterranean diet among adults is effective in reducing the risk of cardiovascular diseases, such as coronary heart disease and stroke, and overall mortality.[16,17] Studies in Spain, Greece, and the United States have now also found that greater maternal adherence to the Mediterranean diet in pregnancy was associated with lower markers of offspring adiposity, including BMI-z-score, waist circumference, waist-to-height ratio, skinfold thicknesses, as well as lower blood pressure in offspring during childhood (~4–7 years old).[18,19] Therefore, the Mediterranean diet during pregnancy is likely not only of benefit to the mother's long-term health, but also that of her child.

- Dietary Inflammatory Index

The Dietary Inflammatory Index (DII) is a method of classifying the overall inflammatory potential of a diet. It is a validated score that includes 45 food parameters that influence circulating inflammatory biomarkers.[20] The DII is inversely correlated with the Mediterranean diet score, that is, those with greater adherence to the Mediterranean diet will have a lower DII.[21,22] A more negative score is optimal as it represents a less pro-inflammatory (or, more anti-inflammatory) diet.

There have been several studies examining associations of maternal DII in pregnancy with offspring size at birth, with disparate results. The Healthy Start Study from Colorado observed that higher DII scores in mothers with obesity during pregnancy were associated with greater neonatal adiposity, specifically birth weight, fat mass, and percent fat mass.[23] The newborn epigenetics study (NEST), a racially and ethnically diverse cohort in North Carolina, did not observe associations of maternal energy-adjusted DII scores with birth anthropometry.[24] However, a 2021 meta-analysis of 24,861 mother–child dyads in seven European cohorts observed that a higher energy-adjusted DII during pregnancy was associated with an increased risk of low birth weight and being small for gestational age.[25] Similarly, the Massachusetts-based Project Viva cohort found that higher DII scores were associated with lower birth weight for gestational age z-score in infants born to mothers with obesity.[26]

Although low infant birth weight is generally associated with lower attained size and obesity risk, it is independently associated with greater cardiometabolic risk in later life.[27,28] In addition, rapid weight gain in infancy, especially among those with low birth weight, is associated with greater odds of being classified as having overweight and obesity in childhood[29] and adulthood.[30] In Project Viva, children 3 to 10 year old who were exposed to the highest versus lowest quartile of DII in utero had faster weight gain and in higher BMI-z-scores in mid-childhood (**Fig. 2**).[22] Further, children exposed in utero to low adherence to a Mediterranean-type diet also experienced faster growth rates in childhood, whereas adherence to the Alternate Healthy Eating Index for Pregnancy (AHEI-P) was not associated with offspring growth rates.[22] An additional study in Project Viva observed that combined exposure to a pro-inflammatory diet in utero and in early childhood was associated with higher adiposity in all children.[31]

Thus, it is possible that maternal dietary inflammation, like other pro-inflammatory exposures including cigarette smoking and air pollution, predicts the specially pernicious offspring growth pattern of poor fetal growth followed by rapid postnatal growth and higher obesity risk. Although the evidence base remains limited and inconsistent, there is likely no harm in maintaining a low-inflammatory diet during pregnancy. This advice may be especially critical for reproductive-age women with obesity.

- Other dietary patterns

Other measures may capture dietary patterns associated with offspring weight status and growth. In the conditions affecting neurocognitive development and learning in early childhood (CANDLE) study, a maternal dietary pattern during pregnancy represented by fried foods and sugar-sweetened beverages was found to contribute to rapid early childhood growth and increased risk for obesity in offspring at age 4 years.[32] In the Irish randomized control trial of a low glycaemic index diet in pregnancy to prevent macrosomia (ROLO) study, a randomized control trial (RCT) of a low glycemic index diet in pregnancy to prevent macrosomia, a low glycemic diet in pregnancy was not observed to impact offspring body composition 5 years after the intervention.[33] The ALPHABET consortium across Europe observed a higher maternal Dietary Approaches to Stop Hypertension (DASH) score, characterized by reduced intakes of saturated and total fat and sodium restriction of less than 2300 mg per day during pregnancy was associated with a lower odds of offspring overweight and obesity (OWOB) in late-childhood and was not associated with early- childhood or mid-childhood OWOB.[34] Relative to other dietary patterns, maternal DASH score and associations with offspring adiposity and childhood obesity are understudied.

### Nutritional Exposures During Infancy and Later Obesity Risk

We highlight the following nutritional exposures associated with the development of excess adiposity in early childhood: breastfeeding, complementary feeding timing and quality, sugar-sweetened beverage intake, and fruit juice intake.

### Breastfeeding

Breastfeeding has many health benefits for mother and child, including improved cognitive development and lower risk for atopic diseases. There is evidence that infant exposure to breast milk, and thereby, to a variety of flavors from the maternal diet, may promote greater dietary variety and quality later in life.[35] Breastmilk itself may promote healthy infant growth through nutritional cues in the breastmilk, such as human milk oligosaccharides, which are natural prebiotics that shape the infant gut microbiome.

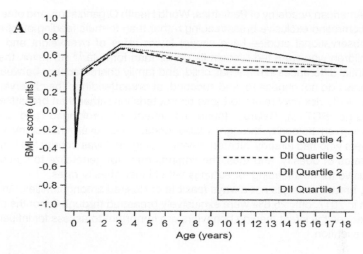

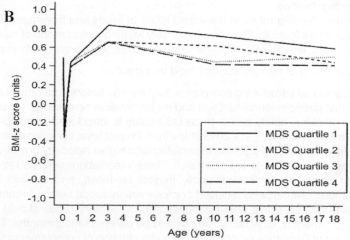

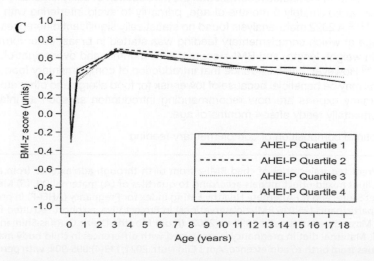

Thus, the American Academy of Pediatrics, World Health Organization, and other expert bodies recommend exclusive breastfeeding rather than formula feeding of infants.[36]

Many observational studies have shown lower rates of overweight and obesity among children who were fed breastmilk rather than formula.[14] However, there may be substantial differences in maternal, child, and family characteristics between those that do versus do not choose to, and succeed, at breastfeeding. The observed differences in obesity risk may relate to these characteristics rather than breastfeeding itself. A large RCT in Belarus found no effect of prolonged and exclusive breastfeeding on adiposity through adolescence.[37] However, that study included only mothers who had already initiated breastfeeding, and was conducted in a setting with low rates of obesity, and thus, the findings may not generalize to comparisons with exclusive formula feeding, or settings with higher obesity rates.

Further, breastfeeding is not always feasible or desired among families. Among infants born in 2017, only 25.6% were exclusively breastfed through 6 months of age.[38] Thus, other healthy infant feeding behaviors are important to assess for influences on obesity prevention.

### Complementary feeding

Complementary feeding refers to the introduction of foods and beverages other than breast milk or infant formula. The complementary feeding period is one of rapid growth and development, and therefore, a time when good nutrition is especially important.[39]

- Optimal timing of complementary food introduction

Experts agree that introducing complementary feeding before 4 months of age is too early given that gastrointestinal function and motor development are not yet sufficiently mature. Nonetheless, nearly one in three US infants is introduced to complementary foods before age 4 months.[40] In a 2019 study from Project Viva, complementary feeding initiated before 4 months of age was associated with higher adiposity in mid-childhood in both breastfed and formula-fed children.[41] These associations persisted into adolescence, with higher waist circumference, truncal fat mass, and skinfold thickness observed among children who received complementary foods before 4 months.[41]

An ongoing debate exists about whether complementary foods should be introduced at 4 to 5 months, or whether they should be delayed until 6 months. The American Academic of Pediatrics recommends the introduction of complementary foods to infants at approximately 6 months of age, primarily to avoid interfering with breastfeeding.[40,42] A 2022 meta-analysis found no statistically significant differences related to the age at which complementary feeding was started in breastfed or formula-fed infants in weight, length, and BMI z-scores at 12 months, and overweight/obesity at 3 years.[43] However, given evidence that introduction of complementary foods before 6 months may be beneficial because of lower risk for food allergy and other atopic diseases, many experts are now recommending introduction as soon as infants are developmentally ready after 4 months of age.

- Optimal composition of complementary feeding

**Fig. 2.** Predicted trajectories of child BMI-z from birth through adolescence from adjusted linear splines mixed-effect models according to quartiles of (*A*) maternal DII, (*B*) Mediterranean Diet Score, and (*C*) Alternate Healthy Eating Index for Pregnancy (AHEI-P) in pregnancy in 1459 participants (25,016 BMI-z observations) in Project Viva, a cohort recruited from the Boston, Massachusetts, area in 1999 to 2002. (*From* Monthé-Drèze C, Rifas-Shiman SL, Aris IM, et al. Maternal diet in pregnancy is associated with differences in child body mass index trajectories from birth to adolescence. Am J Clin Nutr. 2021;113(4):895-904; with permission.)

There are limited data to suggest that the quality of complementary foods introduced in infancy influences obesity risk. A systematic review performed to inform the 2020 to 2025 Dietary Guidelines for Americans generally found no relation between types and amounts of complementary foods and beverages, including meat, cereal, and foods with different fats, with growth, size, body composition, and/or risk of malnutrition, overweight, or obesity.[44] Nevertheless, evidence is growing that patterns of complementary feeding behaviors in infancy have been found to predict later diet quality, which itself may be important for obesity and cardiometabolic risk. In the Project Viva cohort, infants with a dietary pattern characterized by the introduction of more foods, especially those with stronger flavors, as well as delayed introduction of sweets and fruit juice and longer exposure to breast milk, had healthier diet quality scores at around age 3 years.[45]

Given the high nutrient density of vegetables but low overall consumption in childhood, a "vegetable-first" approach to complementary feeding has been proposed.[46] In an RCT, infants randomized to receive vegetables only (n = 61) versus a combination of fruit and vegetables (control, n = 56) for a duration of 4 weeks, starting from the first day of complementary feeding at 4 to 6 months of age, had higher intake and greater acceptance of vegetables at 9 months, and no difference in iron status.[47] Early exposure to vegetables, as well as the timing, variety, and consistency of vegetable introduction during the weaning period, increases the likelihood of vegetable acceptance and consumption in childhood.[48]

- Sugar-sweetened beverages

As summarized by the US Dietary Guidelines Advisory Committee, avoiding the consumption of sugar-sweetened beverages (SSB) by children younger than age 2 years is important for several reasons.[14] First, the energy provided by such beverages displaces "room" for energy from nutritious complementary foods and beverages, leading to potential nutrient deficiencies. Second, limited evidence suggests that SSB consumption by infants and young children is associated with the subsequent risk of child overweight. Lastly, intake of SSB in early life may set the stage for a greater intake of SSB later in life, with potentially adverse health risks. Accordingly, children should avoid consuming beverages with added sugar.

- Fruit juice

Consumption of 100% fruit juice may also be detrimental to optimal health. In the Project Viva cohort, higher fruit juice intake at 1 year of age was associated not only with higher fruit juice intake, but also with greater sugar-sweetened beverage intake and higher BMI-z-score in early-childhood and mid-childhood.[49] It may be that fruit juice is especially harmful in younger children. For example, a meta-analysis showed that fruit juice intake during ages 1 to 6 years was significantly associated with a higher change in BMI [50]; however, in children older than 6 years, fruit juice consumption was not associated with weight gain.[51]

Most of these studies did not include direct assessments of adiposity, and it is possible that higher BMI reflects higher lean mass as well as fat mass. In our own work in Project Viva, we confirmed that higher fruit juice intake at 1 year was associated with persistently greater abdominal adiposity measured directly by dual-energy x-ray absorptiometry, in particular, the metabolically pernicious visceral adiposity, in mid-childhood and early adolescence.[52] There is now a widespread consensus, which has subsequently informed national guidelines that fruit juice should not be consumed by infants ≤12 month old and should be limited to ≤4 ounces per day in children over 12 months old.[53]

## Mechanisms of Intergenerational Obesity

Developmental exposures such as diet likely influence long-term obesity risk through a variety of mechanisms, including changes to offspring epigenetics, microbiome, and inflammation.

- Epigenetics

Epigenetics, literally "above the genes," relates to changes in gene activity that do not involve changes in DNA sequence. Early-life nutrition can influence epigenetic differences that are linked to health later in life.[54] Nutritional status early in pregnancy has been linked to persistent epigenetic changes in offspring.[55] Further, evidence is emerging regarding paternal diet and physical activity that may influence offspring health via alterations in the sperm epigenome.[56]

- Microbiome

The human microbiome is the environment of microbial communities found on the skin and in the oral, gastrointestinal, respiratory, and urinary tracts. Changes in the microbiome have been linked widely to a variety of human diseases, including obesity, over the life course. The maternal microbiome "seeds" the infant microbiome[57] at birth and perhaps even prenatally. In addition, maternal obesity and poor diet can alter breastmilk composition, and thereby, restructure the infant gastrointestinal microbiome.[58] Alteration of the composition of the infant gut microbiota may contribute to the programming of metabolism.[59] There is also evidence that the interaction of maternal dietary factors with early-life epigenetic mechanisms and the gut microbiome contributes to offspring obesity in adulthood (**Fig. 3**).[60]

- Inflammation

Diet is a potential contributor to systemic inflammation, which in pregnant women may influence the fetus' physiologic development. Further, oxidative stress and

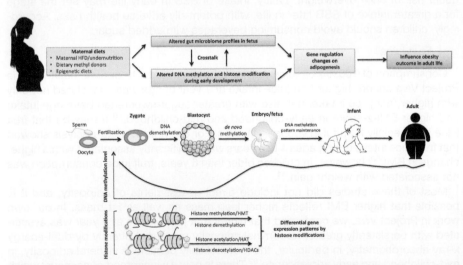

**Fig. 3.** The interaction of maternal dietary factors with early-life epigenetic mechanism and the gut microbiome in the regulation of obesity in adult life. (*From* Li Y. Epigenetic Mechanisms Link Maternal Diets and Gut Microbiome to Obesity in the Offspring. Front Genet. 2018;9.)

inflammation impair placental circulation and thus fetal growth. For example, fructose may induce inflammation in adipocytes, driving its obesogenic effects.

## SUMMARY

Nutritional exposures during the first thousand days of development are associated with adiposity and obesity risk throughout later childhood and adolescence, perhaps tracking throughout life. We have reviewed here evidence that poor maternal dietary quality, as well as the timing and composition of complementary foods and beverages in infancy, can influence risks for childhood obesity.

### Future Directions

The nutritional factors we reviewed here may be directly and successfully intervened upon for obesity prevention. For example, in an RCT among mothers of young children, those in the intervention arm had a significant reduction in caloric beverage intake themselves as well as a significant increase in limit setting for 100% fruit juice in their children.[61]

Despite the abundance of observational research on this topic, future investigation that will translate into direct changes in clinical care is warranted. Specifically, trials during pregnancy and even preconception will further investigate the causality between maternal nutrition and obesity in offspring. Obesity care and management will be best informed by research that focuses on critical intervention elements associated with clinically important, patient-centered, and longer-term health and weight outcomes in the mother and child.

It is also important to note that not only individual-level interventions, but also policy changes are likely needed to sustainably improve these behaviors.[62,63] Childhood obesity, and the developmental risk factors for obesity reviewed in this article, are disproportionately prevalent among low-income, Black and Hispanic populations. As but one example, there is a higher prevalence of early introduction of complementary foods among Black infants and infants of mothers and households with lower socioeconomic status.[40] These populations are at higher risk for childhood obesity, and evidence suggests that improving early-life risk factors may eliminate such obesity disparities.[64] As structural factors such as neighborhood characteristics may influence diet quality and thereby obesity and cardiometabolic risk,[65] effective solutions may also need to address these larger structures and systemic inequities.

## CLINICS CARE POINTS

- Clinicians should understand that developmental contributions to obesity occur through intricate mechanisms and include a multitude of early-life risk factors, many beyond the patient's control.

- Clinicians can screen for obesity risk in children by assessing exposure to early-life factors including maternal obesity.

- Clinicians caring for individuals who are or may become pregnant can target the promotion of healthy eating through the consumption of
  - Low inflammatory diet, including avoidance of SSB and fewer fried foods
  - Mediterranean diet

- Clinicians may counsel parents with infants to
  - Delay complementary feeding in the first 4 months of life.
  - Introduce a variety of complementary foods, especially vegetables, those with stronger tastes, and potential allergens, after 4 months of age.

> ○ Avoid providing fruit juice to children younger than 12 months and limit it to less than 4 ounces per day in children 12 months and older.
> ○ Avoid giving children beverages with added sugars.

## DISCLOSURE

The authors have no commercial or financial conflicts of interest to disclose.

## REFERENCES

1. Fryar CD, Carroll MD, Afful J. Prevalence of overweight, obesity, and severe obesity among children and adolescents aged 2–19 Years: United States, 1963–1965 through 2017–2018. National Center for Health Statistics 2020.
2. Guo SS, Wu W, Chumlea WC, et al. Predicting overweight and obesity in adulthood from body mass index values in childhood and adolescence. Am J Epidemiol 2002;76(3):653–8.
3. Jensen ET, Dabelea D. Type 2 diabetes in youth: new lessons from the search study. Curr Diabetes Rep 2018;18(6):36.
4. Aris IM, Fleisch AF, Oken E. Developmental origins of disease: emerging prenatal risk factors and future disease risk. Curr Epidemiol Rep 2018;5(3):293–302.
5. Hu J, Aris IM, Lin PID, et al. Longitudinal associations of modifiable risk factors in the first 1000 days with weight status and metabolic risk in early adolescence. Am J Clin Nutr 2020;113(1):113–22.
6. Miller AL, Lumeng JC. Pathways of association from stress to obesity in early childhood. Obesity 2018;26(7):1117–24.
7. Hawkins SS, Oken E, Gillman MW. Early in the life course: time for obesity prevention. In: Handbook of life course health development. Cham, Switzerland: Springer International Publishing; 2018. p. 169–96.
8. Voerman E, Santos S, Golab BP, et al. Maternal body mass index, gestational weight gain, and the risk of overweight and obesity across childhood: An individual participant data meta-analysis. PLoS Med 2019;16(2):e1002744.
9. Heslehurst N, Vieira R, Akhter Z, et al. The association between maternal body mass index and child obesity: A systematic review and meta-analysis. PLoS Med 2019;16(6):e1002817.
10. Perng W, Hajj H, Belfort MB, et al. Birth size, early life weight gain, and midchildhood cardiometabolic health. J Pediatr 2016;173:122–30.e1.
11. Pitkin RM. Folate and neural tube defects. Am J Clin Nutr 2007;85(1):285S–8S.
12. Means RT. Iron deficiency and iron deficiency anemia: implications and impact in pregnancy, fetal development, and early childhood parameters. Nutrients 2020;12(2):447.
13. Rodriguez-Diaz E, Pearce EN. Iodine status and supplementation before, during, and after pregnancy. Best Pract Res Clin Endocrinol Metabol 2020;34(4):101430.
14. Dietary Guidelines Advisory Committee. Scientific report of the 2020 dietary guidelines advisory committee: advisory report to the secretary of agriculture and the secretary of health and human services. USDA; 2020.
15. Lecorguillé M, Teo S, Phillips CM. Maternal dietary quality and dietary inflammation associations with offspring growth, placental development, and DNA methylation. Nutrients 2021;13(9):3130.
16. Fung TT, Rexrode KM, Mantzoros CS, et al. Mediterranean diet and incidence and mortality of coronary heart disease and stroke in women. Circulation 2009;119(8):1093–100.

17. Ahmad S, Moorthy MV, Demler OV, et al. Assessment of risk factors and bio-markers associated with risk of cardiovascular disease among women consuming a mediterranean diet. JAMA Netw Open 2018;1(8):e185708.
18. Fernández-Barrés S, Romaguera D, Valvi D, et al. Mediterranean dietary pattern in pregnant women and offspring risk of overweight and abdominal obesity in early childhood: the INMA birth cohort study. Pediatr Obes 2016;11(6):491–9.
19. Chatzi L, Rifas-Shiman SL, Georgiou V, et al. Adherence to the mediterranean diet during pregnancy and offspring adiposity and cardiometabolic traits in child-hood. Pediatr Obes 2017;12(S1):47–56.
20. Shivappa N, Steck SE, Hurley TG, et al. Designing and developing a literature-derived, population-based dietary inflammatory index. Publ Health Nutr 2014; 17(8):1689–96.
21. Casas R, Castro-Barquero S, Crovetto F, et al. Maternal dietary inflammatory in-dex during pregnancy is associated with perinatal outcomes: results from the IMPACT BCN Trial. Nutrients 2022;14(11):2284.
22. Monthé-Drèze C, Rifas-Shiman SL, Aris IM, et al. Maternal diet in pregnancy is associated with differences in child body mass index trajectories from birth to adolescence. Am J Clin Nutr 2021;113(4):895–904.
23. Moore BF, Sauder KA, Starling AP, et al. Proinflammatory diets during pregnancy and neonatal adiposity in the healthy start study. J Pediatr 2018;195:121–7.e2.
24. McCullough LE, Miller EE, Calderwood LE, et al. Maternal inflammatory diet and adverse pregnancy outcomes: Circulating cytokines and genomic imprinting as potential regulators? Epigenetics 2017;12(8):688–97.
25. Chen LW, Aubert AM, Shivappa N, et al. Associations of maternal dietary inflam-matory potential and quality with offspring birth outcomes: An individual partici-pant data pooled analysis of 7 European cohorts in the ALPHABET consortium. PLoS Med 2021;18(1):e1003491.
26. Sen S, Rifas-Shiman SL, Shivappa N, et al. Dietary inflammatory potential during pregnancy is associated with lower fetal growth and breastfeeding failure: results from project viva. J Nutr 2016;146(4):728–36.
27. Yun J, Jung YH, Shin SH, et al. Impact of very preterm birth and post-discharge growth on cardiometabolic outcomes at school age: a retrospective cohort study. BMC Pediatr 2021;21(1):373.
28. Knop MR, Geng T, Gorny AW, et al. Birth weight and risk of type 2 diabetes mel-litus, cardiovascular disease, and hypertension in adults: a meta-analysis of 7 646 267 participants from 135 studies. J Am Heart Assoc 2018;7(23):e008870.
29. Taveras EM, Rifas-Shiman SL, Belfort MB, et al. Weight status in the first 6 months of life and obesity at 3 years of age. Pediatrics 2009;123(4):1177–83.
30. Zheng M, Lamb KE, Grimes C, et al. Rapid weight gain during infancy and sub-sequent adiposity: a systematic review and meta-analysis of evidence. Obes Rev 2018;19(3):321–32.
31. Sen S, Rifas-Shiman SL, Shivappa N, et al. Associations of prenatal and early life dietary inflammatory potential with childhood adiposity and cardiometabolic risk in Project Viva. Pediatr Obes 2018;13(5):292–300.
32. Hu Z, Tylavsky FA, Kocak M, et al. Effects of maternal dietary patterns during pregnancy on early childhood growth trajectories and obesity risk: the CANDLE study. Nutrients 2020;12(2):465.
33. Callanan S, Yelverton CA, Geraghty AA, et al. The association of a low glycaemic index diet in pregnancy with child body composition at 5 years of age: A second-ary analysis of the ROLO study. Pediatr Obes 2021;16(12):e12820.

34. Chen LW, Aubert AM, Shivappa N, et al. Maternal dietary quality, inflammatory potential and childhood adiposity: an individual participant data pooled analysis of seven European cohorts in the ALPHABET consortium. BMC Med 2021; 19(1):33.

35. Trabulsi JC, Mennella JA. Diet, sensitive periods in flavour learning, and growth. Int Rev Psychiatr 2012;24(3):219–30.

36. Breastfeeding. Available at: https://www.who.int/health-topics/breastfeeding.

37. Martin RM, Kramer MS, Patel R, et al. Effects of promoting long-term, exclusive breastfeeding on adolescent adiposity, blood pressure, and growth trajectories: a secondary analysis of a randomized clinical trial. JAMA Pediatr 2017;171(7): e170698.

38. CDC. Breastfeeding Report Card. Centers for Disease Control and Prevention. 2020. Available at: https://www.cdc.gov/breastfeeding/data/reportcard.htm. Accessed November 24, 2021.

39. Fewtrell M, Bronsky J, Campoy C, et al. Complementary feeding: a position paper by the european society for paediatric gastroenterology, hepatology, and nutrition (ESPGHAN) Committee on Nutrition. J Pediatr Gastroenterol Nutr 2017;64(1).

40. Chiang KV. Timing of introduction of complementary foods — United States, 2016–2018. MMWR Morb Mortal Wkly Rep 2020;69. Available at: https://www.cdc.gov/mmwr/volumes/69/wr/mm6947a4.htm.

41. Gingras V, Aris IM, Rifas-Shiman SL, et al. Timing of complementary feeding introduction and adiposity throughout childhood. Pediatrics 2019;144(6):e20191320.

42. American Academy of Pediatrics Committee on Nutrition. Complementary Feeding. In: Kleinman RE, Greer FR, editors. Pediatric Nutrition. 8th ed. Itasca, IL: American Academy of Pediatrics; 2019. p. 163–86.

43. Verga MC, Scotese I, Bergamini M, et al. Timing of complementary feeding, growth, and risk of non-communicable diseases: systematic review and meta-analysis. Nutrients 2022;14(3):702.

44. English LK, Obbagy JE, Wong YP, et al. Types and amounts of complementary foods and beverages consumed and growth, size, and body composition: a systematic review. Am J Clin Nutr 2019;109:956S–77S.

45. Switkowski KM, Gingras V, Rifas-Shiman SL, et al. Patterns of complementary feeding behaviors predict diet quality in early childhood. Nutrients 2020; 12(3):810.

46. Nekitsing C, Hetherington MM. Implementing a 'vegetables first' approach to complementary feeding. Curr Nutr Rep 2022;11(2):301–10.

47. Rapson JP, von Hurst PR, Hetherington MM, et al. Starting complementary feeding with vegetables only increases vegetable acceptance at 9 months: a randomized controlled trial. Am J Clin Nutr 2022;116:111–21.

48. Johnson SL. Developmental and environmental influences on young children's vegetable preferences and consumption. Adv Nutr 2016;7(1):220S–31S.

49. Sonneville KR, Long MW, Rifas-Shiman SL, et al. Juice and water intake in infancy and later beverage intake and adiposity: Could juice be a gateway drink? Obesity 2015;23(1):170–6.

50. Shefferly A, Scharf RJ, DeBoer MD. Longitudinal evaluation of 100% fruit juice consumption on BMI status in 2–5-year-old children. Pediatr Obes 2016;11(3): 221–7.

51. Auerbach BJ, Wolf FM, Hikida A, et al. Fruit juice and change in BMI: A Meta-analysis. Pediatrics 2017;139(4):e20162454.

52. Wu AJ, Aris IM, Rifas-Shiman SL, et al. Longitudinal associations of fruit juice intake in infancy with DXA-measured abdominal adiposity in mid-childhood and early adolescence. Am J Clin Nutr 2021;114(1):117–23.

53. U.S. Department of Agriculture, U.S. Department of Health and Human Services. Dietary guidelines for Americans, 2020-2025. DietaryGuidelines.gov 2020;164.

54. Kappil M, Wright RO, Sanders AP. Developmental origins of common disease: epigenetic contributions to obesity. Annu Rev Genom Hum Genet 2016;17(1): 177–92.

55. Waterland RA, Kellermayer R, Laritsky E, et al. Season of conception in rural gambia affects DNA methylation at putative human metastable epialleles. Whitelaw E, ed. PLoS Genet 2010;6(12):e1001252.

56. Schagdarsurengin U, Steger K. Epigenetics in male reproduction: effect of paternal diet on sperm quality and offspring health. Nat Rev Urol 2016;13(10): 584–95.

57. Gomez de Agüero M, Ganal-Vonarburg SC, Fuhrer T, et al. The maternal microbiota drives early postnatal innate immune development. Science 2016; 351(6279):1296–302.

58. Catalano PM, Shankar K. Obesity and pregnancy: mechanisms of short term and long term adverse consequences for mother and child. BMJ 2017;360:j1.

59. Mulligan CM, Friedman JE. Maternal modifiers of the infant gut microbiota: metabolic consequences. J Endocrinol 2017;235(1):R1–12.

60. Li Y. Epigenetic mechanisms link maternal diets and gut microbiome to obesity in the offspring. Front Genet 2018;9.

61. Nezami BT, Lytle LA, Ward DS, et al. Effect of the Smart Moms intervention on targeted mediators of change in child sugar-sweetened beverage intake. Publ Health 2020;182:193–8.

62. Grummon AH, Taillie LS, Golden SD, et al. Sugar-sweetened beverage health warnings and purchases: a randomized controlled trial. Am J Prev Med 2019; 57(5):601–10.

63. Mason AE, Schmidt L, Ishkanian L, et al. A brief motivational intervention differentially reduces sugar-sweetened beverage (SSB) consumption. Ann Behav Med 2021;55(11):1116–29.

64. Taveras EM, Gillman MW, Kleinman KP, et al. Reducing racial/ethnic disparities in childhood obesity: the role of early life risk factors. JAMA Pediatr 2013;167(8): 731–8.

65. Aris IM, Rifas-Shiman SL, Jimenez MP, et al. Neighborhood child opportunity index and adolescent cardiometabolic risk. Pediatrics 2021;147(2). e2020018903.

# Obesity, Chronic Stress, and Stress Reduction

Donald Goens, MD[a], Nicole E. Virzi, MS[b], Sarah E. Jung, MA[c],
Thomas R. Rutledge, PhD[c], Amir Zarrinpar, MD, PhD[a,c],*

## KEYWORDS

- Insulin resistance • Cardiovascular disease • Metabolic syndrome
- Nonalcoholic fatty liver disease • Caloric restriction
- Mindfulness-based interventions • Circadian rhythms • Sleep

## KEY POINTS

- The current obesity epidemic is the result of the misalignment between human biology and the modern food environment, which has led to unhealthy eating patterns and behaviors and an increase in metabolic diseases.
- This has been caused by the shift from a "leptogenic" to an "obesogenic" food environment, characterized by the availability of unhealthy food and the ability to eat at any time of day due to advances in technology.
- Stress eating is a common response to chronic stress that can contribute to weight gain and obesity and can be addressed through stress reduction strategies such as mindfulness-based interventions.
- The increase in light at night, shift work, and the availability of high-caloric foods at abnormal times can lead to chronic stress and circadian dyssynchrony, which has negative impacts on metabolism and can increase the risk of obesity and other diseases.
- One dietary approach to address circadian dysregulation is time-restricted eating (TRE), which involves restricting food intake to specific periods of the day to synchronize the body's internal clock with the external environment.

## INTRODUCTION

Few health problems capture the dynamic interaction between human biology and the environment better than the current obesity epidemic. Although circadian and appetite biological systems were aligned well with the demands of the premodern world to

[a] Division of Gastroenterology, UC San Diego, 9500 Gilman Drive, La Jolla, CA 92093, USA;
[b] Department of Clinical Psychology, San Diego State University/University of California, San Diego Joint Doctoral Program, 6363 Alvarado Court, San Diego, CA 92120, USA; [c] VA San Diego Health Sciences, 3350 La Jolla Village Drive, San Diego, CA 92161, USA
* Corresponding author. Division of Gastroenterology, UC San Diego, 9500 Gilman Drive, La Jolla, CA 92093.
E-mail address: azarrinp@ucsd.edu

Gastroenterol Clin N Am 52 (2023) 347–362
https://doi.org/10.1016/j.gtc.2023.03.009
0889-8553/23/Published by Elsevier Inc.
gastro.theclinics.com

promote survival in unstable food environments, these same systems are now misaligned with the modern food environment to instead promote obesity, metabolic diseases, and eating disorders.[1] This article will provide an overview of ways in which this biology-environment interaction has shifted in the last half-century to predispose individuals to develop metabolic diseases related to overnutrition and unhealthy eating patterns and behaviors, and to highlight validated treatments to reverse these trends.

Consider some of the most important food environment changes occurring in recent decades. In the "leptogenic" food environment characterizing the Western world prior to the mid-20th century, food was unprocessed, high in fiber, nutrient dense, and available only at limited times.[2] The premodern food environment was characterized by high energy demands for obtaining and preparing food and lighting constraints that limited eating to daytime and early evening hours. Culture played a complimentary role by encouraging social and family-oriented eating patterns that partly constrained both food choices and food quantities.

In just a few decades, however, centuries of biologically, socially, and culturally regulated aspects of eating and appetite were replaced by an "obesogenic" environment.[2] Food became hyperpalatable, calorie dense, and fiber and nutrient poor. Advances in food technology further made these premade foods available ubiquitously. Combined with similar advances in commercial electricity and multimedia entertainment, these changes enabled eating across day and nighttime hours to become not only possible but desirable and even normative.[3] With rapid changes in society, food and eating themselves assumed new meanings. Traditionally tied to family meals and cultural events, food evolved to become a form of self-expression, a source of entertainment, the focal point of holidays, and a means of coping with stress.[4] The latter form of coping, described further in the subsections later in this discussion, became widespread as the type of stress we experienced in society gradually transformed from mostly acute stress to primarily chronic stress. These physical changes in the food environment, coupled with behavioral and psychological changes in eating patterns and preferences, may help explain both the rapid rise of obesity in recent decades and the difficulties sustaining weight loss with conventional behavioral treatments (**Fig. 1**).[5] As a result of these interactive changes, our circadian and appetite regulatory systems are disrupted by the modern food environment, with the sobering result being that an estimated 88% of Americans were metabolically unhealthy in 2018.[6]

## CLINICS CARE POINTS

- The modern food environment is contributing to the obesity epidemic and related metabolic diseases.
- Food has become more processed, calorie-dense, and lacking in nutrients compared to the premodern environment.
- Changes in food technology, commercial electricity, and multimedia entertainment have enabled eating at all hours of the day and night.
- Food has also taken on new meanings, such as a form of self-expression and a means of coping with stress.
- These changes in the food environment and eating patterns have disrupted circadian and appetite regulatory systems, leading to an estimated 88% of Americans being metabolically unhealthy in 2018.

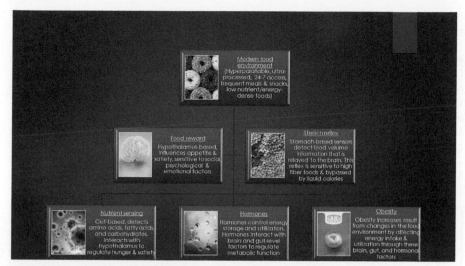

**Fig. 1.** Psychophysiological mechanisms contributing to the obesity epidemic.

## STRESS EATING AND EMOTIONAL EATING

Stress eating or emotional eating is a maladaptive behavioral response to stress. While some people may undereat and/or lose weight under stressful conditions, approximately 70% of individuals tend to overeat and/or gain weight in response to stress.[7] Stress eating also typically involves ingesting calorically dense and highly palatable foods, also known as "comfort foods." In conjunction with the overabundance of food and a modern, sedentary lifestyle, stress eating behavior plays an important role in unintended weight gain, metabolic health, and the continuing obesity epidemic.

The traditional, physiological model of stress includes the "fight or flight" mode in response to acute (ie, life threatening) stress. In this model, acute stress triggers a cascade of sympathetic hormones that redirects bodily and organ functioning away from metabolic and appetitive mechanisms, such as food intake and digestion.[8] Instead of the acute stress most often faced by our premodern ancestors, in the modern world individuals are more likely to face stressors that are long-term, cumulative, and psychosocial in nature – that is, chronic stress. Chronic stress instigates an HPA-axis-regulated endocrine response, in particular the release of cortisol, which induces overeating of energy-dense foods.[9] Eating these "comfort foods"—those that are high in fat and carbohydrate content—may reduce the chronic-stress activation of the HPA-axis.[10] Thus, stress eating or emotional eating can be fundamentally understood as a coping mechanism to chronic stress.

Men and women respond differently to stress. Women are more likely to use food as a coping mechanism, whereas men tend to use nicotine or alcohol.[11,12] The association between stress-related eating and obesity is also stronger among women than men.[13] Women also are more likely than men to engage in dietary restraint, which can be defined as the self-regulatory behavior of restraining caloric intake to lose or maintain weight, due to societal pressures to be thin.[14] Dietary restraint, especially among those who have a tendency to overeat, may trigger compensatory eating, and thus beget a cycle of overeating.[15] Being overweight may also increase the risk of stress-eating behavior, as the stress related to weight stigma may be a trigger.[16]

Additionally, in the absence of adaptive stress coping mechanisms, such as physical exercise, one may be more likely to engage in stress eating.[17]

Since chronic stress is a key factor in stress-eating, stress reduction strategies are essential for successful treatment. Mindfulness, both a key component of Acceptance Commitment Therapy (ACT) and Dialectical Behavior Therapy (DBT), encourages regulating eating habits by increasing awareness to internal hunger and satiety cues and to sensory responses while eating.[18] Guided meditations to increase awareness and identify eating triggers is also a key element in mindfulness-based interventions. Mindfulness-based approaches are effective in addressing dysregulated eating in both subclinical and clinical populations.[19]

## CLINICS CARE POINTS

- Stress eating or emotional eating is a coping mechanism for chronic stress and is characterized by the ingestion of calorically dense and highly palatable foods.
- Stress eating behavior plays a role in unintended weight gain and the obesity epidemic.
- Chronic stress can trigger the release of cortisol, which can induce overeating of energy-dense foods.
- Women are more likely than men to use food as a coping mechanism for stress and to engage in dietary restraint.
- Being overweight may increase the risk of stress-eating behavior due to weight stigma.
- Stress reduction strategies, such as mindfulness-based approaches, can be effective in addressing dysregulated eating in both subclinical and clinical populations.

## PATHOLOGICAL EATING AND EATING DISORDERS

In some cases, stress or emotional eating can lead to binge eating disorder (BED). BED is characterized by recurrent episodes of binge eating (BE; ie, occurring once per week over a 3-month period) during which individuals consume large amounts of food within a distinct period of time (ie, 2 hours) and experience a sense of loss of control over their eating. Those with BED are markedly distressed by BE episodes but refrain from using extreme compensatory behaviors (ie, self-induced vomiting, laxative misuse) between episodes.[20] Though not central to the diagnosis, BE episodes tend to occur during the evening hours.[21,22] BED is the most commonly diagnosed eating disorder, with lifetime prevalence rates of 3.5% for women and 2.0% for men.[23] Most individuals with BED are either overweight (BMI: 25–29.9) or obese (BMI: 30+).[24] The diagnosis is associated with numerous psychological and medical comorbidities, including overweight and obesity.[23]

Though the eating pattern exhibited by individuals with BED is distinct from those of anorexia and bulimia nervosa, the three major eating disorders share the same underlying psychopathology: an over-evaluation of the importance of shape and weight—and an individual's corresponding ability to control these factors—when determining one's self-worth. Across presentations, this emphasis leads to attempts to restrain or reduce one's eating, the severity of which differs by diagnosis.[25] The front-line treatment of eating disorders, including BED, is cognitive-behavioral therapy-enhanced (CBT-E),[24] a time-limited, transdiagnostic, yet individualized treatment of eating disorder psychopathology. When used to treat BED, CBT-E consists of 20 treatment sessions across 20 weeks and can be administered in either an individual or group format.

BED treatment consists of 4 distinct stages.[25] Stage one involves intensive twice-weekly sessions during which the provider constructs an individualized client case conceptualization, provides psychoeducation about treatment, and introduces the client to the main tenets of CBT-E: weekly in-session weight assessments and the establishment and ongoing self-monitoring of a regular eating pattern (ie, 3 meals and 3 snacks per day) to disrupt attempts at dietary restraint. Within the CBT-E framework, these attempts—and subjective "failures" to maintain this restraint—are posited as the practice that perpetuates binge eating episodes. Stage 2 is a transitionary stage during which the provider assesses client momentum and self-monitoring records in order to detect any barriers to weekly weighing and/or adherence to a regular eating pattern. Stage 3 consists of 8 weekly sessions of individualized treatment during which the provider and client work collaboratively to evaluate the negative consequences of the overemphasis on shape and weight, bolster the relative importance of other domains when assessing self-worth (eg, relationships, school, work, hobbies) and address other potential BED maintenance factors, including self-imposed dietary rules, event or mood-related changes in eating, negative body image, low self-esteem, clinical perfectionism, and interpersonal problems. The fourth and final stage of treatment consists of 2 biweekly sessions that prepare the client for future success by reviewing the maintenance of treatment gains, identifying realistic goals for continued improvement, and developing a plan for any anticipated obstacles. Typically, a follow-up session occurs approximately 20 weeks after treatment completion to review the client progress. CBT for BEDs yields transdiagnostic remission rates of no more than 50%, rendering it only marginally more efficacious than, if not equal to, other treatments for eating disorders.[26,27] However, it remains the most extensively studied and evidence-informed treatment of EDs to date.[28]

## CLINICS CARE POINTS

---

- Binge eating disorder (BED) is characterized by recurrent episodes of binge eating and a sense of loss of control over eating, occurring at least once per week over a 3-month period.

- BED is the most commonly diagnosed eating disorder, with a lifetime prevalence of 3.5% for women and 2.0% for men.

- Most individuals with BED are either overweight or obese.

- The underlying psychopathology of BED, as well as other eating disorders, is an overevaluation of the importance of shape and weight in determining self-worth.

- The front-line treatment of BED is cognitive-behavioral therapy-enhanced (CBT-E), which consists of 4 stages and 20 treatment sessions over 20 weeks.

- CBT-E can be administered in either an individual or group format and aims to disrupt attempts at dietary restraint, evaluate the negative consequences of an overemphasis on shape and weight, bolster the relative importance of other domains in assessing self-worth and address other potential BED maintenance factors.

- CBT-E yields transdiagnostic remission rates of no more than 50% and is the most extensively studied and evidence-informed treatment of eating disorders.

---

## CIRCADIAN CLOCK AND METABOLISM

A particularly modern source of chronic stress is the increase in light at night, shift work, and the availability of high-caloric foods in abnormal feeding times. These sources of chronic stress can lead to circadian dyssynchrony which has particularly dire metabolic consequences.[29] The human body functions with an endogenous time-keeping system driven by internal molecular clock mechanisms and environmental entrainment cues such as light and feeding. The term circadian, derived from Latin "circa" (about) and "diem" (day), was first introduced in the 1950s as a means of defining this system. Mammalian innate physiology is influenced by rhythms organized with near 24-h periodicity.[30–32] This circadian clock is an integral component of human function, with about 80% of all protein-coding genes displaying circadian expression,[33] including the majority of genes encoding pharmaceutical drug targets.[34] Alterations in the circadian clock can lead to states of disequilibrium with implications for aging and disease risk on a molecular level.[35] Indeed, specific polymorphisms in circadian clock genes (eg, CRYPTOCHROME genes, PERIOD genes, CLOCK) are associated with obesity and poor weight loss in response to various therapies including bariatric surgery.[36,37]

The influence of circadian rhythms on metabolism has been an area of extensive investigation. Animal models with disruptions in circadian rhythms lead to metabolic pathophysiology.[32] Various environmental cues can augment endogenous timekeeping. The most significant modulator is light,[38] but others such as food intake independently alter peripheral body circadian rhythms, particularly of metabolically important organs such as the intestines, liver, and muscles.[39] When behaviors (sleeping, physical activity, eating/drinking) are mistimed within the normal 24-h day cycle this can lead to circadian misalignment. One way which the interplay between metabolism and circadian misalignment has been studied is by examining the impact of shift work on body metabolism.

## CLINICS CARE POINTS

- Chronic stress, such as that caused by light at night, shift work, and abnormal feeding times, can lead to circadian dyssynchrony, which has negative consequences for metabolism.
- The human body has an endogenous timekeeping system (circadian clock) that is influenced by internal molecular mechanisms and external cues such as light and feeding.
- Alterations in the circadian clock can contribute to the development of aging and disease.
- Specific genetic variations in circadian clock genes have been linked to obesity and poor weight loss in response to various therapies, including bariatric surgery.
- The influence of circadian rhythms on metabolism has been widely studied, and disruptions in these rhythms can lead to metabolic pathophysiology.
- Environmental cues, including light and food intake, can alter the circadian rhythms of metabolically important organs such as the intestines, liver, and muscles.
- Mistiming behaviors such as sleeping, physical activity, and eating can lead to circadian misalignment, which has been studied in the context of shift work and its impact on body metabolism.

## SHIFT WORK AND OBESITY AND OBESITY-RELATED DISEASES

Shift work is a particularly modern source of chronic stress that can disrupt the body's natural circadian rhythms. Shift-based workers often engage in atypical sleep/wake cycles based on the scheduling needs of their occupation. The misalignment caused by shift-work has been linked to negative consequences for metabolism and disease risk. This form of circadian disruption has been associated with adverse health events, including cardiovascular disease, and metabolic syndrome.[29] There is a strong association between shift work and risk of overweight and obesity.[40] Night shift work in particular is associated with the increased risk of obesity/overweight and shift workers had a higher frequency of developing abdominal obesity rather than other obesity types.[41] Having ever worked a night shift is associated with increased risk for metabolic syndrome; higher cumulative years of night shifts was associated with progressively higher risk.[42]

Studies evaluating the association between sleep/duration and obesity-related disorders, in particular nonalcoholic fatty liver disease (NAFLD), have yielded varying results. Studies have shown that sleep duration <5 hours[43,44] and <6 hours[45] increased the risk of NAFLD among women; sleep duration <5 hours increased the risk of NAFLD and obesity in men compared to >7 hours which was associated with lower risk for NAFLD/obesity.[46] However, long sleep duration (>9 hours) was associated with a modestly increased risk of NAFLD in both men and women.[47] Poor sleep quality was associated with increased risk for NAFLD among both men and women[44]; and poor sleep quality predicted up to 20% of variability in liver stiffness among obese men and women with NAFLD.[48] Overall, although there are associations between sleep variability and increased risk for metabolic derangements, the specifics of this interplay require further investigation. Still, these relationships between shift work and sleep variability with obesity exemplifies the impact circadian dysregulation can have on metabolism.

## CLINICS CARE POINTS

- Shift work is a modern source of chronic stress that can disrupt the body's natural circadian rhythms and lead to negative consequences for metabolism and disease risk.

- Shift work has been associated with an increased risk of overweight and obesity, particularly among those working night shifts.

- Shift work has also been linked to an increased risk of metabolic syndrome.

- The relationship between sleep variability and increased risk for metabolic derangements, including obesity and NAFLD, is not fully understood but requires further investigation.

- It is important to consider the role of circadian rhythms in the development and management of chronic stress, especially among shift workers, in order to minimize negative health outcomes.

## THERAPEUTIC APPROACH: TIME-RESTRICTED EATING

The impact of shift work on metabolism and the risk of obesity and related disorders highlights the importance of addressing circadian dysregulation. One approach that has shown promise in this regard is time-restricted eating (TRE), which Involves restricting food intake to specific periods of the day in order to synchronize the body's internal clock with the external environment. TRE refers to the dietary intervention of limiting food consumption to a specific time window each day. The goal of TRE is the correction of circadian dyssynchrony by aligning feeding times to more active periods of central circadian rhythms. TRE is one of the many modalities of intermittent fasting, which encompasses dietary interventions that limit the timing, rather than content, of food intake.[30,49]

Early studies investigating the timing of food intake have shown that many individuals do not eat 3 discrete meals a day but rather are constantly grazing with an expanded window of caloric consumption.[3] Several studies have investigated the effects of TRE on metabolism-related health outcomes. Some key findings from extended duration (>4 weeks) randomized-controlled trials are summarized in **Table 1**. In all, the weight loss outcomes from TRE tend to be modest with only 2% to 3% TBWL in long-term clinical trials.[30] However, these clinical trials demonstrate that TRE can lead to improvements in insulin sensitivity, blood pressure, and oxidative stress in men with prediabetes[50]; improved blood glucose and insulin sensitivity in overweight adults with type 2 diabetes mellitus[51]; weight loss in overweight women[52]; weight loss and improved fasting blood glucose in obese men and women when combined with a commercial weight loss program[53]; weight loss with improved diastolic blood pressure and improved mood[54]; and significantly greater loss of fat in overweight/obese individuals when combined with concurrent exercise training.[55] Yet, some studies have found that TRE does not improve metabolic outcomes despite causing weight loss. For example, one study noted that TRE led to a reduction in fat mass in patients with NAFLD, but did not alter liver stiffness, insulin sensitivity, or LDL/HDL.[56] Another study showed that TRE reduced weight and frequency of eating but did not improve metabolic endpoints such as A1C, insulin sensitivity, or lipid measures.[57] One RCT of middle-aged women found that TRE increased fasting glucose and insulin resistance despite causing weight loss.[58]

In contrast to some studies that have found TRE to have modest benefits on metabolic outcomes, other RCTs have observed no such effects. A recent trial found no difference between groups in the primary outcome of weight change from baseline, nor in secondary outcomes such as waist circumference, insulin sensitivity, and serum lipids.[59] However, it is worth noting that this study did not adequately track food intake and the authors reported that the control group voluntarily restricted their food intake, which may complicate the interpretation of the results. Another RCT found no significant difference in weight change or secondary metabolic outcomes between the TRE group and the control group, which followed a consistent-meal timed diet with 3 structured meals and allowed for light snacking in between.[60]

Like other dietary and behavioral interventions, the success of patients using TRE will likely depend heavily on their adherence to the prescribed eating schedule. Moreover, it is not clear whether these benefits are due to the change in eating schedule itself or to the resulting caloric restriction that occurs when people adhere to this schedule,[61–63] or whether they are particularly beneficial to shift workers. Only a single study has investigated the effects of TRE on shift workers.[64] Early results from a study of firefighters who work 24-h shifts concluded that a 10-h TRE protocol significantly increased quality of life metrics, and in patients with cardiometabolic risk factors, decreased VLDL, and improved hemoglobin A1c and diastolic blood pressure.

More studies are needed to determine the optimal duration and timing of TRE that would increase the chances of desired metabolic outcomes and to better understand its effects on metabolism-related health outcomes. Mouse studies suggest that changes in the gut microbiome may play a role in the metabolic effects of time-restricted diets.[65,66] For example, certain methods that mimic the changes in the microbiome caused by TRE improve glucose tolerance without affecting mouse weights.[67] However, our understanding of the relationship between chronic stress, circadian disruption, and metabolism is incomplete, and further research may identify new therapeutic targets for reversing the negative metabolic effects of chronic stress.

**Table 1**
Randomized control trials on time-restricted eating

| Article | Intervention | Control | Population | Key Findings |
|---|---|---|---|---|
| Jamshed et al,[54] 2022 | TRE (7:00–15:00) with energy restriction diet and exercise counseling for 14 wk | Energy restriction diet and exercise counseling | Men and women aged 25–75 y with obesity following in weight management clinic at the University of Alabama at Birmingham hospital (N = 90) | TRE was more effective for losing weight and improving diastolic blood pressure and mood than eating over a window of 12 or more hours at 14 wk. |
| Sutton et al,[50] 2018 | TRE (6-h eating window, dinner before 15:00) for 5 wk followed by 7 wk washout and crossover | 12-h eating period with matched food intake | Men with prediabetes (N = 12) | TRE did not improve weight loss but improved insulin sensitivity, β cell responsiveness, blood pressure, oxidative stress, and appetite. |
| Che et al,[51] 2021 | TRE (8:00–18:00) for 12 wk | Unrestricted eating | Overweight men and women with type 2 diabetes (N = 60) | TRE led to significant decreases in body weight, A1C, and in hyperlipidemia |
| Domaszewski et al,[52] 2022 | TRE (12:00–20:00) for 6 wk | Unrestricted eating | Overweight or obese women over age 60 (N = 45) | TRE led to weight loss (approximately 2 kg) with decreases in BMI and weight, with 88% of participants adherent to the TRE diet |
| Peeke, et al,[53] 2021 | TRE (10 h) starting after dinner between 17:00 and 20:00) on a commercial weight loss program diet with a snack at fasting hour 12 for 8 wk | TRE (12 h) starting after dinner between 17:00 and 20:00) on a commercial weight loss program diet | Obese men and women (N = 60) | Those on 10 h TRE diet + fasting snack had slightly more weight loss (11 kg compared to 9 kg), with a significant reduction in fasting blood glucose only in the 10 hr TRE study arm |

(continued on next page)

**Table 1**
*(continued)*

| Article | Intervention | Control | Population | Key Findings |
|---|---|---|---|---|
| Kotarsky et al,[55] 2021 | TRE (12:00–20:00) for 8 wk combined with aerobic and resistance training | Normal diet combined with aerobic and resistance training | Overweight and obese men and women (N = 21) | TRE led to more weight loss, specifically greater loss of fat mass |
| Cai et al,[56] 2019 | TRE (8 h eating window) for 12 wk | 80% of energy needs consumed via otherwise unrestricted diet | Men and women aged 18–65 y with NAFLD (N = 271) | TRE led to a reduction in body weight and fat mass and serum triglycerides |
| Chow et al,[57] 2020 | TRE (8 h eating window) for 12 wk | Unrestricted eating | Obese men and women (N = 20) | TRE led to reduced weight and fat mass, without impact on metabolic markers |
| Isenmann et al,[62] 2021 | TRE (12:00–20:00) for 14 wk | Macronutrient-based diet | Overweight or obese (class I) adults aged 20–40 years old exercising at least twice per week (N = 35) | Both TRE and macronutrient-based diet led to weight loss, with higher adherence in the TRE group |
| Liu et al,[59] 2022 | TRE (8:00–16:00) with calorie restriction for 12 mo | Calorie-restricted diet alone | Men and women with obesity (N = 118) | TRE with calorie restriction did not lead to significant changes in body weight, fat, or metabolic risk factors compared to calorie restriction alone |
| Lowe et al,[60] 2002 | TRE (12:00–20:00) for 12 wk | 3 structured meals per day without time restriction | Overweight or obese men and women aged 18–64 (N = 116) | TRE did not lead to greater weight loss or improvement in secondary metabolic endpoints compared to structured meal intake |

| Study | Intervention | Comparator | Population | Outcome |
|---|---|---|---|---|
| Lin et al,[58] 2022 | TRE (8 h eating window) with low-calorie diet for 8 wk | Low-calorie diet | Overweight or obese women aged 40–65 (N = 63) | TRE with low-calorie diet led to more weight loss and decease in diastolic blood pressure compared to low-calorie diet alone, but higher fasting glucose and insulin resistance were noted in the TRE arm |
| Phillips et al,[63] 2021 | TRE (12 h eating window) for 6 mo | Standard dietary advice with unrestricted eating | Adults with eating duration >14 h and one component of metabolic syndrome | TRE did not lead to a significant difference in weight loss achieved with standard dietary advice |
| Thomas et al,[61] 2022 | TRE (10 h eating window) starting within 3 h of waking with daily caloric restriction for 12 wk | Daily caloric restriction | Overweight or obese men and women (N = 81) | TRE did not lead to any difference in weight loss at 12 or 39 wk or metabolic markers |

## CLINICS CARE POINTS

---

- Time-restricted eating (TRE) involves limiting food intake to specific periods of the day to synchronize the body's internal clock with the external environment.

- TRE is a form of intermittent fasting that limits the timing of food intake rather than the content.

- TRE has been shown to have modest weight loss effects in long-term clinical trials, with a 2% to 3% reduction in total body weight loss (TBWL).

- TRE has been linked to improvements in insulin sensitivity, blood pressure, and oxidative stress in men with prediabetes; improved blood glucose and insulin sensitivity in overweight adults with type 2 diabetes mellitus; weight loss in overweight women; weight loss and improved fasting blood glucose in obese men and women when combined with a commercial weight loss program; and significant fat loss in overweight/obese individuals when combined with concurrent exercise training.

- TRE may be of particular benefit to those who are shift workers.

- More research is needed to determine the optimal duration and timing of TRE, its effects on metabolism-related health outcomes, and whether it is particularly beneficial for shift workers.

- Further research is needed to understand the relationship between chronic stress, circadian disruption, and metabolism and to identify potential therapeutic targets for reversing the negative metabolic effects of chronic stress.

---

## SUMMARY

Environmental factors, including diet and stress, can contribute to the development of obesity. Stress-related eating patterns, such as consuming high-calorie foods in excess and eating late at night, may contribute to weight gain. Disruptions to the body's natural circadian rhythms, such as those experienced by shift workers, may also contribute to obesity and metabolic syndrome. While more research is needed to determine the effectiveness of time-restricted eating for obesity management, stress reduction and mindfulness techniques, as well as cognitive-behavioral therapy, have been found to be helpful in addressing disordered eating behaviors, including Binge Eating Disorder.

## DISCLOSURES

A. Zarrinpar is a co-founder, acting chief medical officer, and equity-holder in Endure Biotherapeutics. He is supported by the VA Merit BLR&D Award I01 BX005707, and NIH R21 MH117780, R01 HL148801, R01 EB030134, R01 HL157445, and U01 CA265719. All authors receive institutional support from NIH P30 DK120515, P30 DK063491, P30 CA014195, P50 AA011999, and UL1 TR001442.

## REFERENCES

1. Schnabel L., Kesse-Guyot E., Alles B., et al., Association Between Ultraprocessed Food Consumption and Risk of Mortality Among Middle-aged Adults in France, *JAMA Intern Med*, 179, 2019, 490–498.
2. Swinburn B, Egger G, Raza F. Dissecting obesogenic environments: the development and application of a framework for identifying and prioritizing environmental interventions for obesity. Prev Med 1999;29:563–70.

3. Gill S, Panda S. A Smartphone App Reveals Erratic Diurnal Eating Patterns in Humans that Can Be Modulated for Health Benefits. Cell Metabol 2015;22(5): 789–98.

4. Allison DB, Heshka S. Emotion and eating in obesity? A critical analysis. Int J Eat Disord 1993;13:289–95.

5. Hall K.D., Farooqi I.S., Friedman J.M., et al., The energy balance model of obesity: beyond calories in, calories out, Am J Clin Nutr, 115, 2022, 1243–1254.

6. Araujo J, Cai J, Stevens J. Prevalence of Optimal Metabolic Health in American Adults: National Health and Nutrition Examination Survey 2009-2016. Metab Syndr Relat Disord 2019;17:46–52.

7. Epel E, Jimenez S, Brownell K, et al. Are stress eaters at risk for the metabolic syndrome? Ann N Y Acad Sci 2004;1032:208–10.

8. Torres SJ, Nowson CA. Relationship between stress, eating behavior, and obesity. Nutrition 2007;23:887–94.

9. Dallman MF, Pecoraro N, Akana SF, et al. Chronic stress and obesity: a new view of "comfort food. Proc Natl Acad Sci U S A 2003;100:11696–701.

10. Dallman MF. Stress-induced obesity and the emotional nervous system. Trends Endocrinol Metabol: TEM (Trends Endocrinol Metab) 2010;21:159–65.

11. Conway TL, Vickers RR Jr, Ward HW, et al. Occupational stress and variation in cigarette, coffee, and alcohol consumption. J Health Soc Behav 1981;22:155–65.

12. Mehlum L. Alcohol and stress in Norwegian United Nations peacekeepers. Mil Med 1999;164:720–4.

13. Laitinen J, Ek E, Sovio U. Stress-related eating and drinking behavior and body mass index and predictors of this behavior. Prev Med 2002;34:29–39.

14. Smith JM, Serier KN, Belon KE, et al. Evaluation of the relationships between dietary restraint, emotional eating, and intuitive eating moderated by sex. Appetite 2020;155:104817.

15. Ouwens MA, van Strien T, van der Staak CP. Tendency toward overeating and restraint as predictors of food consumption. Appetite 2003;40:291–8.

16. Mouchacca J, Abbott GR, Ball K. Associations between psychological stress, eating, physical activity, sedentary behaviours and body weight among women: a longitudinal study. BMC Publ Health 2013;13:828.

17. Steptoe A, Lipsey Z, Wardle J. Stress, hassles and variations in alcohol consumption, food choice and physical exercise: A diary study. Br J Health Psychol 1998; 3:51–63.

18. Afari N., Herbert M.S., Godfrey K.M., et al., Acceptance and commitment therapy as an adjunct to the MOVE! programme: a randomized controlled trial, Obes Sci Pract, 5, 2019, 397–407.

19. Corsica J, Hood MM, Katterman S, et al. Development of a novel mindfulness and cognitive behavioral intervention for stress-eating: a comparative pilot study. Eat Behav 2014;15:694–9.

20. American psychiatric association. Washington, DC: American Psychiatric Association Publishing; 2022. p. 1, online resource.

21. Masheb RM, Grilo CM. Eating patterns and breakfast consumption in obese patients with binge eating disorder. Behav Res Ther 2006;44:1545–53.

22. Harvey K, Rosselli F, Wilson GT, et al. Eating patterns in patients with spectrum binge-eating disorder. Int J Eat Disord 2011;44:447–51.

23. Hudson JI, Hiripi E, Pope HG Jr, et al. The prevalence and correlates of eating disorders in the National Comorbidity Survey Replication. Biol Psychiatry 2007; 61:348–58.

24. Fairburn CG. Cognitive behavior therapy and eating disorders. New York: Guilford Press; 2008. p. 324, xii.

25. Murphy R, Straebler S, Cooper Z, et al. Cognitive behavioral therapy for eating disorders. Psychiatr Clin North Am 2010;33:611–27.

26. Moberg LT, Solvang B, Saele RG, et al. Effects of cognitive-behavioral and psychodynamic-interpersonal treatments for eating disorders: a meta-analytic inquiry into the role of patient characteristics and change in eating disorder-specific and general psychopathology in remission. J Eat Disord 2021;9:74.

27. Atwood ME, Friedman A. A systematic review of enhanced cognitive behavioral therapy (CBT-E) for eating disorders. Int J Eat Disord 2020;53:311–30.

28. Agras WS, Fitzsimmons-Craft EE, Wilfley DE. Evolution of cognitive-behavioral therapy for eating disorders. Behav Res Ther 2017;88:26–36.

29. Scheer FA, Hilton MF, Mantzoros CS, et al. Adverse metabolic and cardiovascular consequences of circadian misalignment. Proc Natl Acad Sci U S A 2009;106:4453–8.

30. Petersen MC, Gallop MR, Flores Ramos S, et al. Complex physiology and clinical implications of time-restricted eating. Physiol Rev 2022;102:1991–2034.

31. Golombek DA, Rosenstein RE. Physiology of circadian entrainment. Physiol Rev 2010;90:1063–102.

32. Zarrinpar A, Chaix A, Panda S. Daily Eating Patterns and Their Impact on Health and Disease. TEM (Trends Endocrinol Metab) 2016;27:69–83.

33. Mure LS, Le HD, Benegiamo G, et al. Diurnal transcriptome atlas of a primate across major neural and peripheral tissues. Science 2018;359:eaao0318.

34. Zhang R, Lahens NF, Ballance HI, et al. A circadian gene expression atlas in mammals: implications for biology and medicine. Proc Natl Acad Sci U S A 2014;111:16219–24.

35. Lopez-Otin C, Kroemer G. Hallmarks of Health. Cell 2021;184:33–63.

36. Valladares M, Obregon AM, Chaput JP. Association between genetic variants of the clock gene and obesity and sleep duration. J Physiol Biochem 2015;71:855–60.

37. Torrego-Ellacuria M, Barabash A, Matia-Martin P, et al. Influence of CLOCK Gene Variants on Weight Response after Bariatric Surgery. Nutrients 2022;14:3472.

38. Wright KP Jr, McHill AW, Birks BR, et al. Entrainment of the human circadian clock to the natural light-dark cycle. Curr Biol 2013;23:1554–8.

39. Manella G, Sabath E, Aviram R, et al. The liver-clock coordinates rhythmicity of peripheral tissues in response to feeding. Nat Metab 2021;3:829–42.

40. Wang F, Zhang L, Zhang Y, et al. Meta-analysis on night shift work and risk of metabolic syndrome. Obes Rev 2014;15:709–20.

41. Sun M, Feng W, Wang F, et al. Meta-analysis on shift work and risks of specific obesity types. Obes Rev 2018;19:28–40.

42. Vyas MV, Garg AX, Iansavichus AV, et al. Shift work and vascular events: systematic review and meta-analysis. BMJ 2012;345:e4800.

43. Kim CW, Yun KE, Jung HS, et al. Sleep duration and quality in relation to non-alcoholic fatty liver disease in middle-aged workers and their spouses. J Hepatol 2013;59:351–7.

44. Bernsmeier C, Weisskopf DM, Pflueger MO, et al. Sleep Disruption and Daytime Sleepiness Correlating with Disease Severity and Insulin Resistance in Non-Alcoholic Fatty Liver Disease: A Comparison with Healthy Controls. PLoS One 2015;10:e0143293.

45. Imaizumi H, Takahashi A, Tanji N, et al. The Association between Sleep Duration and Non-Alcoholic Fatty Liver Disease among Japanese Men and Women. Obesity facts 2015;8:234–42.

46. Hsieh SD, Muto T, Murase T, et al. Association of short sleep duration with obesity, diabetes, fatty liver and behavioral factors in Japanese men. Intern Med 2011;50: 2499–502.

47. Liu C, Zhong R, Lou J, et al. Nighttime sleep duration and risk of nonalcoholic fatty liver disease: the Dongfeng-Tongji prospective study. Ann Med 2016;48: 468–76.

48. Marin-Alejandre BA, Abete I, Cantero I, et al. Association between Sleep Disturbances and Liver Status in Obese Subjects with Nonalcoholic Fatty Liver Disease: A Comparison with Healthy Controls. Nutrients 2019;11:322.

49. Saran AR, Dave S, Zarrinpar A. Circadian Rhythms in the Pathogenesis and Treatment of Fatty Liver Disease. Gastroenterology 2020;158:1948–1966 e1941.

50. Sutton E.F., Beyl R., Early K.S., et al., Early Time-Restricted Feeding Improves Insulin Sensitivity, Blood Pressure, and Oxidative Stress Even without Weight Loss in Men with Prediabetes, *Cell Metabol*, 27, 2018, 1212–1221 e1213.

51. Che T, Yan C, Tian D, et al. Time-restricted feeding improves blood glucose and insulin sensitivity in overweight patients with type 2 diabetes: a randomised controlled trial. Nutr Metab 2021;18:88.

52. Domaszewski P, Konieczny M, Pakosz P, et al. Effect of a Six-Week Intermittent Fasting Intervention Program on the Composition of the Human Body in Women over 60 Years of Age. Int J Environ Res Public Health 2020;17:4138.

53. Peeke PM, Greenway FL, Billes SK, et al. Effect of time restricted eating on body weight and fasting glucose in participants with obesity: results of a randomized, controlled, virtual clinical trial. Nutr Diabetes 2021;11:6.

54. Jamshed H., Steger F.L., Bryan D.R., et al., Effectiveness of Early Time-Restricted Eating for Weight Loss, Fat Loss, and Cardiometabolic Health in Adults With Obesity: A Randomized Clinical Trial, *JAMA Intern Med*, 182, 2022, 953–962.

55. Kotarsky CJ, Johnson NR, Mahoney SJ, et al. Time-restricted eating and concurrent exercise training reduces fat mass and increases lean mass in overweight and obese adults. Physiol Rep 2021;9:e14868.

56. Cai H, Qin YL, Shi ZY, et al. Effects of alternate-day fasting on body weight and dyslipidaemia in patients with non-alcoholic fatty liver disease: a randomised controlled trial. BMC Gastroenterol 2019;19:219.

57. Chow L.S., Manoogian E.N.C., Alvear A., et al., Time-Restricted Eating Effects on Body Composition and Metabolic Measures in Humans who are Overweight: A Feasibility Study, *Obesity*, 28, 2020, 860–869.

58. Lin YJ, Wang YT, Chan LC, et al. Effect of time-restricted feeding on body composition and cardio-metabolic risk in middle-aged women in Taiwan. Nutrition 2022; 93:111504.

59. Liu D, Huang Y, Huang C, et al. Calorie Restriction with or without Time-Restricted Eating in Weight Loss. N Engl J Med 2022;386:1495–504.

60. Lowe DA, Wu N, Rohdin-Bibby L, et al. Effects of Time-Restricted Eating on Weight Loss and Other Metabolic Parameters in Women and Men With Overweight and Obesity: The TREAT Randomized Clinical Trial. JAMA Intern Med 2020;180:1491–9.

61. Thomas EA, Zaman A, Sloggett KJ, et al. Early time-restricted eating compared with daily caloric restriction: A randomized trial in adults with obesity. Obesity 2022;30:1027–38.

62. Isenmann E, Dissemond J, Geisler S. The Effects of a Macronutrient-Based Diet and Time-Restricted Feeding (16:8) on Body Composition in Physically Active Individuals-A 14-Week Randomised Controlled Trial. Nutrients 2021;13:3122.

63. Phillips NE, Mareschal J, Schwab N, et al. The Effects of Time-Restricted Eating versus Standard Dietary Advice on Weight, Metabolic Health and the Consumption of Processed Food: A Pragmatic Randomised Controlled Trial in Community-Based Adults. Nutrients 2021;13:1042.

64. Manoogian ENC, Zadourian A, Lo HC, et al. Feasibility of time-restricted eating and impacts on cardiometabolic health in 24-h shift workers: The Healthy Heroes randomized control trial. Cell Metabol 2022;34:1442–56.e7.

65. Zarrinpar A, Chaix A, Yooseph S, et al. Diet and feeding pattern affect the diurnal dynamics of the gut microbiome. Cell Metabol 2014;20:1006–17.

66. Dantas Machado AC, Brown SD, Lingaraju A, et al. Diet and feeding pattern modulate diurnal dynamics of the ileal microbiome and transcriptome. Cell Rep 2022;40:111008.

67. Russell B.J., Brown S.D., Siguenza N., et al., Intestinal transgene delivery with native E. coli chassis allows persistent physiological changes, *Cell*, 185, 2022, 3263–3277 e3215.

# Health Complications of Obesity

## 224 Obesity-Associated Comorbidities from a Mechanistic Perspective

Michele M.A. Yuen, MBBS (HK), MRCP (UK), FRCP (Edin), FHKCP, FHKAM (Medicine), MPH (HK)[a,b,*]

### KEYWORDS

- Obesity-associated comorbidities • Inflammation • Oxidative stress
- Growth-promoting adipokines • Insulin resistance • Endothelial dysfunction
- RAAS and SNS activations • Mechanical effects

### KEY POINTS

- Obesity is associated with 224 distinct comorbidities.
- These obesity-associated comorbidities transverse multiple specialties.
- Development of these comorbidities is driven by various mechanistic changes that are seen when excessive adipose tissue accumulates in the body.

## INTRODUCTION
### Background

Obesity is associated with a wide range of comorbidities that transverse multiple specialties in clinical medicine. The development of these comorbidities is driven by various mechanistic changes that are seen when excess adipose tissue accumulates in the body. This review will discuss obesity-associated comorbidities (OACs) in the context of these mechanistic changes.

### Method

The list of OACs in this review is generated from work by the Obesity Comorbidity Collaborative (OCC). In brief, an initial list of 198 OACs in adults was retrieved from the title review of published articles in the English language in Pubmed using Medical Subject Headings (MeSH) terms and filters. A second set of searches was performed

[a] Department of Medicine, Obesity, Metabolism and Nutrition Institute, Massachusetts General Hospital; [b] University of Hong Kong, 102 Pokfulam Road, Pok Fu Lam, Hong Kong
* Corresponding author. Department of Medicine, Queen Mary Hospital, 102 Pokfulam Road, Pok Fu Lam, Hong Kong.
E-mail address: micheleyuen@gmail.com

Gastroenterol Clin N Am 52 (2023) 363–380
https://doi.org/10.1016/j.gtc.2023.03.006
0889-8553/23/© 2023 Elsevier Inc. All rights reserved.

using MeSH terms specific to individual OACs from the initial list to retrieve articles for full review. Details of the article searches strategies are outlined in **Fig. 1**. The final list consists of 224 distinct OACs (Supplement Table). For purpose of this review, further searches with respect to the pathogenesis of each comorbidity were performed, and the predominant mechanistic change was identified. The OACs, categorized by mechanistic changes, are listed in **Table 1**.

### Overview of Mechanistic Changes in Obesity

Chronic inflammation and oxidative stress are predominant features in obesity, which are mediated by various proinflammatory adipokines and are attributable to

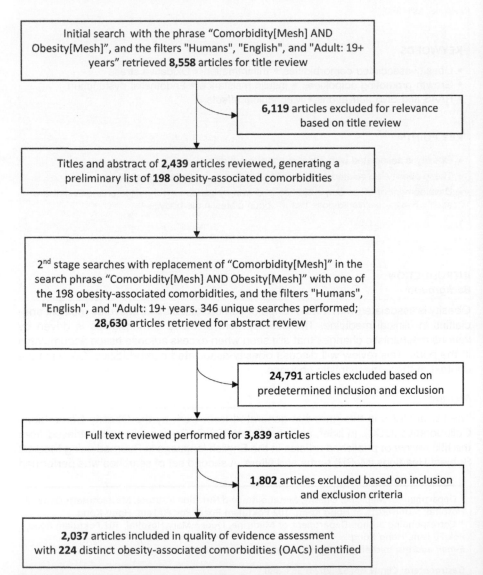

**Fig. 1.** Flowchart for retrieval of articles for the generation of the list of obesity-associated comorbidities (based on work by the obesity comorbidity collaborative).

**Table 1**
Obesity-associated comorbidities (OAC) in relation to mechanistic changes (n = 224)

| | | | |
|---|---|---|---|
| Inflammation/Oxidative Stress | | | 112 |
| Standalone mechanism | | | 59 |
| Orthopedics | 4 | *Chronic leg pain*<br>*Fracture of clavicle*<br>*Fracture of hip*<br>*Fracture of lower extremities*<br>*Fracture of spine*<br>*Fracture of upper extremities*<br>*Lower back pain* | • Osteoarthritis (hips)<br>• Osteoarthritis (knees)<br>• Osteoporosis<br>• Osteoarthritis (hands)<br>• Rotator cuff tendonitis<br>• Sciatica<br>• Upper extremity tendonitis |
| Obstetrics | 7 | *Abruptio placentae*<br>*Disordered childbirth*<br>*Genital tract infection*<br>*Maternal DVT* | • Maternal PE<br>• Maternal sepsis<br>• Maternal thrombosis |
| Dermatology | 6 | *Alopecia*<br>*Atopic dermatitis*<br>*Dermatophytes* | • Hidradenitis suppurativa<br>• Psoriasis<br>• Pyoderma gangrenosum |
| ENT | 5 | *Allergic rhinitis*<br>*Chronic rhinosinusitis*<br>*Nasal obstruction* | • Otitis media (eosinophilic)<br>• TMJ disorder |
| Hematology | 4 | *Anti-phospholipid syndrome*<br>*Deep vein thrombosis* | • Leukemia<br>• Venous thromboembolism |
| Infection | 3 | *Multiple bladder infections*<br>*Tonsillitis* | • Upper respiratory tract infection |
| Offspring | 3 | *Offspring asthma*<br>*Offspring autism* | • Offspring epilepsy |
| Oral and maxillofacial | 3 | *Edentulism*<br>*Gingivitis* | • Periodontitis |
| Rheumatology | 3 | *Fibromyalgia* | • Rheumatoid arthritis |

*(continued on next page)*

**Table 1**
*(continued)*

| | | |
|---|---|---|
| Urogenital | • Psoriatic arthritis<br>• Benign prostatic hypertrophy<br>• Lower urinary tract symptoms | • Urinary tract infections | 3 |
| Endocrinology | • Insulin resistance | • Hypothyroidism | 2 |
| Geriatrics | • Cerebral atrophy | • Cognitive impairment | 2 |
| Neurology | • Chronic pain syndrome | • Multiple sclerosis | 2 |
| Ophthalmology | • Cataract | • Glaucoma | 2 |
| Vascular | • Abdominal aortic aneurysm | • Thrombophlebitis | 2 |
| Psychiatry | • Depression | • Negative affects (distress, anger, disgust, fear and shame) | 2 |
| GI/Hepatology | • Colonic diverticulosis | • *Pancreatitis* | 1 |
| Cardiovascular | • Carotid atherosclerosis | | 1 |
| Gynecology | • Uterine leiomyomata | | 1 |
| Micronutrient | • Iron deficiency | | 1 |
| Respiratory | • Chronic bronchitis | | 1 |
| Transplant | • Solid organ graft dysfunction | | 1 |

**Inflammation/Oxidative Stress + Growth-Promoting Adipokines** — 26

| | | |
|---|---|---|
| Oncology | • Anaplastic thyroid carcinoma<br>• Cholangiocarcinoma<br>• Colorectal adenocarcinoma<br>• Endometrial cancer<br>• Cutaneous melanoma<br>• Epithelial ovarian cancer<br>• Esophageal SqCC carcinoma<br>• Extrahepatic bile duct cancer<br>• Gallbladder cancer<br>• Gastric cardia adenocarcinoma<br>• Glioma<br>• Inflammatory breast cancer | • Invasive ductal carcinoma of breast<br>• Meningioma<br>• Pancreatic adenocarcinoma<br>• Papillary thyroid carcinoma<br>• Prostatic adenocarcinoma<br>• Renal cell carcinoma<br>• T1 endometrioid cancer<br>• T2 invasive endometrial cancer<br>• Urothelial cell carcinoma | 21 |

| Category | | | |
|---|---|---|---|
| Hematology | • MGUS<br>• Multiple myeloma | • Non-Hodgkin's lymphoma<br>• WM and plasmacytoma | 4 |
| GI/Hepatology | • Colorectal adenoma | | 1 |
| Dermatology | • Acrochordons | • Acanthosis nigricans | 1 |
| Inflammation/Oxidative Stress + Insulin Resistance | | | 20 |
| Endocrinology | • Dyslipidemia<br>• Hypercholesterolemia<br>• Hypertriglyceridemia | • Prediabetes<br>• Thyroid nodule<br>• Type 2 diabetes mellitus | 6 |
| GI/Hepatology | • Gallstone disease | • *NASH*<br>• *NASH-associated cirrhosis* | 1 |
| Dermatology | • Acrochordons<br>• Acanthosis nigricans | • Lichen sclerosus | 3 |
| Obstetrics | • Gestational diabetes mellitus<br>• PPROM | • Preterm delivery | 3 |
| Reproductive | • Secondary hypogonadism (M) | • Sexual dysfunction (F) | 2 |
| Geriatric | • Frailty | | 1 |
| Gynecology | • Menstrual irregularities | | 1 |
| Neurology | • Peripheral neuropathy | | 1 |
| Offspring | • Offspring obesity | | 1 |
| Oncology | • Follicular thyroid carcinoma | | 1 |
| Cardiovascular | • Heart Failure | | 1 |
| Inflammation/Oxidative Stress + Endothelial Dysfuntion | | | 7 |
| Cardiovascular | • Acute myocardial infarction<br>• Coronary artery disease<br>• *Heart failure* | • Stable angina<br>• Unstable angina | 4 |
| Obstetrics | • Eclampsia<br>• Gestational hypertension | • Preeclampsia | 3 |
| Mechanical Effect | | | 68 |
| Mechanical (Direct loading Effect of Excess Adiposity) | | | 48 |

*(continued on next page)*

**Table 1**
*(continued)*

| Orthopedic | Chronic leg pain<br>Fracture of clavicle<br>Fracture of hip<br>Fracture of lower extremities<br>Fracture of spine<br>Fracture of upper extremities | • Intervertebral disc disorders<br>• Lower back pain<br>• Osteoarthritis (hips)<br>• Osteoarthritis (knees)<br>• Osteoporotic fracture | 11 |
|---|---|---|---|
| Dermatology | Cellulitis<br>Elephantiasis nostras verrucosa<br>Intertrigo<br>Keratosis pilaris | • Lymphedema<br>• Plantar hyperkeratosis<br>• Striae distensae | 7 |
| GI/Hepatology | Erosive esophagitis<br>GERD<br>GERD-associated asthma | • Hiatal hernia<br>• Barrett's esophagus | 5 |
| Respiratory | Asthma<br>Atelectasis | • EIB<br>• Obstructive sleep apnea | 4 |
| Urogenital | Nocturia<br>Overactive bladder | • Stress urinary incontinence (F)<br>• Urge urinary incontinence (F) | 4 |
| ENT | *Otitis media (eosinophilic)*<br>Primary CSF rhinorrhea | • Temporal bone encephalocele | 2 |
| Neurology | Meralgia paresthetica | • Ulnar nerve compression | 2 |
| Traumatology | Fall-related injuries | • Increased risk of injuries | 2 |
| Obstetrics | Peripheral edema | • Postepidural hypotension | 2 |
| Oncology | Esophageal adenocarcinoma | • Gastric high-grade dysplasia | 2 |
| General surgery | Ventral hernia | | 1 |
| Cardiovascular | Peripheral artery disease | | 1 |
| Geriatrics | Pressure ulcer | | 1 |

| Category | Complication | |
|---|---|---|
| Gynecology | • Fecal incontinence (female) | 1 |
| Neonatology | • Neonatal complications | 1 |
| Reproductive | • Poor semen quality | 1 |
| Vascular | • Venous insufficiency | 1 |
| Ophthalmology | • *Glaucoma* | |
| Transplant | • *Solid organ graft dysfunction* | |
| **Mechanical (Ectopic distribution of fat with end-organ damage and dysfunction)** | | |
| Renal | • Albuminuria<br>• Chronic kidney disease<br>• Diabetic nephropathy<br>• End-stage renal failure<br>• Glomerulonephritis<br>• Nephrosclerosis<br>• Proteinuria | 20<br>7 |
| Cardiovascular | • Atrial fibrillation<br>• Diastolic dysfunction<br>• Heart failure<br>• Left atrial enlargement | 4 |
| GI/Hepatology | • NAFLD<br>• NASH<br>• NASH-associated cirrhosis<br>• Pancreatitis | 4 |
| Neurology | • Carpal tunnel syndrome | 1 |
| Oncology | • Hepatocellular carcinoma | 1 |
| Ophthalmology | • Macular degeneration | 1 |
| Endocrinology | • Osteoporosis | 1 |
| Urology | • Kidney stone | 1 |
| **RAA System and SNS activations** | | |
| Cardiovascular | • Stroke, hemorrhagic<br>• Hypertension<br>• Left ventricular hypertrophy | 5<br>3 |
| Dermatology | • Hyperhidrosis | 1 |
| Gynecology | • Premenstrual syndrome | |
| Transplant | • *Solid organ graft dysfunction* | 1 |

(continued on next page)

**Table 1**
*(continued)*

| Others (Include impaired immunity, altered sex hormones, altered brain structure, elevated cortisol, increased uric acid production or secondary to one or more comorbidities) | | 18 |
|---|---|---|
| Dermatology | • Erysipelas<br>• Folliculitis | • Onychomycosis<br>• Tinea cruris | 4 |
| Cardiovascular | • Stroke, ischemic<br>• Stroke, mixed | • Sudden cardiac death | 3 |
| Reproductive | • Subfertility (F), IVF<br>• Subfertility (F), natural | • Erectile dysfunction | 3 |
| Obstetrics | • Postpartum hemorrhage<br>• Postterm birth | • Spontaneous abortion | 3 |
| Psychiatry | • Manic episode | • Stress | 2 |
| Rheumatology | • Gout | • Hyperuricemia | 2 |
| Micronutrient | • Vitamin D deficiency | | 1 |
| Gynecology | • *Menstrual irregularities*<br>• *Premenstrual syndrome* | • *Uterine leiomyomata* | |
| Urogenital | • *Lower urinary tract symptoms* | • *Kidney stone* | |
| Infection | • *Multiple bladder infections* | | |
| Unknown | | | 21 |
| Psychiatry | • Anti-social personality disorder<br>• Anxiety<br>• ADHD | • Avoidant personality disorder<br>• Panic disorder | 5 |
| Oncology | • Appendix carcinoid tumor<br>• Pancreatic NET | • Peritoneal cancer<br>• Transitional cell carcinoma | 4 |
| Neurology | • Idiopathic headache<br>• Migraine headaches | • Pseudotumor cerebri | 3 |

| Obstetric | • Cervical incompetence | • Polyhydramnios | 2 |
|---|---|---|---|
| Social work | • Low self-esteem | • Perceived vulnerability | 2 |
| ENT | • Meniere's disease | | 1 |
| GI/Hepatology | • Gallbladder polyps | | 1 |
| Gynecology | • Dyspareunia | | 1 |
| Infection | • Multiple yeast infections | | 1 |
| Micronutrient | • Thiamine deficiency | | 1 |

Listed by discipline in descending order of the number of comorbidities within that discipline. For OAC that have more than one pathogenesis, the condition is listed under the primary mechanism and again in *italic* under the secondary mechanism(s). Each comorbidity is counted once only under the primary mechanism. *Abbreviations:* ADHD, attention deficit hyperactivity disorder; CSF, cerebrospinal fluid; DVT, deep vein thrombosis; EIB, exercise-induced bronchoconstriction; ENT, ear; F, female; GI, gastrointestinal or gastroenterology; IVF, in vitro fertilization; M, male; MGUS, monoclonal gammopathy of undetermined significance; NAFLD, nonalcoholic fatty liver disease; NASH, nonalcoholic steatohepatitis; NET, neuroendocrine tumor; nose, throat or otolaryngology; PE, pulmonary embolism; PPROM, premature preterm rupture of membrane; SqCC, squamous cell carcinoma; TMJ, temporomandibular joint; WM, Waldenstrom macroglobulinemia.

approximately 50.0% (n = 112) of all OACs in this review. Elevated levels of growth-promoting adipokines, insulin resistance, and endothelial dysfunction are additionally present in close to half (n = 53) of these inflammation and oxidative stress-related conditions. A second feature is the mechanical effects of excess adiposity on the body, which accounts for approximately 30.4% (n = 68) of all OACs. This can manifest as a direct loading effect (21.4%, n = 48) or as an infiltrative effect into ectopic sites with resulting end-organ damage and dysfunction (8.9%, n = 20). A third feature in obesity is heightened activities of the renin-angiotensin-aldosterone system (RAAS) and sympathetic nervous system (SNS), which accounts for approximately 2.2% (n = 5) of all OACs. Finally, 8.0% of OACs (n = 18) can be attributed to a mixture of changes including impaired immunity, altered sex hormones, altered brain structure, hypercortisolemia, and elevated uric acid production. Potential mechanistic changes for 9.4% of OACs (n = 21) remain unknown. An overview of the mechanistic changes in obesity and the number of comorbidities attributable to each change is given in **Fig. 2**.

## INFLAMMATION AND OXIDATIVE STRESS IN OBESITY

Obesity is associated with chronic inflammation, which is mediated through a complex array of adipokines. Key changes observed include the elevation of tumor necrosis factor-alpha (TNF-$\alpha$) and interleukin-6 (IL-6), increased leptin resistance as well as a reduction in adiponectin. TNF-$\alpha$ is a pro-inflammatory cytokine, and elevation in the expression of its mRNA has been demonstrated in fat biopsy samples from human subjects with obesity.[1] The role of IL-6 in inflammation is more controversial. While muscle-derived IL-6 has anti-inflammatory properties,[2] adipocyte-derived IL-6 is pro-inflammatory.[3] Obesity is associated with increased expression of adipocyte-derived IL-6 and IL-6 receptor, which correlates positively with markers of macrophage infiltration and low-grade inflammation.[3,4] IL-6 has also been demonstrated to induce the production of C-reactive protein in human hepatocytes,[5] which may be an intermediary or marker of inflammatory disease processes.[6] Adiponectin, an anti-inflammatory factor produced by adipocytes, is down-regulated in obesity.[7] Leptin is proinflammatory. Its signaling informs the brain of nutritional sufficiency and promotes weight reduction.[8] Positive correlation between leptin levels and body mass index (BMI) suggests leptin resistance in obesity, and elevated leptin levels promote inflammation.[9] Oxidative stress in obesity is evident by increased production of reactive oxygen species (ROS) in adipose tissue of obese mice, augmented expression of NADPH oxidase, and decreased expression of antioxidative enzymes.[10] Chronic inflammation and oxidative stress are implicated in orthopedic, obstetric, dermatologic, otorhinolaryngological and even psychiatric comorbidities of obesity (see **Table 1**).

### Inflammation, Oxidative Stress, and Insulin Resistance

Chronic inflammation and oxidative stress predisposes to insulin resistance, which is implicated in metabolic diseases including type 2 diabetes,[11] hypercholesterolemia,[12] and hypertriglyceridemia.[12] TNF-$\alpha$, for instance, appears to have a central role in insulin resistance and has been shown to interfere with normal insulin signaling by reducing tyrosine phosphorylation of insulin receptor in skeletal muscles.[13] Reactive oxygen species (ROS) are another causative factor of insulin resistance in the peripheral tissues. ROS affects insulin receptor signal transduction through various mechanisms and ultimately leads to a reduction in the expression of GLUT4 transporters, the main glucose transporter in the cellular membrane of peripheral insulin-sensitive

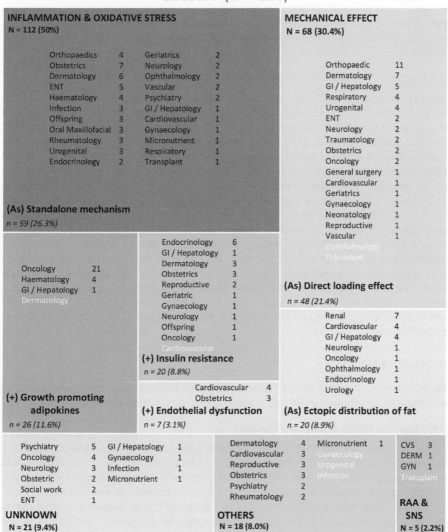

**Fig. 2.** Mechanistic changes in obesity and the number of OACs by discipline associated with each mechanism.

tissues.[14] Insulin resistance also contributes to the whole spectrum of fatty liver disease from nonalcoholic steatosis to cirrhosis,[15] and is implicated in dermatologic conditions (such as acanthosis nigricans[16] and acrochordons)[17] and even frailty[18] (see **Table 1**).

## Inflammation, Oxidative Stress, and Endothelial Dysfunction

Chronic Inflammation and oxidative stress have been connected to endothelial dysfunction by way of increased expression of cell-surface adhesion molecules and impaired endothelium-dependent vascular relaxation.[19] Endothelial dysfunction is an early step in the pathogenesis of atherosclerosis and its related conditions, including stable and unstable angina,[20] acute myocardial infarction,[21] coronary artery disease,[22] and ischemic stroke.[23] In addition to cardiovascular disorders, endothelial dysfunction is also responsible for the spectrum of hypertensive diseases during pregnancy, including gestational hypertension, preeclampsia and eclampsia (see **Table 1**).[24]

### Inflammation, Oxidative Stress, and Growth-Promoting Adipokines

Growth promoting properties of adipokines such as insulin-like growth factor 1 (IGF-1) and leptin, and changes in sex hormones create a pro-tumorigenic environment and have been implicated in the pathogenesis of various obesity-associated cancers. Over 20 distinct cancers have been linked to growth-promoting adipokines and changes in sex hormones (see **Table 1**). Colonic cancer, for instance, has been linked to an elevation in IGF-1, a by-product of insulin resistance and hyperinsulinemia, in *in vitro* studies.[25] Increased insulin is also suspected to be one of the underlying etiologies for pancreatic cancer, which is increased 1.1- to 1.6-fold in overweight and 1.2- to 3.5-fold in obesity.[26–29] Stimulation of the leptin receptor supported stem cell-like properties in breast cancer cells *in vitro*, thereby preserving their self-renewal ability and facilitating recurrence and metastasis.[30] Elevated leptin level has also been implicated in papillary, follicular and anaplastic thyroid cancer, among other etiologies in obesity-associated thyroid cancers.[31,32] Increased adiposity further leads to an increase in aromatase activity and reduced sex-hormone binding globulin (SHBG), which increases the pool of bioactive estrogen. Elevated estrogen level is linked to endometrial[33] and epithelial ovarian cancer[34] in women and prostate cancer[35] in men.

## MECHANICAL EFFECTS

The mechanical effects of obesity refer to (1) direct loading effect of excess adiposity or (2) ectopic distribution of fat with resulting end-organ damage and dysfunction.

### Direct Loading Effect of Excess Adiposity

The shear presence of regional excess adiposity can cause a direct obstructing effect. For instance, fat deposition in the neck region, which narrows the upper airways, and central obesity, which reduces lung volume, increases pharyngeal collapsibility, and reduces caudal traction on the upper airway, predispose to the development of obstructive sleep apnea (OSA).[36] Increased intraabdominal adiposity is associated with increased transient lower esophageal sphincter relaxation, disruption in the esophagogastric junction pressure, and increased gastroesophageal pressure gradient, which predispose to gastroesophageal reflux disease (GERD),[37,38] and to erosive esophagitis and Barrett's esophagus.[39] By extension, esophageal adenocarcinoma and gastric adenocarcinoma, which are in part attributable to GERD, are also more prevalent in obesity.[39,40] Increased intrathoracic adiposity and chronic inflammation, among other factors (eg, GERD), is attributable to obesity-associated asthma.[41]

Excess adiposity affects joint loading pattern as well, which stimulates the inflammatory process in cartilages and bones and predispose to osteoarthritis (OA) in both weight-bearing joints, including the knees and hips, and non-weight-bearing joints like the hands.[42] Individuals suffering from obesity might further experience a change in the center of gravity, which predisposes to injuries[43] and fractures, especially fractures of clavicle, upper extremities, hip and lower extremities.[44]

Mechanical effects of obesity also give rise to various dermatologic conditions. Increased skinfolds, for instance, leads to localized occlusive effects with increased heat and moisture, which along with skin-on-skin friction, increases the risk of intertrigo and hidradenitis suppurativa.[16] The loading effect of obesity on the lower extremities increases the risks of stasis-related skin disorders including cellulitis,[45] lymphedema and elephantiasis nostras verrucose (ENV).[46] The loading effect on the soles increases plantar hyperkeratosis.[16] The stretching effects of obesity increases risks of striae distensae.[16]

Direct loading of obesity can also lead to neurogenic pain conditions such as ulnar nerve compression[47] and meralgia paresthetica.[48] The latter condition is attributable to the compressive effect of increased abdominal fat on the lateral femoral cutaneous nerve.[48] Increased intraabdominal pressure is also implicated in various urologic conditions including nocturia,[49] overactive bladder,[50] and stress and urge urinary incontinence in women.[51,52] Other obesity-associated comorbidities related to the direct loading effect of obesity are listed in **Table 1**.

### Ectopic Distribution of Fat with End-Organ Damage and Dysfunction

Ectopic fat deposition in obesity commonly occurs in the liver, kidneys, pancreas, and heart. Ectopic fat in the liver causes nonalcoholic fatty liver disease (NAFLD), which has the potential of progressing to nonalcoholic steatohepatitis (NASH), cirrhosis and eventually hepatocellular carcinoma (HCC).[15,53] In the kidneys, ectopic fat deposition can lead to the phenomenon of "fatty kidney," which predisposes to albuminuria/proteinuria, glomerulonephritis, chronic kidney disease and end-stage renal failure.[54] Peri-and intrapancreatic fat deposition is postulated to be part of the pathogenesis of acute pancreatitis in obesity, although increased lipolysis secondary to insulin resistance and low-grade inflammation may also play a role.[55,56] Fat deposition in the heart is associated with left atrial enlargement,[57] which can lead to atrial fibrillation,[57] while increased epicardial adipose tissue impacts ventricular contractility[58] and might be a major contributory factor to nonischemic heart failure in overweight and obesity.[59] Other obesity-associated comorbidities associated with ectopic fat deposition are listed in **Table 1**.

## RENIN–ANGIOTENSIN–ALDOSTERONE SYSTEM AND SYMPATHETIC NERVOUS SYSTEM ACTIVATIONS

Activities of both the RAAS and SNS increase with increasing adiposity and may underlie the development of hypertension in obesity.[60,61] Shifting of diuresis and natriuresis to favor high blood pressure in obesity may be an additional contributory factor.[62] Hypertension and other hemodynamic changes in obesity adds to the development of left ventricular hypertrophy.[63] The combined effect of these changes, along with atherosclerosis, might be a plausible explanation for the increased risk of sudden cardiac death in obesity.[64] Hyperhidrosis is another condition attributable to increased RAAS and SNS activities.[65] Finally, RAAS activation may be partially responsible for some of the symptoms constituting premenstrual syndrome, which is more prevalent in obesity.[66]

## OTHERS AND UNKNOWN MECHANISM

Other mechanistic changes underlying the development of OACs include impaired immunity, altered sex hormones, altered brain structure, elevated cortisol, and increased uric acid production. Some conditions can be secondary to one or more other comorbidities. The remaining obesity-associated comorbidities range from psychiatric disorders, most notably anxiety, and panic disorders, to headache disorders, to thiamine deficiency, and to cervical incompetence and polyhydramnios in pregnancy, among others. The mechanistic links between these conditions and obesity remain to be fully elucidated. It is possible that these conditions share common disease processes with obesity or that obesity leads to a disruption in homeostasis in the body that predispose to these conditions. While it is difficult to prove causative relations between excess adiposity and these conditions, improvement or reversal of these disorders with weight reduction is indirect proof that obesity is responsible for these conditions.

## SUMMARY

The primary aim of this review is to provide an overview of the spectrum of OACs and to summarize the possible mechanistic changes connecting these abnormalities with excess adiposity. The perspective in this review is highly simplified to facilitate discussion. The full interactive map between different mechanistic pathways and the OACs is complex. Some OACs are caused by multiple mechanisms, some may develop secondary to other OACs, and some may arise from interactions between multiple OACs. Separate reviews will be needed to fully map out all the mechanistic changes in each individual OAC. Further evaluation of the strength of association between obesity and these comorbidities along with a systematic evaluation of the quality of data that support these associations are warranted to provide further depth into this topic. As our understanding of obesity continues to grow, new mechanistic changes in obesity may be identified and the list of OACs is expected to evolve. Ongoing efforts to review and summarize these comorbidities will be useful to expand understanding of obesity and to identify knowledge gaps to guide further research.

## CLINICS CARE POINTS

- Obesity is associated with multiple comorbidites transversing almost all specialities in clinical medicine.
- Clinicians managing individuals with obesity should maintain a high index of suspicion to screen for and then manage these comorbidities appropriately.

## ACKNOWLEDGMENTS

Special thanks to Joseph Brancale[1] and Nitya Kadambi[1] and the Obesity Comorbidity Collaborative for their contributions to the generation of the list of obesity-associated comorbidities.

## DISCLOSURE

No potential competing interest.

## SUPPLEMENTARY DATA

Supplementary data related to this article can be found online at https://doi.org/10.1016/j.gtc.2023.03.006.

## REFERENCES

1. Kern PA, Saghizadeh M, Ong JM, et al. The expression of tumor necrosis factor in human adipose tissue. Regulation by obesity, weight loss, and relationship to lipoprotein lipase. J Clin Invest 1995;95(5):2111–9.

2. Nara H, Watanabe R. Anti-Inflammatory Effect of Muscle-Derived Interleukin-6 and Its Involvement in Lipid Metabolism. Int J Mol Sci 2021;13(18):22.
3. Sindhu S, Thomas R, Shihab P, et al. Obesity Is a Positive Modulator of IL-6R and IL-6 Expression in the Subcutaneous Adipose Tissue: Significance for Metabolic Inflammation. PLoS One 2015;10(7):e0133494.
4. Weisberg SP, McCann D, Desai M, et al. Obesity is associated with macrophage accumulation in adipose tissue. J Clin Invest 2003;112(12):1796–808.
5. Castell JV, Gomez-Lechon MJ, David M, et al. Recombinant human interleukin-6 (IL-6/BSF-2/HSF) regulates the synthesis of acute phase proteins in human hepatocytes. FEBS Lett 1988;232(2):347–50.
6. Ansar W, Ghosh S. C-reactive protein and the biology of disease. Immunol Res 2013;56(1):131–42.
7. Ouchi N, Walsh K. Adiponectin as an anti-inflammatory factor. Clin Chim Acta 2007;380(1–2):24–30.
8. Rosenbaum M, Leibel RL. 20 years of leptin: role of leptin in energy homeostasis in humans. J Endocrinol 2014;223(1):T83–96.
9. Considine RV, Sinha MK, Heiman ML, et al. Serum immunoreactive-leptin concentrations in normal-weight and obese humans. N Engl J Med 1996;334(5):292–5.
10. Furukawa S, Fujita T, Shimabukuro M, et al. Increased oxidative stress in obesity and its impact on metabolic syndrome. J Clin Invest 2004;114(12):1752–61.
11. Kahn SE, Hull RL, Utzschneider KM. Mechanisms linking obesity to insulin resistance and type 2 diabetes. Nature 2006;444(7121):840–6.
12. Klop B, Elte JW, Cabezas MC. Dyslipidemia in obesity: mechanisms and potential targets. Nutrients 2013;5(4):1218–40.
13. Cheung AT, Ree D, Kolls JK, et al. An in vivo model for elucidation of the mechanism of tumor necrosis factor-alpha (TNF-alpha)-induced insulin resistance: evidence for differential regulation of insulin signaling by TNF-alpha. Endocrinology 1998;139(12):4928–35.
14. Hurrle S, Hsu WH. The etiology of oxidative stress in insulin resistance. Biomed J 2017;40(5):257–62.
15. Loomba R, Friedman SL, Shulman GI. Mechanisms and disease consequences of nonalcoholic fatty liver disease. Cell 2021;184(10):2537–64.
16. Darlenski R, Mihaylova V, Handjieva-Darlenska T. The Link Between Obesity and the Skin. Front Nutr 2022;9:855573.
17. Shah R, Jindal A, Patel N. Acrochordons as a cutaneous sign of metabolic syndrome: a case-control study. Ann Med Health Sci Res 2014;4(2):202–5.
18. Cleasby ME, Jamieson PM, Atherton PJ. Insulin resistance and sarcopenia: mechanistic links between common co-morbidities. J Endocrinol 2016;229(2):R67–81.
19. Stenvinkel P. Endothelial dysfunction and inflammation-is there a link? Nephrol Dial Transplant 2001;16(10):1968–71.
20. Powell-Wiley TM, Poirier P, Burke LE, et al. Obesity and Cardiovascular Disease: A Scientific Statement From the American Heart Association. Circulation 2021;143(21):e984–1010.
21. Rajendran K, Devarajan N, Ganesan M, et al. Obesity, Inflammation and Acute Myocardial Infarction - Expression of leptin, IL-6 and high sensitivity-CRP in Chennai based population. Thromb J 2012;10(1):13.
22. Van Gaal LF, Mertens IL, De Block CE. Mechanisms linking obesity with cardiovascular disease. Nature 2006;444(7121):875–80.

23. Kernan WN, Inzucchi SE, Sawan C, et al. Obesity: a stubbornly obvious target for stroke prevention. Stroke 2013;44(1):278–86.

24. Spradley FT, Palei AC, Granger JP. Increased risk for the development of pre-eclampsia in obese pregnancies: weighing in on the mechanisms. Am J Physiol Regul Integr Comp Physiol 2015;309(11):R1326–43.

25. Lahm H, Suardet L, Laurent PL, et al. Growth regulation and co-stimulation of human colorectal cancer cell lines by insulin-like growth factor I, II and transforming growth factor alpha. Br J Cancer 1992;65(3):341–6.

26. Stolzenberg-Solomon RZ, Schairer C, Moore S, et al. Lifetime adiposity and risk of pancreatic cancer in the NIH-AARP Diet and Health Study cohort. Am J Clin Nutr 2013;98(4):1057–65.

27. Fryzek JP, Schenk M, Kinnard M, et al. The association of body mass index and pancreatic cancer in residents of southeastern Michigan, 1996-1999. Am J Epidemiol 2005;162(3):222–8.

28. Berrington de Gonzalez A, Sweetland S, Spencer E. A meta-analysis of obesity and the risk of pancreatic cancer. Br J Cancer 2003;89(3):519–23.

29. Lin Y, Kikuchi S, Tamakoshi A, et al. Obesity, physical activity and the risk of pancreatic cancer in a large Japanese cohort. Int J Cancer 2007;120(12):2665–71.

30. Zheng Q, Banaszak L, Fracci S, et al. Leptin receptor maintains cancer stem-like properties in triple negative breast cancer cells. Endocr Relat Cancer 2013;20(6):797–808.

31. Kim WG, Cheng SY. Mechanisms Linking Obesity and Thyroid Cancer Development and Progression in Mouse Models. Horm Cancer 2018;9(2):108–16.

32. Masone S, Velotti N, Savastano S, et al. Morbid Obesity and Thyroid Cancer Rate. A Review of Literature. J Clin Med 2021;27(9):10.

33. Onstad MA, Schmandt RE, Lu KH. Addressing the Role of Obesity in Endometrial Cancer Risk, Prevention, and Treatment. J Clin Oncol 2016;34(35):4225–30.

34. Dai L, Song K, Di W. Adipocytes: active facilitators in epithelial ovarian cancer progression? J Ovarian Res 2020;13(1):115.

35. Parikesit D, Mochtar CA, Umbas R, et al. The impact of obesity towards prostate diseases. Prostate Int 2016;4(1):1–6.

36. Schwartz AR, Patil SP, Laffan AM, et al. Obesity and obstructive sleep apnea: pathogenic mechanisms and therapeutic approaches. Proc Am Thorac Soc 2008;5(2):185–92.

37. Wu JC, Mui LM, Cheung CM, et al. Obesity is associated with increased transient lower esophageal sphincter relaxation. Gastroenterology 2007;132(3):883–9.

38. Pandolfino JE, El-Serag HB, Zhang Q, et al. Obesity: a challenge to esophagogastric junction integrity. Gastroenterology 2006;130(3):639–49.

39. Alexandre L, Long E, Beales IL. Pathophysiological mechanisms linking obesity and esophageal adenocarcinoma. World J Gastrointest Pathophysiol 2014;5(4):534–49.

40. Karczewski J, Begier-Krasinska B, Staszewski R, et al. Obesity and the Risk of Gastrointestinal Cancers. Dig Dis Sci 2019;64(10):2740–9.

41. Baffi CW, Winnica DE, Holguin F. Asthma and obesity: mechanisms and clinical implications. Asthma Res Pract 2015;1:1.

42. Reyes C, Leyland KM, Peat G, et al. Association Between Overweight and Obesity and Risk of Clinically Diagnosed Knee, Hip, and Hand Osteoarthritis: A Population-Based Cohort Study. Arthritis Rheumatol. Aug 2016;68(8):1869–75.

43. Corbeil P, Simoneau M, Rancourt D, et al. Increased risk for falling associated with obesity: mathematical modeling of postural control. IEEE Trans Neural Syst Rehabil Eng 2001;9(2):126–36.

44. Rinonapoli G, Pace V, Ruggiero C, et al. Obesity and Bone: A Complex Relationship. Int J Mol Sci 2021;22(24). https://doi.org/10.3390/ijms222413662.

45. Cranendonk DR, Lavrijsen APM, Prins JM, et al. Cellulitis: current insights into pathophysiology and clinical management. Neth J Med 2017;75(9):366–78.

46. Damstra RJ, Dickinson-Blok JL, Voesten HG. Shaving Technique and Compression Therapy for Elephantiasis Nostras Verrucosa (Lymphostatic Verrucosis) of Forefeet and Toes in End-Stage Primary Lymphedema: A 5 Year Follow-Up Study in 28 Patients and a Review of the Literature. J Clin Med 2020;9(10). https://doi.org/10.3390/jcm9103139.

47. Descatha A, Leclerc A, Chastang JF, et al. Incidence of ulnar nerve entrapment at the elbow in repetitive work. Scand J Work Environ Health 2004;30(3):234–40.

48. Deal CL, Canoso JJ. Meralgia paresthetica and large abdomens. Ann Intern Med 1982;96(6 Pt 1):787–8.

49. Moon S, Chung HS, Yu JM, et al. The Association Between Obesity and the Nocturia in the U.S. Population. Int Neurourol J 2019;23(2):169–76.

50. Hagovska M, Svihra J, Bukova A, et al. The Relationship between Overweight and Overactive Bladder Symptoms. Obes Facts 2020;13(3):297–306.

51. Osborn DJ, Strain M, Gomelsky A, et al. Obesity and female stress urinary incontinence. Urology 2013;82(4):759–63.

52. Swenson CW, Kolenic GE, Trowbridge ER, et al. Obesity and stress urinary incontinence in women: compromised continence mechanism or excess bladder pressure during cough? Int Urogynecol J 2017;28(9):1377–85.

53. Rajesh Y, Sarkar D. Molecular Mechanisms Regulating Obesity-Associated Hepatocellular Carcinoma. Cancers 2020;12(5). https://doi.org/10.3390/cancers12051290.

54. Kambham N, Markowitz GS, Valeri AM, et al. Obesity-related glomerulopathy: an emerging epidemic. Kidney Int 2001;59(4):1498–509.

55. Wiese ML, Aghdassi AA, Lerch MM, et al. Excess Body Weight and Pancreatic Disease. Visc Med 2021;37(4):281–6.

56. Cho SK, Huh JH, Yoo JS, et al. HOMA-estimated insulin resistance as an independent prognostic factor in patients with acute pancreatitis. Sci Rep 2019;9(1):14894.

57. Lavie CJ, Pandey A, Lau DH, et al. Obesity and Atrial Fibrillation Prevalence, Pathogenesis, and Prognosis: Effects of Weight Loss and Exercise. J Am Coll Cardiol 2017;70(16):2022–35.

58. Rayner JJ, Banerjee R, Holloway CJ, et al. The relative contribution of metabolic and structural abnormalities to diastolic dysfunction in obesity. Int J Obes (Lond) 2018;42(3):441–7.

59. Ebong IA, Goff DC Jr, Rodriguez CJ, et al. Mechanisms of heart failure in obesity. Obes Res Clin Pract 2014;8(6):e540–8.

60. DeMarco VG, Aroor AR, Sowers JR. The pathophysiology of hypertension in patients with obesity. Nat Rev Endocrinol 2014;10(6):364–76.

61. Kalil GZ, Haynes WG. Sympathetic nervous system in obesity-related hypertension: mechanisms and clinical implications. Hypertens Res 2012;35(1):4–16.

62. Kotsis V, Stabouli S, Papakatsika S, et al. Mechanisms of obesity-induced hypertension. Hypertens Res 2010;33(5):386–93.

63. Avelar E, Cloward TV, Walker JM, et al. Left ventricular hypertrophy in severe obesity: interactions among blood pressure, nocturnal hypoxemia, and body mass. Hypertension 2007;49(1):34–9.

64. Duflou J, Virmani R, Rabin I, et al. Sudden death as a result of heart disease in morbid obesity. Am Heart J 1995;130(2):306–13.

65. Wolosker N, Krutman M, Kauffman P, et al. Effectiveness of oxybutynin for treatment of hyperhidrosis in overweight and obese patients. Rev Assoc Med Bras (1992) 2013;59(2):143–7.

66. Halbreich U. The etiology, biology, and evolving pathology of premenstrual syndromes. Psychoneuroendocrinology 2003;28(Suppl 3):55–99.

# The Effects of Obesity on Health Care Delivery

Amanda Velazquez, MD, DABOM[a], Caroline M. Apovian, MD, FACN, DABOM[b],*

## KEYWORDS

- Obesity • Health care • Implications • Health delivery

## KEY POINTS

- Obesity is a chronic disease with physiologic, physical, social, and economic implications on health care delivery.
- As the prevalence of obesity in the United States continues to rise, so do its effects on health care delivery.
- Currently, the health care system is ill-equipped to appropriately prevent, care for, and treat obesity.
- Inadequate care of patients with obesity by our healthcare system has far-reaching consequences, from delayed diagnosis to poor access to indicated treatments.

## INTRODUCTION

The US rates of obesity continue to rise—half of the adult population will be living with obesity by 2030. The worldwide coronavirus disease 2019 (COVID-19) pandemic has rapidly transformed the delivery of health care, and yet the health care system is utterly unprepared to meet patient needs.[1] US health care systems are still ill-equipped in many regards to appropriately prevent, care for, and treat obesity.[2,3] One majorly problematic challenge is the continued perception of obesity as a personal failure and not as a disease.[4] Despite new therapy options emerging, tools to treat obesity are still underutilized.[4] Of those who qualify for bariatric surgery, only about 1% of those patients will undergo the procedure each year in the United States.[5]

Obesity is reshaping health care delivery in part due to its prevalence in the United States and the physiologic, physical, social, and economic conditions related to weight.[6] Literature is scarce when it comes to the implications of obesity on health care delivery, but this article reviews the existing evidence compiled in addition to expert opinion.

[a] Department of Surgery, Center for Weight Management and Metabolic Health, Cedars Sinai Medical Center, 8635 West 3rd Street, West Tower, Suite 795, Los Angeles, CA 90048, USA; [b] Center for Weight Management and Wellness, Brigham and Women's Hospital, Harvard Medical School, 221 Longwood Avenue, RFB 490, Boston, MA 02115, USA
* Corresponding author. 221 Longwood Avenue, RFB 490, Boston, MA 02115, USA.
*E-mail address:* capovian@partners.org

Gastroenterol Clin N Am 52 (2023) 381–392
https://doi.org/10.1016/j.gtc.2023.03.007
0889-8553/23/© 2023 Elsevier Inc. All rights reserved.

**gastro.theclinics.com**

## DISCUSSION
### Physiologic Implications

#### Weight-related medical conditions

The physiology of obesity cannot be oversimplified to overeating and underexpenditure of energy. Excess body weight is a risk factor for the three leading causes of death in the United States: coronary artery disease, cancer, and COVID-19.[7] Obesity is a chronic, complex disease, and its pathogenesis impacts numerous organ systems.[8] The literature equates obesity's pathogenesis to the aging process of the human body, which is multifactorial in origin.[9]

On cellular level, adiposopathy ("sick fat") leads to excessive energy storage in the form of fat.[10] This is due to several physiologic contributors, including oxidative stress, mitochondrial dysfunction, immune dysfunction, chronic low-grade inflammation, and metabolic dysfunction. Unfortunately, to date, the initial physiologic inflammatory triggers that kick-start this cascade are unclear.[4]

On a macro level, it is well established that obesity is multifactorial in origin. The interplay of variables leads to dysregulation of the body's energy balance that promotes energy storage. This is unique to every individual and establishes a setpoint for an equilibrium body weight where the body wants to physiologically remain. Obesity ultimately defends obesity.[11]

Currently, obesity is not a curable disease but a chronic, complex medical condition, and existing treatments are underutilized for weight management. As a result, the prevalence of chronic diseases stemming from obesity continues to rise. This reshapes health care delivery from focusing on disease prevention to chronic disease management. For example, excess body weight is the number one risk factor for diabetes. From 2001 to 2020, the prevalence of diabetes has increased by 18%, and it affects 37.3 million American adults.[12] Individuals having multiple chronic diseases are also on the rise, with more than 25% of Americans living with multiple chronic diseases.[13] No specialty of medicine is unaffected by the impact of obesity.

#### Medication dosage

Obesity has a significant impact on the pharmacokinetics and pharmacodynamics of medications. In patients with severe obesity, the increased adiposity influences the properties of drugs, which can impact drug efficacy and toxicity. Obesity is not recognized as a special population by the Food and Drug Administration, and as a result, pharmaceutical companies are not required to perform studies on patients with obesity.[14] With little data on this population, appropriate dosing is becoming a common concern in clinical practice.[15]

The following factors underlie the rate and extent of drug distribution in patients with severe obesity.

- Degree of tissue perfusion
- Binding of drugs to plasma proteins
- Permeability of tissue membranes

In general, the extent to which obesity influences the distribution volume of a drug depends on its lipid solubility. Water content in adipose tissue is 20% to 50% of that found in other tissues. Distribution of drugs may warrant adjusting dosage in proportion to the excess in body weight with the use of a dosing weight correction factor.[16]

#### Laboratory testing

There is insufficient literature on obesity laboratory analysis reference values for both adults and children. The first comprehensive study results were published only in

2020. The study looked at the impact of 3 adiposity measures (body mass index [BMI], waist circumference, and waist-to-height ratio) on 35 biochemical markers in a cohort of healthy children who are of normal weight, overweight, or obese. Of 1332 children and adolescents, ages ranging from approximately 5 to 19 years with BMI 13 to 65 kg/m$^2$, it was found that 70% of routine blood tests, including lipids, liver function, and so forth, were affected by obesity.[17]

For adults, there are a handful of studies evaluating the impact of obesity on laboratory assessments. In the case of determining the cut-points for B-type natriuretic peptide (BNP) in diagnosing acute heart failure, previous investigations had found a cutoff point of BNP to be ≥100 pg/mL to diagnose heart failure. However, there is an inverse relationship between BNP and BMI that was not considered. In the Breathing Not Properly Multinational Study, 1586 patients presented with acute dyspnea at the emergency department (ED). BNP levels were measured on arrival in addition to height and weight data. Two independent cardiologists found that a lower cut-point of BNP (≥54 pg/mL) should be used in patients with severe obesity to preserve sensitivity, whereas a higher cut-point could be used to increase specificity for lean patients (BNP ≥170 pg/mL).[18]

### Physical Implications

### Physical examination

The physical examination of patients with obesity can prove challenging when the tissue layers of adiposity may obscure physical findings. Primary techniques of the physical examination include inspection, palpation, auscultation, and percussion. These are the foundational skills physicians and health care professionals learn in the early stages of training. Still, adaptations to the technique are needed when caring for patients with obesity. For details on this, please refer to **Table 1**. Literature has demonstrated that cardiac, abdominal, and gynecologic examinations on patients with obesity are exceedingly more difficult.[19] A recent 2021 retrospective analysis of 210 patients undergoing arthroscopic procedures looked at the impact of BMI on physical examination maneuvers. They found BMI to impact the accuracy of provocative knee tests, which are routinely performed during a knee physical examination.[20]

Clinicians may not always be inclined to perform a thorough physical examination despite its importance. Some physicians perceive performing a gynecologic examination on a patient with obesity to be "difficult" and "inadequate."[21] It is known that patients with obesity are less likely to undergo routine preventive screenings with mammograms and Papanicolaou tests.[22] A 2018 study analyzing a large cohort of women aged 30 to 64 years showed that increasing BMI was associated with lower risk of cervical precancer and higher risk of cervical cancer, perhaps due to the underdiagnosis of cervical precancer.[23]

### Imaging studies

The quality and interpretability of imaging studies performed on patients with obesity can be affected due to the body habitus of the individual. In a study evaluating 100,622 women, it was found that Mammograms are less accurate among women with obesity.[24] Visualization of the fetus at 18 to 24 weeks was also significantly decreased during fetal anatomy surveys for women with obesity. This study evaluated over 10,000 women with a wide range of BMI, and due to limitations of the ultrasound examination, only 50% of fetal anatomy surveys could be completed during the initial examination.[25] Notably, ultrasound imaging is impacted more than any other imaging modality by adipose tissue obscuring visualization.[26,27]

**Table 1**
**Recommendations for the physical examination of patients with obesity**

| Domain | Recommended Approach |
|---|---|
| Clinical space | • Use large-size gowns<br>• Use wide examination tables that accommodate higher weights<br>• Make available sturdy armless chairs or wide-seated bariatric chairs |
| Vital signs | • Use wide-based scales with adequate weight capacity of >350 lbs with handles for support during weighing<br>• Choose a scale accessible to patients with disabilities<br>• Ensure the scale is located in the office in an area that provides privacy<br>• Use a wall-mounted stadiometer<br>• Use large and extra-large adult and thigh blood pressure cuffs when indicated |
| Phlebotomy | • Use extra-long phlebotomy needles and tourniquets when drawing blood<br>• Make available bariatric phlebotomy chairs[1] |
| Head and neck | • Use a tongue depressor or ask the patient to yawn for oropharynx examination<br>• Have the patient look up to stretch the neck to better visualize thyroid<br>• Ensure the examination table is at 30°–45° incline to improve visualization of JVD[2] |
| Cardiovascular | • If the patient is recumbent, have them raise their arms above their head to spread the chest-wall soft tissue for cardiac examination<br>• If the patient is sitting, ask them to lean forward to bring the heart closer to the chest wall<br>• Make available a handheld Doppler to check pulses if needed[2]<br>• Consider using an electronic stethoscope to improve auscultation of heart sounds and murmurs[3] |
| Lung | • Ensure auscultation occurs directly over exposed skin |
| Abdomen | • To aid in finding the liver edge, consider using the scratch test[2]<br>• If indicated, respectfully ask the patient to help in facilitating examination by retracting their own pannus |
| Chest | • Consider having the patient rest in the lateral decubitus position for breast examination[2]<br>• Respectfully ask the patient to help in facilitating the examination by retracting their own breast |
| Musculoskeletal | • Use power examination tables to help facilitate proper positioning of the patient<br>• If limbs are difficult to lift, consider a medical team member assisting in properly positioning the patient for this examination |
| Genitourinary (female) | • Ensure large vaginal specula are made available[1]<br>• Consider vaginal specula with an integrated battery-operated LED light source<br>• Encourage the patient to take deep breathes to encourage relaxation of body, and in turn, this can help relax pelvic floor muscles and abduct legs |
| Genitourinary (male) | • If indicated, respectfully ask the patient to lift pannus and/or escutcheon |
| Lymphatic | • Ensure palpation occurs directly over exposed skin |
| Skin | • Respectfully ask the patient to help in facilitating examination by retracting their own breasts and pannus to assess intertriginous folds adequately |

(continued on next page)

| Table 1 (continued) | |
| --- | --- |
| Domain | Recommended Approach |
| Neurologic | • Use power examination tables to help facilitate proper positioning of the patient<br>• In performing balance and gait testing, walk along the patient on one side and consider having an additional team member on the patient's other side, to minimize fall risk |
| Psychiatric | • Consider the use of PHQ-9, GAD-7, and ACE-Q screening tools |

*Abbreviations:* ACE-Q, Adverse Childhood Experience questionnaire; GAD-7, General Anxiety Disorder-7; JVD, jugular vein distention; PHQ-9, Patient Health Questionnaire-9.
*Data from Refs.*[19,44,45]

Inadequacies of imaging studies vary in patients with obesity. Limitations by x-ray beam attenuation can lead to reduced image contrast and amplification of noise, resulting in increased exposure time and motion artifacts.[26]

Other diagnostic imaging modalities, such as fluoroscopy, computed tomography (CT), and magnetic resonance imaging (MRI), are constrained by table weight and aperture diameter limits. Industry standards for table weight limits are 350 lbs (158 kg) for fluoroscopy, 450 lbs (204 kg) for CT, and 350 lbs (158 kg) for MRI.[28] For patients weighing up to 550 lbs, a vertical-field open MRI system is warranted.[26] Aperture diameter standard limits are opening of 45 cm for fluoroscopy, 70 cm for CT, and 60 cm diameter for MRI. Some patients may meet table limits with their weight, but their body habitus may not fit the aperture diameter.[29]

About a decade ago, only 10% of US hospitals with EDs owned large-weight-capacity CT scanners.[29] With the increasing need to accommodate patients with obesity, manufacturers recently have started to address these limitations by making "bariatric" CT and MRI machines with higher weight limits. Also, manufacturers have addressed the limitation of aperture diameter.[28]

## Procedures

From the ED to inpatient/outpatient settings, day-to-day procedures are greatly impacted by obesity. Emergency room health care professionals reported a strong correlation of BMI with difficulty in performing venous pressure measurements and conducting procedures such as cannulation and venipuncture. Patient positioning and conducting physical examinations were also challenges.[30] Cases of patients with obesity requiring intensive care during the COVID-19 pandemic also caused issues. It is more difficult to perform intubation or diagnostic imaging with weight limits, and transporting patients with obesity is near impossible when specialized equipment and beds are lacking. The pandemic significantly exposed these shortcomings in the health care system.[31]

## Offices, outpatient clinics, and operating rooms

Practice management must take into consideration the physical environment in which care is delivered. A comfortable and welcoming outpatient and inpatient environment is critical for patients with obesity. There is a pressing need for health care institutions to adapt their facilities to provide a safe and nonbiased space for their patients with obesity.

Clinical settings that are ill-equipped to care for patients with obesity further stigmatize weight. This unnecessary stress and trauma can lead to avoidance of care while negatively impacting care team trust.[32] In addition to emotional and mental effects, there are also safety hazards involved for institutions with unsuitable equipment and facilities for patients with obesity. In 2013, the Pennsylvania Patient Safety Authority conducted an internal review of their database to analyze the extent of adverse events among patients with class III obesity over a 5-year period from 2007 to 2011. They found 10% of adverse event reports, or 1774 incidents, were related to "facility, equipment, or device limitations."[33] Ultimately, this leads to reduced quality care for patients with obesity.[32]

In 2012, the Metabolic and Bariatric Surgery Accreditation and Quality Improvement Program (MBSAQIP) was formed to make notable efforts to accommodate patients with obesity in health care centers. For an institution to receive accreditation from MBSAQIP, it must demonstrate compliance with the standards outlined in the MBSAQIP manual. In 2019, 900 MBSAQIP-accredited centers existed in the United States and Canada. Although this is great progress for delivering better care for patients with obesity, there is a long road ahead for the health care system to properly evolve.[32]

### Social Implications

#### Attitudes and beliefs of health care professionals and patients

A current gap exists between the stigmatizing narrative that obesity is due to a "lack of willpower" and the current scientific knowledge of the complex, pathophysiology of the dysregulation of energy balance.[34] Awareness of obesity as a disease is emerging, but societal weight stigma continues to be insidious, and widespread joint efforts to challenge these biases are lagging. A 2018 study found that approximately 40% to 50% of US adults who are overweight and obese experienced internalized weight bias.[35] Results of the national awareness, care and treatment in obesity management (ACTION) study found one-third of primary care physicians perceived their patients' weight to be completely within their own control.[36]

It creates a vicious cycle when health care professionals carry these negative stereotypes. Patients with obesity ultimately suffer the worst consequences, including low-quality health care, reduced health care utilization, and negative effects on physical and mental health.[35] This only perpetuates the burden of illness among patients with obesity.

#### The chronic disease treatment paradigm

With the rising prevalence of chronic diseases in the United States, the standard of care centers on management through lifestyle modifications, pharmacotherapy, and/or surgical treatments. The focus is on the already present disease(s) and preventing or treating its downstream consequences. This is a reactive approach and often does not address the root causes. There is opportunity for intervention upstream with a focus on obesity.[4]

Obesity is challenging the way health care professionals have traditionally approached patient care, by positioning weight management as the primary goal. Modest weight loss reaching categorical targets of 5%, 10%, or 15% can help significantly improve prediabetes, type-2 diabetes, hyperlipidemia, hypertension, obstructive sleep apnea, and more.[37] With the expansion of available treatments, promise of new options on the horizon, and increased awareness of obesity as a disease, the time is now to adopt an adipose-centric approach to caring for patients living with chronic disease(s).[4]

#### Knowledge and medical training of health care professionals

The social implications of obesity extend beyond the perceptions of clinicians—they also affect the training of health care professionals.[38] Obesity is a part of medical education for physicians, but is not a priority for medical schools' curricula. A 2017 expert review panel found 36% of the 802 multiple-choice questions of all 3 United states

Medical Licensing Examination Step examinations contained obesity-related content, with the majority about weight-related comorbidities, such as type-2 diabetes or obstructive sleep apnea. The focus on obesity as a disease was poorly represented on these examinations, as was the prevention, management, and treatment of obesity.[39]

The American Board of Obesity Medicine (ABOM) was established to improve the education of physicians caring for patients with obesity. ABOM certification indicates that physicians have achieved competency in obesity care and have specialized knowledge of obesity medicine.[40]

Please refer to Rebecca M. Puhl, "Weight Stigma and Barriers to Effective Obesity Care," in this issue.

## Economic Effects

### Direct, indirect, and personal costs

The economic consequences of obesity are notable and can be grouped into three categories: direct, indirect (societal), and personal costs. Direct costs describe the costs needed to pay for the management of obesity and weight-related medical conditions.[41] This may include preventive, diagnostic, and treatment services. In 2019, the US direct medical costs related to obesity were estimated to be $173 billion.[42] The indirect costs include lost productivity in the job setting which can be due to a number of reasons. For example, absence from work, premature death, reduced life expectancy, disability, and unemployment could all lead to lost work.[41] Obesity-related absenteeism in 2019 was found to range from US productivity costs of $3.38 billion ($79 per individual with obesity) to $6.38 billion ($132 per individual with obesity).[42] Finally, personal costs are the most concerning. Patients with obesity encounter weight stigma and discrimination in the workforce, which negatively impacts their health. There is evidence that individuals with obesity report lower salaries and are ranked as less qualified than their counterparts.[34] Also, patients with obesity encounter cost barriers to care services because coverage by health care systems for weight-management services is extremely limited.[43]

Please refer to Chapter 10: *Economic and Social Complications of Obesity* for further details on this topic.

## Case Study

### Case presentation

A 45-year-old female patient with a history of obesity (BMI 40), nephrolithiasis with microscopic hematuria, and irritable bowel syndrome (IBS) presented to the ED in September of 2016 with a chief complaint of "left upper quadrant (LUQ) pain." The pain had been present for 2 years and had significantly worsened in last 2 months. The pain was noted to start after caretaking for her mother, which required manual labor and heavy lifting. It was described as crampy and localized to the left size, with no radiation. Differential at the time was a repeat episode of acute nephrolithiasis versus muscle spasms versus IBS but unlikely without any bowel movement changes. Notably, incidental history was discovered while reviewing systems, and the patient had a history of bilateral axillary lymphadenopathy with normal mammogram from 6 months before presentation.

### Initial workup

A CT abdomen and pelvis routine laboratory testing was ordered. The result was negative, aside from a mildly elevated A1c in prediabetes range. The patient was placed on metformin and discharged home from the ED.

### Subsequent visits and workup

At the end of October 2016, the patient was seen for follow-up in outpatient primary care where she complained of constipation, no bright red blood per rectum (BRBPR), and persistent hematuria. She was instructed to take Miralax and milk of magnesia in addition to undergoing a pelvic ultrasound and abdominal x-ray. Both were negative but for a small fibroid shown on ultrasound. No further follow-up was scheduled.

In January 2017, the patient presented to urgent care with generalized abdominal pain. She was diagnosed with an acute flare of IBS and referred to gastroenterology (GI). GI referred her to the anesthesia pain clinic for a trial of cortisone injections to the abdominal wall. The patient was also referred to gynecology to exclude this as a source of pain, and gynecology supported the diagnosis of musculoskeletal origin. Patient was seen by anesthesia pain for 6 visits over the course of a year through the end of 2017 where she received spinal injections targeting T5–T7 for a diagnosis of "intercostal neuralgia." Despite the injections, pain persisted without relief.

During these years, and again in early 2018, the patient was followed up for her bilateral axillary lymphadenopathy every 6 months with imaging, which was regarded as "reactive."

In April 2018, the patient presented to urgent care again with LUQ pain and was discharged. The subsequent day, she returned to the urgent care for a chief complaint of "back pain" and was discharged. Two months later, the patient presented to an outpatient internal medicine clinic with BRBPR. Blood tests were ordered and found hemoglobin was stable. No follow-up was scheduled.

It was not until October of that year that the patient was referred for a colonoscopy after she reported 4 episodes of BRBPR in 10 months.

The colonoscopy revealed several polyps and a fungating and ulcerated nonobstructing large mass in distal rectum, partially circumferential involving one-third of the lumen circumference and measuring 3.5 × 2.7 × 4.4 cm, in addition to hemorrhoids. The pathology demonstrated numerous tubular adenomas, 1 tubulovillous adenoma, and a rectal invasive adenocarcinoma. With the chest and pelvic CT, a 3-mm nodule, that was not seen previously, was noted, along with multiple enlarged perirectal lymph nodes up to 1.4 cm with central necrosis concerning for local nodal metastases. Ultimately, this patient was diagnosed with stage IIIB cT3N1bM0 distal rectal cancer, and the treatment indicated included surgical resection, chemotherapy, and radiation. At this time, the patient was referred to the hospital's comprehensive weight-management center for assistance in helping the patient to lose weight before undergoing surgical resection.

### Takeaways from the clinical case

Regardless of their weight, every patient deserves to be treated with respect, dignity, and appropriate care in medicine. Obesity is a risk factor for many chronic diseases, including colorectal cancer.[7] This patient was seen by numerous care providers, and although her experiences with the health care system were not witnessed, the lineage of events suggest several areas for improvement in care delivery. As discussed earlier, patients with obesity are less likely to undergo routine preventive screening.[22] Also, performing an abdominal physical examination and medical procedures on this patient population can be perceived by clinicians as "challenging."[19,30] The negative results from abdominal x-ray may have been due to equipment limitations in imaging patients with larger body habitus. Finally, the attitudes and beliefs of the health care providers who cared for this patient may have played a role in her delayed diagnosis.

## SUMMARY

The impacts of obesity on health care delivery are undeniable. Adiposopathy contributes to an individual's increased risk of a multitude of chronic diseases. These conditions are what have become the focus of health care professionals' clinical practice in today's world. With social efforts to abandon the view that obesity is a choice, there is greater possibility in addressing the topic of weight and prioritizing weight management. From a systems level, this hopefully means accelerated advancements in health care facilities and equipment. From an individual level, this involves more systematic bias training and more opportunities for education on obesity management. Ultimately, this will yield higher quality of care for individuals with obesity, improved health outcomes, and cost-savings.

## CLINICS CARE POINTS

---

- The physiologic, physical, social, and economic impacts of obesity on health care delivery are undeniable.

- With the slow response by the health care system to address the needs of patients with obesity, these individuals are enduring far-reaching consequences, from delayed diagnosis to inadequate access to indicated treatments.

- With social efforts to abandon the view that obesity is a choice, there is greater possibility in addressing the topic of weight and prioritizing weight management.

- There are changes occurring on an individual and systems level in response to the obesity epidemic, both of which are equally important to deliver the best quality care to patients with obesity.

---

## DISCLOSURE

Dr Velazquez: Advisory Board for Intellihealth and Weight Watchers; Consultant for Novo Nordisk. Dr Apovian has participated on advisory boards for Abbott Nutrition, Allergan, Inc., Altimmune, Inc., Cowen and Company, LLC, Curavit Clinical Research, Currax Pharmaceuticals, LLC, Echosens North America, Inc., EPG Communication Holdings Ltd., EnteroMedics, Gelesis, Srl., Jazz Pharmaceuticals, Inc., L-Nutra, Inc., NeuroBo Pharmaceuticals, Inc., Novo Nordisk, Inc., Nutrisystem, Pain Script Corporation, Real Appeal, Pursuit By You, Riverview School, Rhythm Pharmaceuticals, Tivity Health, Inc. Xeno Biosciences and Zafgen Inc. Dr Apovian has received research funding from NIH, PCORI, Novo Nordisk and GI Dynamics, Inc. Dr Apovian has participated on advisory boards for Abbott Nutrition, Allergan, Inc., Altimmune, Inc., Cowen and Company, LLC, Curavit Clinical Research, EnteroMedics, EPG Communication Holdings Ltd , Gelesis, Srl., Jazz Pharmaceuticals, Inc., L-Nutra, Inc., NeuroBo Pharmaceuticals, Inc., Novo Nordisk, Inc., Pain Script Corporation, Real Appeal, Riverview School, Rhythm Pharmaceuticals, Roman Health Ventures, Inc., Scientific Intake Ltd. Co., Tivity Health, Inc., Xeno Biosciences and Zafgen Inc. Dr Apovian has received research funding from NIH, PCORI, Novo Nordisk and GI Dynamics, Inc. Dr Apovian has participated on advisory boards for Altimmune, Inc., Cowen and Company, LLC, Currax Pharmaceuticals, LLC, EPG Communication Holdings Ltd., Gelesis, Srl., L-Nutra, Inc., NeuroBo Pharmaceuticals, Inc., Novo Nordisk, Inc., Pain Script Corporation, Pursuit By You, ReShape Lifesciences Inc., Riverview School, Rhythm Pharmaceuticals, and Xeno Biosciences. Dr Apovian has received research funding from the NIH, PCORI and GI Dynamics, Inc.

## REFERENCES

1. Ward ZJ, Bleich SN, Cradock AL, et al. Projected U.S. State-Level Prevalence of Adult Obesity and Severe Obesity. N Engl J Med 2019;381(25):2440–50.
2. Wosik J, Fudim M, Cameron B, et al. Telehealth transformation: COVID-19 and the rise of virtual care. J Am Med Inform Assoc 2020;27(6):957–62.
3. Wolfenden L, Ezzati M, Larijani B, et al. The challenge for global health systems in preventing and managing obesity. Obes Rev 2019;20(Suppl 2):185–93.
4. Lingvay I, Sumithran P, Cohen RV, et al. Obesity management as a primary treatment goal for type 2 diabetes: time to reframe the conversation. Lancet 2022; 399(10322):394–405 [Erratum in: Lancet. 2022 Jan 22;399(10322):358].
5. Gasoyan H, Tajeu G, Halpern MT, et al. Reasons for underutilization of bariatric surgery: the role of insurance benefit design. Surg Obes Relat Dis 2019;15: 146–51.
6. Understanding Complications/Co-morbidities of Obesity In: Rethink Obesity. Available at: https://www.rethinkobesity.global/global/en/weight-and-health/obesity-related-complications.html - section1. Accessed July 1 2022.
7. Leading Causes of Death In: CDC/National Center for Health Statistics Fasts-Stats. 2022. Available at: https://www.cdc.gov/nchs/fastats/leading-causes-of-death.htm. Accessed July 1 2022.
8. AMA. House of Delegates. Recognition of Obesity as a Disease. Resolution 2013; 420(A-13).
9. Kawai T, Autieri MV, Scalia R. Adipose tissue inflammation and metabolic dysfunction in obesity. Am J Physiol Cell Physiol 2021;320(3):C375–91.
10. De Lorenzo A, Gratteri S, Gualtieri P, et al. J Transl Med 2019;17:169.
11. Garvey WT. Is Obesity or Adiposity-Based Chronic Disease Curable: The Set Point Theory, the Environment, and Second-Generation Medications. Endocr Pract 2022;28(2):214–22.
12. By the Numbers: Diabetes in America In: National Diabetes Statics Report, 2022. 2022. Available at: https://www.cdc.gov/diabetes/health-equity/diabetes-by-the-numbers.html. Accessed July 1 2022.
13. Chronic Disease Prevention and Management In: National Conference of State Legislatures. 2013. Available at: https://www.ncsl.org/documents/health/chronic dtk13.pdf. Accessed July 1 2022.
14. Polso AK, Lassiter JL, Nagel JL. Impact of hospital guideline for weight-based antimicrobial dosing in morbidly obese adults and comprehensive literature review. J Clin Pharm Ther 2014;39(6):584–608.
15. Smit C, De Hoogd S, Brüggemann RJM, et al. Obesity and drug pharmacology: a review of the influence of obesity on pharmacokinetic and pharmacodynamic parameters. Expert Opin Drug Metab Toxicol 2018;14(3):275–85.
16. Deutschman CS, Neligan PJ. Evidence-based practice of critical care. ©. Elsevier Inc 2016. https://doi.org/10.1016/C2009-0-37460-7.
17. Higgins V, Omidi A, Tahmasebi H, et al. Marked Influence of Adiposity on Laboratory Biomarkers in a Healthy Cohort of Children and Adolescents. J Clin End Met 2020;105(4):e1781–97.
18. Daniels LB, Clopton P, Bhalla V, et al. How obesity affects the cut-points for B-type natriuretic peptide in the diagnosis of acute heart failure. Results from the Breathing Not Properly Multinational Study. Am Heart J 2006;151(5):999–1005.
19. Silk AW, McTigue KM. Reexamining the physical examination for obese patients. JAMA 2011;305(2):193–4.

20. Gilat R, Mitchnik IY, Moriah A, et al. The impact of body mass index on the accuracy of the physical examination of the knee. Int Orthop 2022;46(4):831–6.

21. Ferrante JM, Fyffe DC, Vega ML, et al. Family physicians' barriers to cancer screening in extremely obese patients. Obesity 2010;18(6):1153–9.

22. Ferrante JM, Chen PH, Crabtree BF, et al. Cancer screening in women. Am J Prev Med 2007;32(6):525–31.

23. Clarke MA, Fetterman B, Cheung LC, et al. Epidemiologic Evidence That Excess Body Weight Increases Risk of Cervical Cancer by Decreased Detection of Precancer. J Clin Oncol 2018;36(12):1184–91.

24. Elmore JG, Carney PA, Abraham LA, et al. The association between obesity and screening mammography accuracy. Arch Intern Med 2004;164(10):1140–7.

25. Dashe JS, McIntire DD, Twickler DM. Maternal obesity limits the ultrasound evaluation of fetal anatomy. J Ultrasound Med 2009;28(8):1025–30.

26. Deutschman CS, Neligan PJ. Evidence-based practice of critical care. Second Edition. Philadelphia, PA: Elsevier Inc; 2016.

27. From the American Association of Neurological Surgeons (AANS), American Society of Neuroradiology (ASNR), Cardiovascular and Interventional Radiology Society of Europe (CIRSE), Canadian Interventional Radiology Association (CIRA), Congress of Neurological Surgeons (CNS), European Society of Minimally Invasive Neurological Therapy (ESMINT), European Society of Neuroradiology (ESNR), European Stroke Organization (ESO), Society for Cardiovascular Angiography and Interventions (SCAI), Society of Interventional Radiology (SIR), Society of NeuroInterventional Surgery (SNIS), and World Stroke Organization (WSO), Sacks D, Baxter B, Campbell BCV, et al. Multisociety Consensus Quality Improvement Revised Consensus Statement for Endovascular Therapy of Acute Ischemic Stroke. Int J Stroke 2018;13(6):612–32.

28. Uppot RN. Impact of Obesity on Medical Imaging In: Obesity Causes, Consequences, Therapies, Policies Vol14, 3. 2014. Available at: https://healthmanagement.org/c/healthmanagement/issuearticle/impact-of-obesity-on-medical-imaging -:~:text=Industry%20standard%20table%20weight%20limits%20are%20450lbs%20%5B204kg%5D,the%20patient%E2%80%99s%20girth%20may%20exceed%20the%20aperture%20diameter. Accessed July 7 2022.

29. Ginde AA, Foianini A, Renner DM, et al. The challenge of CT and MRI imaging of obese individuals who present to the emergency department: a national survey. Obesity 2008;16(11):2549–51.

30. Kam J, Taylor DM. Obesity significantly increases the difficulty of patient management in the emergency department. Emerg Med Australas 2010 Aug;22(4):316–23.

31. Coronovarius (COVID-19) & Obesity In: World Obesity. Available at: https://www.worldobesity.org/news/statement-coronavirus-covid-19-obesity. Accessed on: July 7 2022.

32. MBSAQIP Standards Manual. 2019. Available at: https://www.facs.org/quality-programs/accreditation-and-verification/metabolic-and-bariatric-surgery-accreditation-and-quality-improvement-program/standards/. Accessed July 10 2022.

33. Gardner, LA. Class III Obese Patients: Is Your Hospital Equipped to Address Their Needs?, Vol. 10, No. 1, 2013. Available at: Class III Obese Patients: Is Your Hospital Equipped to Address Their Needs?. Accessed on July 10 2022.

34. Rubino F, Puhl RM, Cummings DE, et al. Joint international consensus statement for ending stigma of obesity. Nat Med 2020;26(4):485–97.

35. Puhl RM, Himmelstein MS, Quinn DM. Internalizing weight stigma: prevalence and sociodemographic considerations in US adults. Obesity 2018;26:167–75.
36. Kaplan LM, Golden A, Jinnett K, et al. Perceptions of Barriers to Effective Obesity Care: Results from the National ACTION Study. Obesity 2018;26(1):61–9.
37. Ryan DH, Yockey SR. Weight Loss and Improvement in Comorbidity: Differences at 5%, 10%, 15%, and Over. Curr Obes Rep 2017;6(2):187–94.
38. Butsch WS, Kushner RF, Alford S, et al. Low priority of obesity education leads to lack of medical students' preparedness to effectively treat patients with obesity: results from the U.S. medical school obesity education curriculum benchmark study. BMC Med Educ 2020;20(1):23.
39. Kushner RF, Butsch WS, Kahan S, et al. Obesity Coverage on Medical Licensing Examinations in the United States. What Is Being Tested? Teach Learn Med 2017; 29(2):123–8.
40. Our History: The ABOM Story. 2022. Available at: https://www.abom.org/history/. Accessed on July 10 2022.
41. Chu DT, Minh Nguyet NT, Dinh TC, et al. An update on physical health and economic consequences of overweight and obesity. Diabetes Metab Syndr 2018; 12(6):1095–100.
42. Consequences of Obesity. 2022. Available at: https://www.cdc.gov/obesity/basics/consequences.html. Accessed on July 11 2022.
43. Kahan S, Look M, Fitch A. The benefit of telemedicine in obesity care. Obesity 2022;30(3):577–86.
44. Creating a Comfortable and Welcoming Office Environment for Patients with High Body Weight." UCONN Rudd Center for Food Policy and Obesity. 2020. Available at: Creating a Comfortable and Welcoming Office Environment (uconnruddcenter.org) .Accessed on July 15 2022
45. Kalinauskienė E, Razvadauskas H, Morse DJ, et al. A Comparison of Electronic and Traditional Stethoscopes in the Heart Auscultation of Obese Patients. Medicina (Kaunas) 2019;55(4):94.

# Obesity and Viral Infections

Priya Jaisinghani, MD[a],*, Rekha Kumar, MD[b]

## KEYWORDS

- COVID-19 • SARS-CoV-2 • Obesity • Mortality • Body mass index (BMI)
- Cytokine storm • Inflammatory

## KEY POINTS

- In the United States, there have been more than 95 million cases of COVID-19.
- Obesity is a risk factor for severe clinical course in patients with COVID-19, possibly due to underlying immune and inflammatory changes, pulmonary system impairments and cooccurring obesity-related conditions that are also risk factors for COVID-19.
- There is a need for intensive COVID-19 management as obesity severity increases and also promotion of COVID-19 prevention strategies in those living with obesity including continued vaccine prioritization, masking and timely booster dosages.

## BACKGROUND

COVID-19 is the name of the disease caused by severe acute respiratory syndrome coronavirus 2 (SARS-CoV-2), which recently triggered a rapidly emerging global pandemic.[1] The source of the pneumonia outbreak was in Wuhan, China in late 2019.[2] The virus was found to be a member of the beta coronavirus family, in the same species as SARS-CoV and SARS-related CoVs that have been seen in bats.[3,4] According to the World Health Organization, as of September 2022, there have been more than 611 million cases, resulting in more than 6 million deaths worldwide. In the United States itself, there have been more than 95 million cases of COVID-19 that have resulted in 1,050,631 deaths.[5]

## COVID-19 CLINICAL SPECTRUM

A virus surface spike protein mediates SARS-CoV-2 entry into cells. The SARS-CoV-2 spike protein binds to its receptor human ACE2 through its receptor-binding domain and is proteolytically activated by human proteases. Coronavirus entry into host cells is an important determinant of viral infectivity and pathogenesis.[6,7]

Patients with COVID-19 can range from being asymptomatic to having critical illness. According to the NIH, patients with mild illness are individuals who have fever, cough,

[a] Division of Endocrinology, Diabetes and Metabolism, New York University Grossman School of Medicine, New York, NY, USA; [b] Division of Endocrinology, New York-Presbyterian Hospital and Weill Cornell Medical Center, New York, NY, USA
* Corresponding author. 160 West 26th Street, 2nd Floor, NY, NY 10001.
E-mail address: priya.jaisinghani@nyulangone.org

Gastroenterol Clin N Am 52 (2023) 393–402
https://doi.org/10.1016/j.gtc.2023.03.012
0889-8553/23/© 2023 Elsevier Inc. All rights reserved.

sore throat, malaise, headache, muscle pain, nausea, vomiting, diarrhea, loss of taste, and smell but who do not have shortness of breath, dyspnea, or abnormal chest imaging. Those with moderate illness show evidence of lower respiratory disease during clinical assessment or imaging and an oxygen saturation ($SpO_2$) greater than or equal to 94% on room air. Individuals with an $SpO_2$ less than 94% on room air, a ratio of arterial partial pressure of oxygen to fraction of inspired oxygen ($Pao_2/Fio_2$) less than 300 mm Hg, a respiratory rate greater than 30 breaths/min, or lung infiltrates greater than 50% are considered to have severe illness. Those who progress to respiratory failure, septic shock, and/or multiple organ dysfunction have critical illness.[8–11]

Increased plasma concentrations of proinflammatory cytokines including interleukin-6 (IL-6), IL-10, granulocyte colony-stimulating factor (G-CSF), monocyte chemoattractant protein (MCP) 1A, tumor necrosis factor alpha (TNFα), and others are present in more severe cases and are associated with a worse prognosis.[12,13]

Elevated lactate dehydrogenase, ferritin, D-dimer, and creatine kinase elevation are also associated with severe disease. Elevated D-dimer and fibrinogen are consistent with thrombosis and pulmonary embolism in severe disease.[14]

## HOW DOES COVID-19 AFFECT PATIENTS WITH OBESITY

The large number of people infected with COVID-19 combined with the wide spectrum of disease severity led to investigation of whether various phenotypes and baseline biomarkers are associated with a higher risk of infection and critical illness. Initial data on COVID-19 implicated several factors associated with worse disease severity including older age and comorbidities such as diabetes and hypertension.[2,3]

Because of the close relationship between these conditions and metabolic syndrome, it was hypothesized that obesity may also be a risk factor for worse clinical outcomes. There were then studies looking at presenting characteristics and outcomes of US patients requiring hospitalization for COVID-19. A study looking at 12 major New York City hospitals included 5700 patients (median age, 63 years [interquartile range, 52–75; range, 0–107 years]; 39.7% women). The most common comorbidities were hypertension (3026; 56.6%), obesity (1737; 41.7%), and diabetes (1808; 33.8%).[15]

Petrilli and colleagues noted any increase in body mass (body mass index [BMI]>40, odds ratio [OR] 1.8, confidence interval [CI] 1.8–3.4) to be one of the strongest risk factors for hospital admission in patients among age, heart failure, and chronic kidney disease. Although early descriptive COVID-19 studies did not report on the direct association of obesity with disease severity, BMI was found to be higher in those with development of critical illness in COVID-19.[4,5] Petrilli and colleagues found the strongest risks for critical illness besides age were associated with heart failure (OR 1.9, CI 1.4–2.5), BMI greater than 40 (OR 1.5, CI 1.0–2.2), and male sex (OR 1.5, CI 1.3–1.8).[16] It was also later reported that in adults with COVID-19 a nonlinear relationship was found between BMI and COVID-19 severity. The lowest risk was BMI near the threshold between healthy weight and overweight and then increasing risk with higher BMI.[17]

Emerging data also showed that obesity is an independent predictor of intensive care unit (ICU) admission, mechanical ventilation, and death.[17–20] Risk for invasive mechanical ventilation increased over the full range of BMIs possibly because of impaired lung function associated with higher BMI.[21] Although only some studies found an increased risk of ICU admission in obese patients younger than 60 years, Hajifathalian and colleagues found this association to hold true across all age groups including adults older than 60 years specifically.[1,22]

Multiple studies went on to confirm that obesity is a major risk factor for COVID-19 disease severity and significantly affects disease presentation, development of critical illness, need for hospitalization, critical care requirements, and mortality.[23] The Centers for Disease Control and Prevention (CDC) assessed 148,494 adults with a COVID-19 diagnosis during an emergency department or inpatient visit at 238 US hospitals during March to December 2020; 28.3% were found to be overweight and 50.8% were found to have obesity. Overweight and obesity were risk factors for invasive mechanical ventilation, and obesity was a risk factor for hospitalization and death, particularly among adults younger than 65 years. The CDC recognized obesity as a risk factor for severe COVID-19. The Advisory Committee on Immunization Practices considers obesity to be a high-risk medical condition for COVID-19 vaccine prioritization.[17,24]

Early global studies looking at risk factors for clinical course of illness and mortality also noted similar trends. A retrospective study assessing the clinical course and risk factors for mortality of adult inpatients with COVID-19 in Wuhan, China[25] showed that among the 191 patients included in this study, 137 were discharged and 54 died in the hospital. Of the patients with comorbidities (48%), hypertension was the most common (58 [30%] patients), followed by diabetes (36 [19%] patients) and coronary heart disease (15 [8%] patients). Multivariable regression showed increasing odds of in-hospital death associated with older age (OR $1 \cdot 10$, 95% CI $1 \cdot 03$–$1 \cdot 17$, per year increase; $P = 0 \cdot 0043$), higher Sequential Organ Failure Assessment (SOFA) score ($5 \cdot 65$, $2 \cdot 61$–$12 \cdot 23$; $P < 0 \cdot 0001$), and D-dimer greater than 1 µg/mL ($18 \cdot 42$, $2 \cdot 64$–$128 \cdot 55$; $P = 0 \cdot 0033$) on admission. The potential risk factors of older age, high SOFA score, and D-dimer greater than 1 µg/mL could help clinicians to identify patients with poor prognosis at an early stage. There were also temporal changes in laboratory markers from illness onset in patients hospitalized with COVID-19. Markers such as D-dimer, IL-6, lactate dehydrogenase, and troponin among others were more elevated in nonsurvivors than survivors.

## PATHOGENESIS RELATED TO OBESITY

COVID-19 leads to fast activation of innate immune cells, especially in patients developing severe disease.[26] Circulating neutrophil numbers are consistently higher in survivors of COVID-19 than in nonsurvivors, whereas the infection also induces lymphocytopenia that affects mostly the CD4$^+$ T cells.[27] Levels of many proinflammatory effector cytokines, such as TNF$\alpha$, IL-1$\beta$, IL-6, IL-8, G-CSF and granulocyte-macrophage colony-stimulating factor, and chemokines, such as MCP1, inducible protein-10, and macrophage inflammatory protein 1$\alpha$, reflect innate immunity and are elevated in patients with COVID-19.[12] The SARS-CoV-2 infection can drive an uncontrolled inflammatory response, leading to a cytokine response in the host.[28] Levels of such markers are higher in those who are critically ill and also associated with increased mortality.[12,29–31] The most important mediators of cytokine storm in COVID-19 disease are IL-6, IL-10, and TNF$\alpha$.[3] On the contrary, it was noted that in COVID-19 cases that were postulated to be milder such as those with anosmia tended to have lower IL-6 levels and lower cytokine storm.[32] The inflammatory response in COVID-19 can lead to more clinical complications such as development of acute respiratory distress syndrome, cardiac injury, thromboembolic disease, and disseminated intravascular coagulation rather than the direct viral cytopathic injury alone.[1,33,34]

Likewise, obesity, a common metabolic disease affecting 41.8% of the United States from 2017 to March 2020 (NHANES, 2021) and a risk factor for other chronic diseases such as type 2 diabetes, heart disease, and some cancer,[35] can lead to a state of chronic inflammation termed "metaflammation."[36–39] This state is characterized by a sustained proinflammatory response from the immune system and adipose tissue secreting proinflammatory markers such as TNF$\alpha$, IL-1, and IL-6, leading to oxidative stress.[40,41] This metaflammation also contributes to the pathogenesis of several obesity-related conditions, such as type 2 diabetes mellitus, cardiovascular disease, and nonalcoholic fatty liver disease.[23,31,42]

Patients with obesity also often have respiratory dysfunction due to alterations in respiratory mechanisms, increased airway resistance, impaired gas exchange, and low lung volume and muscle strength. Thus, they are also predisposed to hypoventilation-associated pneumonia, pulmonary hypertension, and cardiac stress. Many of the obesity-related conditions such as diabetes mellitus and cardiovascular disease are considered to result in increased vulnerability to pneumonia-associated organ failures.[23]

For these underlying reasons, obesity is a recognized risk factor for severe COVID-19 possibly related to chronic inflammation, impaired lung function, and cooccurring obesity-related conditions, which are also risk factors for COVID-19.[21,43] Early in the pandemic, a study by Stefan and colleagues noted that 85% of the patients with obesity required mechanical ventilation and 62% of the patients with obesity died versus patients without obesity of whom 64% required mechanical ventilation and 36% died.[23]

More than 900,000 adult COVID-19 hospitalizations occurred in the United States between the beginning of the pandemic and November 18, 2020. Models estimate that 271,800 (30.2%) of these hospitalizations were attributed to obesity.[44] Although children diagnosed with COVID-19 are less likely to develop severe illness compared with adults, children diagnosed with obesity may suffer worse outcomes from COVID-19. A study found that in patients with obesity younger than 18 years, having obesity was associated with a 3.07 times higher risk of hospitalization and a 1.42 times higher risk of severe illness (ICU admission, invasive mechanical ventilation, or death) when hospitalized.[45]

There are also changes in the innate immune response to COVID-19 in individuals with obesity. In mice with obesity, it has been shown that there is increased expression of ACE2, the receptor facilitating COVID-19 infection. Alveolar macrophage metabolism is altered in the lung environment of those with obesity, with baseline chronic inflammation affecting early microbial containment. Circulating bone marrow–derived monocytes can be affected by obesity-related metabolic stressors such as poor blood glucose control and hyperlipidemia.[22,31,46–49]

Thus, the immune dysregulation and systemic inflammation seen in those living with obesity, combined with impairments in the cardiovascular, respiratory, metabolic, and thrombotic pathways that characterize COVID-19, may potentiate critical illness.[50,51] Similarly, worst outcomes in those with obesity were also observed with the H1N1 influenza virus where weight was found to affect risk for hospitalization, mechanical ventilation, and death, independent of other comorbidities.[52]

## COVID-19: OBESITY AND DISPARITIES

Evidence emerged from studies throughout the pandemic that some racial and ethnic minorities as well as socioeconomically disadvantaged groups are bearing a disproportionate burden of illness and death due to disparities in testing, treatment, and overall access to care. According to the CDC, data from 2018 to 2020 showed that non-Hispanic Black adults had the highest prevalence of self-reported obesity

(40.7%), followed by Hispanic adults (35.2%), and non-Hispanic White adults (30.3%). Hispanic and non-Hispanic Black adults have a higher prevalence of obesity and are more likely to suffer worse outcomes from COVID-19.[53]

Azar and colleagues conducted a study in a large California health care system in which African American had 2.7 times the odds of hospitalization after adjusting for age, sex, comorbidities, and income compared with non-Hispanic White patients.[54-58]

Many of the disparities have also contributed to risk factors such as obesity and type 2 diabetes in racial and monitory groups. Disparities include access to care, biases on the part of the patients and providers due to prior negative experiences, distrust of the medical community, neighborhood design, access to healthy, afford-able foods and beverages, access to safe and convenient places for physical activity, and so forth; this further highlights the need to address social determinants of health particularly in populations disproportionately affected by obesity and more likely to have worse outcomes from COVID-19.[17]

These findings should not be used to further stigmatize a patient population that already suffers from biases but rather understand this important link and continue to treat patients with obesity thoroughly.

## COVID-19 VACCINES AND OBESITY

To combat the immense toll on global public health, vaccines against COVID-19 were developed. According to the vaccine safety and efficacy information for the Pfizer, Moderna, and Johnson & Johnson formulations, these vaccines showed a similar efficacy in both individuals with and without obesity. However, there have been conflicting studies. Clinical trials that assessed BMI and central obesity showed that induced antibody titers are lower in individuals with obesity when compared with healthy weight individuals; this highlights a potential early waning of vaccine-induced antibodies linked to obesity.[59,60] Further studies investigating the clinical implications of the association between obesity and lower antibody titers will need to be conduct-ed to understand the effectiveness and durability of these vaccines in individuals with obesity; this will become especially important, as boosters are being adminis-tered with the purpose of ensuring and sustaining long, lasting protection against COVID-19.

Multiple studies have shown that a booster or third dose of an SARS-CoV-2 vaccine helps provide protection, as immunity against this virus wanes.[61-63] One study measured antibody levels to COVID-19 following the Pfizer BNT162b2 mRNA vaccina-tion at baseline, 21 days after first dose, 30 to 40 days after second dose, and 90 to 100 days after second dose and compared between subjects with obesity versus those without. Early antibody titers were essentially equivalent between individuals with obesity versus those without. One and three months after second dose, antibody titers reported for subjects with obesity were significantly lower than those for subjects of healthy weight.[59] These findings were consistent with studies conducted following seasonal influenza virus vaccination.[63,64]

Obesity hinders immune responses to vaccines and infections. These studies, how-ever, only reported a waning of the antibody response and did not address the impli-cations of decreased antibody titers in individuals with obesity clinically. Some studies conducted after COVID-19 vaccinations became widely available suggest that break-through infections were linked to obesity.[65]

In addition, study methods differed across studies including measuring antibody ti-ters at varying time points, using different antibody-measuring kits and different mea-sures of obesity. The sample sizes in the clinical trials mentioned were also smaller compared with the vaccine trials and may not have been entirely representative of the general population of individuals with obesity.

Although the duration of the effectiveness may be shortened postvaccination in those with obesity, it must be highlighted that there is a window of time where protection is observed. More follow-up studies need to be done to assess how different patterns of fat distribution could be affecting immune responses to vaccination, long-term efficacy of the available COVID-19 vaccines, and optimal scheduling for boosters. Studies should also be expanded to include subjects of varying ages including in children with obesity.

At this time the Obesity Society critically evaluated data from published peer-reviewed literature and briefing documents from Emergency Use Authorization applications submitted by Pfizer-BioNTech, Moderna, and Johnson & Johnson and concluded that all 3 vaccines are highly efficacious and that their efficacy is not significantly different in people with and without obesity.[63]

With increasing obesity rates, higher risk of severe viral infection and death by COVID-19, and potentially impaired vaccine-conferred protection and breakthrough infections in those with obesity, it is important to conduct further studies to provide medical treatment plans and vaccine schedules that will induce long-lasting, protective immune responses in patients with obesity.[65–72]

## SUMMARY

Obesity is a risk factor for severe clinical course in patients with COVID-19, possibly due to underlying immune and inflammatory changes along with pulmonary system impairments and cooccurring obesity-related conditions that are also risk factors for COVID-19. These findings highlight the need for intensive COVID-19 management as obesity severity increases but also promotion of COVID-19 prevention strategies in those living with obesity including continued vaccine prioritization and masking and timely booster dosages. Providers should continue to advocate for individuals facing racial and socioeconomic health disparities and stigma to seek medical attention policies to treatment and/or prevention of COVID-19 while also encouraging and supporting a healthy BMI.[17]

## CLINICS CARE POINTS

- Obesity hinders immune responses to vaccines and infections. Studies, however, have only reported a waning of the antibody response and did not address the implications of decreased antibody titers in individuals with obesity clinically.

- More follow-up studies need to be done to assess how different patterns of fat distribution could be affecting immune responses to vaccination, long-term efficacy of the available COVID-19 vaccines, and optimal scheduling for boosters. Studies should also be expanded to include subjects of varying ages including in children with obesity.

- With increasing obesity rates, higher risk of severe viral infection and death by COVID-19, and potentially impaired vaccine-conferred protection and breakthrough infections in those with obesity, it is important to conduct further studies to provide medical treatment plans and vaccine schedules that will induce long-lasting, protective immune responses in patients with obesity.

- Providers should continue to advocate for individuals facing racial and socioeconomic health disparities and stigma to seek medical attention policies to treatment and/or prevention of COVID-19 while also encouraging and supporting a healthy BMI.

## DISCLOSURE

The authors have no disclosures of commercial or financial conflicts of interest for any funding sources.

## REFERENCES

1. Hajifathalian K, Kumar S, Newberry C, et al. Obesity is Associated with Worse Outcomes in COVID-19: Analysis of Early Data from New York City. Obesity 2020;28(9):1606–12.
2. WHO Novel Coronavirus (2019-nCoV) Situation Report 1. (2020). Available at: $$ https://www.who.int/docs/default-source/coronaviruse/situation-reports/20200121-sitrep-1-2019-ncov.pdf?sfvrsn$=$20a99c10_4. Accessed April 01, 2020.
3. Ragab D, Salah Eldin H, Taeimah M, et al. The COVID-19 Cytokine Storm; What We Know So Far. Front Immunol 2020;11:1446.
4. Wacharapluesadee S, Tan CW, Maneeorn P, et al. Evidence for SARS-CoV-2 related coronaviruses circulating in bats and pangolins in Southeast Asia. Nat Commun 2021;12:972.
5. Centers for Disease Control and Prevention. COVID data tracker. Atlanta, GA: US Department of Health and Human Services, CDC; 2022. https://covid.cdc.gov/covid-data-tracker.
6. Li F. Structure, function, and evolution of coronavirus spike proteins. Annu Rev Virol 2016;3:237–61.
7. Perlman S, Netland J. Coronaviruses post-SARS: Update on replication and pathogenesis. Nat Rev Microbiol 2009;7:439–50.
8. COVID-19 Treatment Guidelines Panel. Coronavirus disease 2019 (COVID-19) treatment guidelines. National Institutes of Health. Available at: https://www.covid19treatmentguidelines.nih.gov/. Accessed September, 25 2022.
9. Zaim S, Chong JH, Sankaranarayanan V, et al. COVID-19 and Multiorgan Response. Curr Probl Cardiol 2020;45(8):100618.
10. YeA WB, Mao J. The pathogenesis and treatment of the 'Cytokine Storm' in COVID-19. J Infect 2020;45(4):372–89.
11. Qin C, Zhou L, Hu Z, et al. Dysregulation of immune response in patients with COVID-19 in Wuhan, China. Clin Infect Dis 2020.
12. Huang C, Wang Y, Li X, et al. Clinical features of patients infected with 2019 novel coronavirus in Wuhan, China. Lancet 2020;395:497–506.
13. Costela-Ruiz VJ, Illescas-Montes R, Puerta-Puerta JM, et al. SARS-CoV-2 infection: The role of cytokines in COVID-19 disease. Cytokine Growth Factor Rev 2020;54:62–75.
14. Koleilat I, Galen B, Choinski K, et al. Clinical characteristics of acute lower extremity deep venous thrombosis diagnosed by duplex in patients hospitalized for coronavirus disease 2019. J Vasc Surg Venous Lymphat Disord 2021;9(1): 36–46.
15. Richardson S, Hirsch JS, Narasimhan M, et al. Presenting Characteristics, Comorbidities, and Outcomes Among 5700 Patients Hospitalized With COVID-19 in the New York City Area. JAMA 2020;323(20):2052–9 [published correction appears in JAMA. 2020 May 26;323(20):2098].
16. Petrilli CM, Jones SA, Yang J, et al. Factors associated with hospital admission and critical illness among 5279 people with coronavirus disease 2019 in New York City: prospective cohort study. BMJ 2020;369:m1966.
17. Kompaniyets L, Goodman AB, Belay B, et al. Body Mass Index and Risk for COVID-19–Related Hospitalization, Intensive Care Unit Admission, Invasive

Mechanical Ventilation, and Death — United States, March–December 2020. MMWR Morb Mortal Wkly Rep 2021;70:355–61.

18. Peng YD, Meng K, Guan HQ, et al. [Clinical characteristics and outcomes of 112 cardiovascular disease patients infected by 2019-nCoV]. Zhonghua Xinxue-guanbing Zazhi 2020;48:E004.

19. Simonnet A, Chetboun M, Poissy J, et al. High prevalence of obesity in severe acute respiratory syndrome coronavirus-2 (SARS-CoV-2) requiring invasive mechanical ventilation. Obesity 2020;28(10):1994.

20. Lighter J, Phillips M, Hochman S, et al. Obesity in patients younger than 60 years is a risk factor for Covid-19 hospital admission. Clin Infect Dis 2020;71(15):896–7.

21. Dixon AE, Peters U. The effect of obesity on lung function. Expert Rev Respir Med 2018;12:755.

22. Sattar N, McInnes IB, McMurray JJV. Obesity a Risk Factor for Severe COVID-19 Infection: Multiple Potential Mechanisms. Circulation 2020;142(1):4–6.

23. Stefan N, Birkenfeld AL, Schulze MB, et al. Obesity and impaired metabolic health in patients with COVID-19. Nat Rev Endocrinol 2020;16(7):341–2.

24. Dooling K, Marin M, Wallace M, et al. The Advisory Committee on Immunization Practices' updated interim recommendation for allocation of COVID-19 vaccine—United States, December 2020. MMWR Morb Mortal Wkly Rep 2021;69:165760.

25. Zhou F, Yu T, Du R, et al. Clinical course and risk factors for mortality of adult inpatients with COVID-19 in Wuhan, China: a retrospective cohort study. Lancet 2020;395(10229):1054–62 [published correction appears in Lancet. 2020 Mar 28;395(10229):1038] [published correction appears in Lancet. 2020 Mar 28;395(10229):1038].

26. Wu F, Zhao S, Yu B, et al. A new coronavirus associated with human respiratory disease in China. Nature 2020;579:265–9.

27. Wang D, Hu B, Hu C, et al. Clinical characteristics of 138 hospitalized patients with 2019 novel coronavirus-infected pneumonia in Wuhan, China. JAMA 2020;323:1061–9.

28. Pedersen SF, Ho YC. A storm is raging. J Clin Invest 2020. https://doi.org/10.1172/JCI137647.

29. Wu C, Chen X, Cai Y, et al. Risk factors associated with acute respiratory distress syndrome and death in patients with coronavirus disease 2019 pneumonia in Wuhan, China. JAMA Intern Med 2020;180:934–43.

30. Schett G, Sticherling M, Neurath MF. COVID-19: risk for cytokine targeting in chronic inflammatory diseases? Nat Rev Immunol 2020;20:271–2.

31. Gleeson LE, Roche HM, Sheedy FJ. Obesity, COVID-19 and innate immunometabolism. Br J Nutr 2021;125(6):628–32.

32. Sanli DET, Altundag A, Kandemirli SG, et al. Relationship between disease severity and serum IL-6 levels in COVID-19 anosmia. Am J Otolaryngol 2021;42(1):102796.

33. Ye Q, Wang B, Mao J. The pathogenesis and treatment of the 'Cytokine Storm' in COVID-19. J Infect 2020;80(6):607–13.

34. Qin C, Zhou L, Hu Z, et al. Dysregulation of immune response in patients with COVID-19 in Wuhan, China. Clin Infect Dis 2020;71(15):762–8.

35. Ghanim H, Aljada A, Hofmeyer D, et al. Circulating mononuclear cells in the obese are in a proinflammatory state. Circulation 2004;110:1564–71.

36. Gregor MF, Hotamisligil GS. Inflammatory mechanisms in obesity. Annu Rev Immunol 2011;29:415–45.

37. Vandanmagsar B, Youm YH, Ravussin A, et al. The NLRP3 inflammasome instigates obesity-induced inflammation and insulin resistance. Nat Med 2011;17: 179–88.
38. Xu C, Lu Z, Luo Y, et al. Targeting of NLRP3 inflammasome with gene editing for the amelioration of inflammatory diseases. Nat Commun 2018;9:4092.
39. Larsen CM, Faulenbach M, Vaag A, et al. Interleukin-1-receptor antagonist in type 2 diabetes mellitus. N Engl J Med 2007;356:1517–26.
40. Divella R, De Luca R, Abbate I, et al. Obesity and cancer: the role of adipose tissue and adipo-cytokines-induced chronic inflammation. J Cancer 2016;7: 2346–59.
41. Wen H, Gris D, Lei Y, et al. Fatty acid-induced NLRP3-ASC inflammasome activation interferes with insulin signaling. Nat Immunol 2011;12:408–15.
42. Wree A, McGeough MD, Peña CA, et al. NLRP3 inflammasome activation is required for fibrosis development in NAFLD. J Mol Med (Berl) 2014;92:1069–82.
43. Popkin BM, Du S, Green WD, et al. Individuals with obesity and COVID-19: a global perspective on the epidemiology and biological relationships. Obes Rev 2020;21:e13128.
44. O'Hearn M, Liu J, Cudhea F, et al. Coronavirus Disease 2019 Hospitalizations Attributable to Cardiometabolic Conditions in the United States: A Comparative Risk Assessment Analysis. J Am Heart Assoc 2021;10(5):e019259.
45. Kompaniyets L, Agathis NT, Nelson JM, et al. Underlying medical conditions associated with severe COVID-19 illness among children. JAMA Netw Open 2021;4:6.
46. Zhu L, She ZG, Cheng X, et al. Association of blood glucose control and outcomes in patients with COVID-19 and pre-existing type 2 diabetes. Cell Metab 2020;31:1068–77.e3.
47. Cavounidis A, Mann EH. SARS-CoV-2 has a sweet tooth. Nature Rev Immunol 2020;20:460.
48. Svedberg FR, Brown SL, Krauss MZ, et al. The lung environment controls alveolar macrophage metabolism and responsiveness in type 2 inflammation. Nat Immunol 2019;20:571–80.
49. Woods PS, Kimmig LM, Meliton AY, et al. Tissue-resident alveolar macrophages Do not rely on glycolysis for LPS-induced inflammation. Am J Respir Cell Mol Biol 2020;62:243–55.
50. Samad F, Ruf W. Inflammation, obesity, and thrombosis. Blood 2013;122: 3415–22.
51. Vilahur G, Ben-Aicha S, Badimon L. New insights into the role of adipose tissue in thrombosis. Cardiovasc Res 2017;113:1046–54.
52. Cruz-Lagunas A, Jimenez-Alvarez L, Ramirez G, et al. Obesity and pro-inflammatory mediators are associated with acute kidney injury in patients with A/H1N1 influenza and acute respiratory distress syndrome. Exp Mol Pathol 2014;97:453–7.
53. Centers for Disease Control and Prevention. (2022).
54. Kristen M JA, Zijun S, Robert JR, et al. Disparities In Outcomes Among COVID-19 Patients In A Large Health Care System In California. Health Aff 2020;39(7): 1253–62.
55. Morgan OW, Bramley A, Fowlkes A, et al. Morbid obesity as a risk factor for hospitalization and death due to 2009 pandemic influenza A(H1N1) disease. PLoS One 2010;5:e9694.
56. Michalakis K, Ilias I. SARS-CoV -2 infection and obesity: common inflammatory and metabolic aspects. Diabetes Metab Syndr 2020;14:469–71.

57. Caussy C, Pattou F, Wallet F, et al. Prevalence of obesity among adult inpatients with COVID-19 in France. Lancet Diabetes Endocrinol 2020;8:562–4.

58. Auld SC, Caridi-Scheible M, Blum JM, et al. ICU and ventilator mortality among critically ill adu.

59. Nasr MC, Geerling E, Pinto AK. Impact of Obesity on Vaccination to SARS-CoV-2. Front Endocrinol 2022;13:898810.

60. Accorsi EK, Britton A, Fleming-Dutra KE, et al. Association Between 3 Doses of mRNA COVID-19 Vaccine and Symptomatic Infection Caused by the SARS-CoV-2 Omicron and Delta Variants. JAMA 2022;327:639–51.

61. Tenforde MW, Patel MM, Gaglani M, et al. Effectiveness of a Third Dose of Pfizer-BioNTech and Moderna Vaccines in Preventing COVID-19 Hospitalization Among Immunocompetent and Immunocompromised Adults - United States, August-December 2021. MMWR Morb Mortal Wkly Rep 2022;71:118–24.

62. Thompson MG, Natarajan K, Irving SA, et al. Effectiveness of a Third Dose of mRNA Vaccines Against COVID-19-Associated Emergency Department and Urgent Care Encounters and Hospitalizations Among Adults During Periods of Delta and Omicron Variant Predominance - VISION Network, 10 States, August 2021-January 2022. MMWR Morb Mortal Wkly Rep 2022;71:139–45.

63. Butsch WS, Hajduk A, Cardel MI, et al. COVID-19 vaccines are effective in people with obesity: A position statement from The Obesity Society. Obesity 2021 Oct; 29(10):1575–9.

64. Malavazos AE, Basilico S, Iacobellis G, et al. Antibody Responses to BNT162b2 mRNA Vaccine: Infection-Naive Individuals With Abdominal Obesity Warrant Attention. Obes (Silver Spring) 2022;30:606–13.

65. Watanabe M, Balena A, Tuccinardi D, et al. Central Obesity, Smoking Habit, and Hypertension are Associated With Lower Antibody Titres in Response to COVID-19 mRNA Vaccine. Diabetes Metab Res Rev 2022;38:e3465.

66. Massetti GM, Jackson BR, Brooks JT, et al. Summary of Guidance for Minimizing the Impact of COVID-19 on Individual Persons, Communities, and Health Care Systems — United States, August 2022. MMWR Morb Mortal Wkly Rep 2022; 71:1057–64.

67. Dinleyici EC, Borrow R, Safadi MAP, et al. Vaccines and Routine Immunization Strategies During the COVID-19 Pandemic. Hum Vaccin Immunother 2021;17: 400–7.

68. Poland GA, Ovsyannikova IG, Kennedy RB. Personalized Vaccinology: A Review. Vaccine 2018;36:5350–7.

69. Ledford H. How Obesity Could Create Problems for a COVID Vaccine. Nature 2020;586:488–9.

70. Frasca D, Reidy L, Cray C, et al. Influence of Obesity on Serum Levels of SARS-CoV-2-Specific Antibodies in COVID-19 Patients. PLoS One 2021;16:e0245424.

71. Ward H, Whitaker M, Flower B, et al. Population Antibody Responses Following COVID-19 Vaccination in 212,102 Individuals. Nat Commun 2022;13:907.

72. Saciuk Y, Kertes J, Mandel M, et al. Pfizer-BioNTech Vaccine Effectiveness Against Sars-Cov-2 Infection: Findings From a Large Observational Study in Israel. Prev Med 2022;155:106947.

# The Effect of Obesity on Gastrointestinal Disease

Jessica E.S. Shay, MD, PhD[a,b], Amandeep Singh, MD, PhD[a,c],*

KEYWORDS

- Barrett's esophagus • Cholelithiasis • Non-alcoholic fatty liver disease
- Nonalcoholic steatohepatitis • Colorectal cancer

KEY POINTS

- Increased abdominal and intragastric pressure due to obesity and central adiposity leads to higher rates of reflux. Similarly, Barrett's esophagus and esophageal adenocarcinoma rates increase with obesity.
- Gallstone disease, pancreatitis and pancreatic adenocarcinoma trend with rising rates of obesity.
- Rates of non-alcoholic fatty liver disease (NAFLD) have increased globally due to rapidly rising rates of obesity. As NAFLD comprises a spectrum of disease from mild steatosis to cirrhosis, it is imperative to ensure patients undergo adequate screening and staging.
- There is a clear increased risk of colorectal cancer as excess weight increases. This risk may be reversible with appropriate weight loss interventions.
- Historically lifestyle changes have met with relatively little sustained success and, as such, bariatric surgery has remained the most successful long-term intervention for weight loss. Key screening pre- and post-operatively is necessary to ensure adequate nutrition and to avoid complications.

## ESOPHAGUS
### Gastroesophageal Reflux Disease

Reflux of caustic gastric contents into the esophagus is prevented by pressure from a combination of the lower esophageal sphincter and the diaphragm.[1] Decreased lower esophageal sphincter tone allows increased regurgitation of acidic contents to encounter esophageal mucosa, which in turn leads to gastroesophageal reflux disease (GERD), one of the most commonly seen gastrointestinal complaints in the United States.[2] Symptoms of GERD include heartburn (chest pyrosis); regurgitation; and less commonly chest pain, chronic cough, belching, and bloating. The incidence

[a] Massachusetts General Hospital, 55 Fruit Street, Wang Building, 5th Floor, Boston, MA 02114, USA; [b] Koch Institute at MIT, Cambridge, MA, USA; [c] Harvard Medical School, 55 Fruit Street, Wang Building, 5th Floor, Boston, MA 02114, USA
* Corresponding author. Massachusetts General Hospital, 55 Fruit Street, Wang Building, 5th Floor, Boston, MA 02114, USA.
E-mail address: ASINGH@mgh.harvard.edu

Gastroenterol Clin N Am 52 (2023) 403–415
https://doi.org/10.1016/j.gtc.2023.03.008
0889-8553/23/© 2023 Elsevier Inc. All rights reserved.
gastro.theclinics.com

of GERD increases with increasing body mass index (BMI) even for patients with normal baseline BMI.[3] This is explained by increased intra-abdominal and intragastric pressure altering the pressure gradient between the abdomen and the chest.

Patients should be referred for esophagogastroduodenoscopy to assess for underlying malignancy, strictures, ulcers, and esophagitis if there are red flag symptoms, such as dysphagia, odynophagia, weight loss, bleeding, and iron deficiency anemia (for which colonoscopy should also be considered). In the absence of red flag signs or symptoms, most patients are successfully treated with an empiric trial of a proton pump inhibitor. Proton pump inhibitor therapy effectively reduces the acidity of gastric contents through inhibition of hydrogen-potassium ATPase in parietal cells of the stomach mucosa.[4] Additionally, lifestyle interventions including decreasing caffeine intake, weight loss, smoking cessation, avoiding late evening meals, and elevating the head-of-bed may be effective in decreasing symptoms of GERD.[5] Endoscopic evaluation should also be considered for patients who do not respond to proton pump inhibitor therapy plus lifestyle interventions.

### Barrett Esophagus

Barrett esophagus (BE) occurs when there is a metaplastic change in the epithelial lining of the esophagus with columnar epithelium extending proximal to the gastroesophageal junction. In a small subset of patients, BE can progress to low-grade dysplasia, followed by high-grade dysplasia, and ultimately esophageal cancer. As such, much emphasis has been placed on adequate screening, endoscopic surveillance, and therapy for dysplastic changes. In this review, we limit our scope to risk factors and screening inclusion.

There is significant evidence to suggest risk factors for BE include white race; male sex; smoking; confirmed family history of BE in a first-degree relative; presence of chronic GERD; age greater than 50; and, importantly, obesity and central adiposity.[6] In fact, central obesity is an independent risk factor for BE and is thought to have mechanical effects through increased intragastric pressure causing acid reflux, and metabolic influences resulting from increased circulating proinflammatory cytokines and signaling molecules and insulin resistance.[7] The American College of Gastroenterology guidelines suggest that screening for BE should be considered in men with chronic (>5 years) and/or frequent (weekly or more) symptoms of GERD and two or more risk factors for BE as listed previously.

### Esophageal Adenocarcinoma

Studies have found increased rates of dysplasia and carcinoma diagnoses in patients who have BE and suffer from excess weight or obesity. Similarly, esophageal adenocarcinoma incidence has increased in the United States, United Kingdom, Australia, and Scandinavian countries over 30 to 40 years along with rates of obesity.[8] There are even data to suggest childhood or adolescent obesity may increase risk of developing esophageal adenocarcinoma.[9] Although studies suggest weight loss can improve symptoms of GERD, there is a lack of data to suggest a similar impact on rates of esophageal adenocarcinoma. This may reflect challenges in cohort size and length of follow-up to see impact of weight loss through diet or surgery.[9]

### PANCREATICOBILIARY
#### Biliary

Obesity is associated with gallstone disease, acute pancreatitis, and pancreatic cancer.[10] There is an increased risk of symptomatic cholelithiasis with rising BMI.

This seems to be multifactorial because of a combination of metabolic factors, dyslipidemia, gallbladder stasis, changes in bile composition, and cholesterol crystallization leading to cholesterol-laden gallstones. This process can actually be accelerated by rapid weight loss, however, rates of elective concomitant cholecystectomies during bariatric surgery have decreased in recent years unless patients report symptomatic cholelithiasis.[10] Management is similar to that of patients who do not have obesity.

Classic symptoms including colicky upper abdominal pain associated with meals and concerning laboratory studies, such as elevated liver function tests, should prompt imaging with abdominal ultrasound. If ultrasound is unrevealing and clinical suspicion remains high, tests with higher sensitivity, such as magnetic resonant cholangiopancreatography or endoscopic ultrasound, are considered. Laparoscopic cholecystectomy remains the mainstay of therapy for patients with symptomatic cholelithiasis. For patients not suitable for surgery, undergoing rapid weight loss, or with recurrent choledocholithiasis, ursodeoxycholic acid is considered.

*Pancreas*

Patients with obesity are more likely to develop severe acute pancreatitis.[10] The reasons are multifactorial and include increasing amounts of pancreatic fat as BMI increases, increased systemic inflammation, and higher rates of gallstone disease.

The rates of pancreatic ductal adenocarcinoma are rising globally.[11] Multiple studies have shown an increased risk of developing pancreatic cancer in individuals as BMI rises with risk increasing in a linear fashion. Other studies have demonstrated the importance of fat distribution with central adiposity and high waist-to-hip ratio correlating with increased rates of pancreatic ductal adenocarcinoma mortality.[12] Because of limited sample sizes and follow-up periods, there is no clear or decisive evidence to suggest bariatric surgery decreases risk of pancreatic cancer. That being said, low-fat dietary intervention does seem to reduce the incidence of pancreatic cancer based on a study in postmenopausal women.[12]

# LIVER
## Introduction/Epidemiology

Nonalcoholic fatty liver disease (NAFLD) is currently thought to impact nearly a quarter of all adults globally.[13] NAFLD is diagnosed when hepatic steatosis exceeds 5% of total liver composition by imaging or biopsy in the absence of other causes of steatosis.[14] NAFLD encompasses a spectrum of disease ranging from simple or "bland" steatosis to nonalcoholic steatohepatitis (NASH), which in turn can progress to fibrosis, cirrhosis, and hepatocellular carcinoma. Approximately 20% of all patients with NAFLD go on to develop NASH.

Patients with NAFLD have an increased overall mortality compared with matched populations. The most common cause of death in patients with NAFLD is cardiovascular disease.[15] Recently, there have been calls to rebrand NAFLD as metabolic-associated fatty liver disease to better characterize the disease and acknowledge the systemic underlying metabolic dysfunction frequently seen in patients with fatty liver and steatohepatitis.

## Histology

Histologically, NAFLD is indistinguishable from alcohol-associated liver disease and thus patient history is critical to making the proper diagnosis. NAFLD is comprised mostly of macrovesicular steatosis (large lipid droplets seen in hepatocytes), whereas

NASH includes findings of NAFLD plus inflammation, ballooning hepatocyte degeneration (zone 3 is a diagnostic feature), and Mallory-Denk bodies.[16,17] Patients with ballooning hepatocyte degeneration found on biopsy are more likely to progress to cirrhosis when compared with patients with NASH histologic features without ballooning, even if inflammation is present.[17] Perisinusoidal or pericellular fibrosis begins in the pericentral region, or zone 3, in a classic "chicken wire" pattern and can progress to bridging fibrosis and cirrhosis.[17]

Because the prevalence of NAFLD and NASH has increased and they have become areas of sustained clinical investigation, attempts have been made to standardize the grading and staging of histologic disease. There are now several scoring systems that include inflammation, fibrosis, steatosis, and ballooning injury.[16] Of these, the Brunt, SAF, and NAFLD Activity Score are most likely to be seen on clinical pathology reports.[17] Fibrosis histologic scoring ranges from stage 0 (no fibrosis) to stage 4 (cirrhosis).[18] More recently, much focus has been directed at the noninvasive assessment of liver fibrosis. Characterizing the amount of fibrosis is particularly relevant, because the degree of fibrosis independently predicts liver-related mortality.[15]

The gold standard for NASH diagnosis and assessment of fibrosis remains liver biopsy. Given the invasive nature and lack of widespread availability, it is genearlly encouraged to reserve biopsy for those patients with NAFLD who are believed to be at higher risk of NASH or advanced fibrosis. In addition, for patients with NAFLD who may also have additional or competing causes of liver disease, biopsy may be warranted. Repeat biopsies are not routinely recommended.[15]

### Noninvasive Evaluation

Although liver biopsy remains the gold standard for diagnosis of NAFLD and assessment of steatosis and fibrosis staging, there is risk of sampling error and approximately 1% risk of complication. Noninvasive blood-based testing methods are widely available with high negative predictive value.[19] Many of these have been validated for NAFLD including aspartate aminotransferase to platelet ratio index, Fibrosis-4 score, and NAFLD fibrosis score (**Table 1**); however, each has varying degrees of accuracy and prognostic ability.[19]

Conventional ultrasonography is widely available and can capture moderate-to-severe hepatic steatosis as demonstrated by increased echogenicity.[20,21] Unfortunately, fibrosis and cirrhosis remain challenging to accurately detect via conventional ultrasound (see **Table 1**).

More recent advances have improved the ability to detect hepatic steatosis and fibrosis through the use of vibration-controlled transient elastography (VCTE).[22] VCTE uses ultrasound-based technology through a handheld transducer that generates a low-frequency elastic shear wave that can measure large volumes of liver tissue, thereby avoiding the sampling error that can occur with liver biopsy.[23] Ultrasound-based VCTE and Fibroscan can generate values for controlled attenuated parameter (CAP) (which estimates steatosis) and stiffness (in kPa, which estimates the degree of fibrosis). Although there is less operator/user variation, there are still circumstances where transient elastography cannot be accurately interpreted (eg, severe central adiposity, congestive hepatopathy, viral hepatitis, alcohol consumption). In addition, VCTE is less accurate at identifying mild-to-moderate fibrosis.

Many of the issues that limit accuracy in VCTE do not apply to magnetic resonance elastography. Magnetic resonance elastography may be more accurate in quantifying liver stiffness and degree of steatosis in patients with BMI greater than 35 kg/m$^2$.[19] Given its limited availability and higher cost, however, magnetic resonance elastography has not been widely adopted into current diagnostic algorithms.

**Table 1**
Noninvasive fibrosis assessment

| | Description | |
|---|---|---|
| APRI | AST, platelet | |
| FIB-4 | Age, AST, ALT, platelet | |
| NAFLD fibrosis score | Age, AST, ALT, platelet, BMI, albumin, presence of impaired glucose tolerance | |
| | *Capability* | *Limitations* |
| Ultrasound | Steatosis, findings of portal hypertension or cirrhosis | Likely to miss mild steatosis; BMI and central adiposity may limit accuracy; no ability to quantify fibrosis |
| VCTE | Uses elastic shear waves generated by handheld transducer to measure steatosis (CAP) and fibrosis (kPa) | Expensive; increased fail rate when detecting mild-to-moderate fibrosis; decreased accuracy in the setting of congestive hepatopathy, viral hepatitis, alcohol consumption |
| Magnetic resonance elastography | Higher accuracy for measuring liver stiffness and steatosis, particularly if BMI >35 | Not widely available; expensive |

*Abbreviations:* ALT, alanine aminotransferase; APRI, aspartate aminotransferase to platelet ratio index; AST, aspartate aminotransferase; CAP, controlled attenuated parameter; FIB-4, fibrosis-4 score.

### Hepatocellular Carcinoma

Many of the systemic metabolic features, such as insulin resistance and obesity, that lead to NAFLD/NASH development are also thought to be risk factors for hepatocellular carcinoma.[24] Indeed, NAFLD is the fastest growing cause of hepatocellular carcinoma in the United States and Europe.[15] The presence of obesity, diabetes mellitus, and NAFLD are some of the largest risk factors for development of hepatocellular carcinoma in US cohorts.[25]

### Interventions

#### Lifestyle interventions

Most clinical societies recommend lifestyle interventions with a goal of 5% to 10% reduction in total body weight for the management of NAFLD and NASH.[26] On a more granular level, a 5% reduction of total body weight can improve hepatic steatosis, whereas more aggressive weight loss of at least 7% reduction can result in improved features of NASH, and more than 10% loss may even allow stability or improvement in fibrosis.[27]

To aid in weight loss, a hypocaloric diet (500–1000 kcal/day deficit lower than baseline consumption) is recommended. Numerous clinical trials demonstrate that a Mediterranean diet leads to improvement in intrahepatic lipid content and liver stiffness measurements.[27] Additional dietary changes, such as limiting carbohydrate and fructose intake, can also improve radiographic evidence of steatosis.[28] Currently, there is insufficient evidence to suggest widespread benefit in following specific high-protein/low-carbohydrate diets or intermittent fasting; however, individual patients may benefit from guided dietary recommendations.

Increased physical activity, even in the absence of weight loss, is beneficial. Regular aerobic exercise was found to decrease intrahepatic lipid content and improve radiographic evidence of steatosis, however without a significant change in alanine aminotransferase.[27,29] Individuals with obesity and NAFLD who walked at least 3 hours per week were found to have lower liver-related mortality.[30] Similarly, resistance training, such as weightlifting, also improved hepatic steatosis and markers of insulin resistance and glucose control despite no change in overall body weight or central adiposity.[28,31] In direct comparison, aerobic exercise is preferred with the most consistent impact on hepatic steatosis and improved liver-related mortality.[28,30]

#### Pharmacologic therapies

Although clinical trials for NASH have increased over recent years and novel therapeutic targets continue to be investigated, there remain few beneficial proven treatments.[28] Currently only vitamin E and pioglitazone are recommended for treatment of NASH.[15] Pioglitazone is a peroxisome proliferator-activated receptor-γ agonist and has been used to improve insulin sensitivity and glycemic control in patients with type 2 diabetes mellitus.[32] Treatment improved liver histology in patients with NASH (with or without type 2 diabetes mellitus); however, associated weight gain may make this option less attractive for many patients.[14]

Vitamin E administration is associated with improved aminotransferases and histologic findings of steatosis and steatohepatitis.[28] As such, 800 IU/day of RRR-α-tocopherol (the version of vitamin E with highest bioavailability) is considered for nondiabetic patients with NASH.[15] Importantly, vitamin E is not recommended for patients with diabetes and NASH or individuals with NASH cirrhosis. In addition, a single randomized control trial demonstrated modest increase rate of prostate cancer in patients prescribed 400 IU RRR-α-tocopherol.[15]

More recently, there has been some encouraging results from glucagon-like peptide 1 receptor agonist therapy with liraglutide and semaglutide. Glucagon-like peptide 1

(GLP-1) receptor agonist therapy can lead to significant weight loss and some trials demonstrate improvement or resolution of NASH on biopsy without progression of fibrosis.[33] With a growing number of GLP-1 agonists, there will likely be more therapeutic options available for improving NASH through this mechanism of action. Other targets currently under clinical trial include farnesoid X receptor agonist therapy and additional peroxisome proliferator-activated receptor agonists among others.

### Bariatric interventions

Because of challenges in achieving and maintaining sustained weight loss, bariatric endoscopic and surgical interventions may be recommended. Although data are limited, patients with NASH who underwent endoscopic gastric balloon placement had significant weight loss and improvement in transaminase levels compared with control patients.[28] Whether these benefits are sustained long term after gastric balloon removal remains to be seen.

Bariatric surgery is associated with an improvement in long-term survival and death from cardiovascular disease, which remains the leading cause of death in patients with NAFLD. Although study results vary slightly, a significant number of patients with NASH undergoing bariatric surgery have subsequent improvement in NASH histology on subsequent biopsies.[15] The safety of bariatric surgery needs to be assessed on an individual basis because although vertical sleeve gastrectomy was associated with 0% mortality in patients with cirrhosis, other surgeries were associated with increasing perioperative mortality as underlying liver disease progressed from NASH to decompensated cirrhosis.[15] In general, these recommendations are largely for

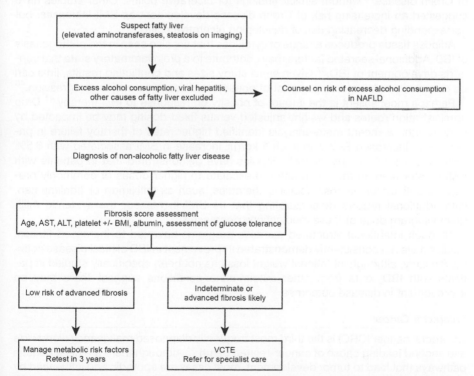

**Fig. 1.** Evaluation flowsheet. ALT, alanine aminotransferase; AST, aspartate aminotransferase. (*Adapted from* Powell et al., 2021; Younossi et al., 2020.)

patients with compensated cirrhosis and evaluation for clinically significant portal hypertension must first be performed because intra-abdominal surgeries can lead to increased mortality in patients with cirrhosis (**Fig. 1**).[34]

## INTESTINE
### Functional Disorders

The small intestine increases capacity to absorb lipid and glucose in obesity. This dietary adaptation may predispose to obesity and development of diabetes.[35] Some population-based studies suggest a relationship between BMI and functional diarrhea, potentially influenced by changes in diet, gut microbiome, and intestinal motility that occur in the setting of obesity and western diets low in fiber, and high in refined carbohydrates and fat.[36] Similarly, there is a strong relationship between BMI and presence of diverticulosis, again perhaps explained by increased methane production because of changes in resident bacterial flora and increased intra-abdominal pressure resulting in increased intraluminal pressure and diverticula formation. In addition to obesity, dietary habits, such as low fiber intake, may also contribute.[36]

### Inflammatory Bowel Disease

Just as the incidence of obesity is increasing globally, so too is the prevalence of inflammatory bowel disease (IBD).[37] The degree to which obesity itself is a risk factor for development of IBD remains unclear and somewhat controversial. Prospective studies have suggested a correlation between adult weight gain and development of Crohn disease[38] without similar findings for ulcerative colitis. Other studies have suggested an increasing risk of Crohn disease development as BMI increases, but corresponding decreasing risk of developing ulcerative colitis.[39]

Adipose tissue produces a range of cytokines that are also seen in the pathogenesis of IBD. Additional secreted factors may contribute to a proinflammatory state that supports development of IBD.[37] Given small study sizes and conflicting results, little can be definitively said regarding impact of obesity on disease severity or progression.[40]

Perhaps most salient is the impact of obesity on response to IBD therapy.[41] Drug administration routes and weight-adjusted versus fixed-dosing may be impacted by body weight. A recent meta-analysis identified higher rates of therapy failure in patients with increased BMI with each 1 kg/m$^2$ increase in BMI associated with 6.5% increased risk of therapy failure.[42] Studies have demonstrated that in patients with BMI greater than 30 there is a need to escalate to higher doses of commonly prescribed anti–tumor necrosis factor-$\alpha$ therapies, such as infliximab or adalimumab, with additional reports demonstrating that as BMI increased, the systemic milligram/kilogram dose of these medications decreased.[40]

Although intentional structured exercise programs have led to increased fitness, studies have not consistently demonstrated improvement in IBD clinical disease activity. Similarly, although intentional weight loss has not been specifically studied in patients with IBD, data from other autoimmune conditions suggest there may be improvement in disease outcomes.[43]

### Colorectal Cancer

Colorectal cancer (CRC) is the third most frequently diagnosed malignancy worldwide and second leading cause of cancer-related death.[44] Although there are clear genetic pathways that lead to tumor development, most cases are sporadic and influenced by environmental and lifestyle factors, such as increased bodyweight, consumption of excess alcohol and processed meat, type 2 diabetes mellitus, and physical inactivity.[45]

Globally, as countries become more industrialized and experience economic transition with adoption of western diet and sedentary lifestyle, there are increasing rates of obesity and CRC.[44] These same factors may also contribute to the rising rates of early onset CRC where a new diagnosis of CRC is made in individuals younger than 50 years of age.[46] In fact, with each 1 kg/m$^2$ increase in BMI, the risk of CRC increases 2% to 3%.[47,48] Importantly, this risk may be mitigated with weight loss.

Although still somewhat controversial, more recent largescale retrospective cohort studies and meta-analyses suggest CRC incidence decreases in patients who undergo bariatric surgery.[49–53] In patients who undergo bariatric surgery, CRC incidence approaches that of the general population, whereas in patients with obesity who do not undergo such interventions, the incidence of CRC remains elevated.[51]

## BARIATRIC INTERVENTIONS INVOLVING THE GASTROINTESTINAL TRACT
### Common Bariatric Surgeries

Bariatric surgery provides consistent sustained weight loss and improvement in comorbid conditions associated with obesity. These procedures include laparoscopic sleeve gastrectomy, Roux-en-Y gastric bypass (RYGB), laparoscopic adjustable gastric banding, and less commonly biliopancreatic diversion with duodenal switch. Most procedures performed today are laparoscopic sleeve gastrectomy and RYGB, with laparoscopic sleeve gastrectomy accounting for nearly two-thirds of all bariatric surgeries.[54] Gastric banding was previously broadly performed because of its short operative time and adjustability; however, complications and limited weight loss because of a lack of the metabolic changes seen in other bariatric procedures, have resulted in it falling out of favor to less than 1% of all bariatric surgeries.[54,55]

### Endoscopic Interventions

Endoscopic bariatric therapies have emerged as potential options for the management of obesity.[56] Current endoscopic interventions include intragastric balloons, gastric aspiration devices, the transpyloric shuttle, endoscopic sleeve gastroplasty, the POSE procedure, TORe, and duodenal resurfacing.[56–58] These techniques, expected outcomes, potential complications, and more are beyond the scope of this article.

### Complications Seen in Clinic

Although routinely counseled to take multivitamin and calcium supplements after bariatric surgery, patients should still undergo regular screening for specific nutritional deficiencies, such as iron, folate, B$_{12}$, calcium, and vitamin D among others.[59] Dysphagia, nausea, vomiting, and abdominal pain should prompt specialist referral because endoscopic evaluation may be warranted to assess for the presence of marginal ulceration at the anastomosis, and stenosis.[60,61] Symptoms of GERD are common after sleeve gastrectomy and gastric banding, whereas the rapid gastric emptying commonly seen in RYGB can improve symptoms of GERD. Reflux symptoms should similarly prompt specialist evaluation to assess for underlying pathology.

Patients who undergo RYGB may experience symptoms of dumping syndrome when consuming high levels of simple carbohydrates, caused by rapid transit of food from the gastric pouch to the small intestine leading to rapid fluid shifts because of high osmolality of the food contents in the lumen.[61] Symptoms vary based on timing with early dumping characterized by abdominal pain, diarrhea, nausea, tachycardia, and possible hypotension soon after ingestion of a meal. Late dumping syndrome occurs a few hours after ingestion and is characterized by fatigue, diaphoresis, and weakness. Both types are largely treated with dietary changes to slow gastric emptying by increasing complex carbohydrates, fiber intake, and protein.[60,61]

## CLINICS CARE POINTS

- Incidence of gastroesophageal reflux disease increases with rising BMI. Although management is largely symptom-based with an emphasis on lifestyle changes, weight loss and use of proton-pump inhibitors, patients with red flag symptoms or who meet criteria for Barrett's esophagus screening should be referred for endoscopic evaluation.

- Non-alcoholic fatty liver disease (NAFLD) comprises a spectrum of disease from simple steatosis to non-alcoholic steatohepatitis (NASH) which can, in turn, progress to fibrosis, cirrhosis and hepatocellular carcinoma. Although liver biopsy remains the gold-standard, non-invasive evaluation is becoming increasingly prevalent, particularly with recent advances in vibration-controlled transient elastography which can estimate both steatosis and fibrosis.

- Weight reduction of 5-10% can improve histologic findings of NAFLD and NASH. Additionally, physical activity – even in the absence of weight loss – can decrease intrahepatic lipid content and lower liver-related mortality. Other interventions include vitamin E and pioglitazone however individual patient characteristics must be taken into consideration. The use of bariatric surgery and anti-obesity medications are increasingly being used for patients with both obesity and NAFLD/NASH.

## REFERENCES

1. Tack J, Pandolfino JE. Pathophysiology of gastroesophageal reflux disease. Gastroenterology 2018;154(2):277–88.
2. Richter JE, Rubenstein JH. Presentation and epidemiology of gastroesophageal reflux disease. Gastroenterology 2018;154(2):267–76.
3. Jacobson BC, Somers SC, Fuchs CS, et al. Body-mass index and symptoms of gastroesophageal reflux in women. N Engl J Med 2006;354(22):2340–8.
4. Maret-Ouda J, Markar SR, Lagergren J. Gastroesophageal reflux disease. JAMA 2020;324(24):2536.
5. Ness-Jensen E, Hveem K, El-Serag H, et al. Lifestyle intervention in gastroesophageal reflux disease. Clin Gastroenterol Hepatol 2016;14(2):175–82.e3. https://doi.org/10.1016/j.cgh.2015.04.176.
6. American Gastroenterological Association Medical Position Statement on the Management of Barrett's Esophagus. Gastroenterology 2011;140(3):1084–91.
7. Chandar AK, Iyer PG. Role of obesity in the pathogenesis and progression of Barrett's esophagus. Gastroenterol Clin N Am 2015;44(2):249–64.
8. El-Serag H. The association between obesity and GERD: a review of the epidemiological Evidence. Dig Dis Sci 2008;53(9):2307–12.
9. Coleman HG, Xie SH, Lagergren J. The epidemiology of esophageal adenocarcinoma. Gastroenterology 2018;154(2):390–405.
10. Cruz-Monserrate Z, Conwell DL, Krishna SG. The impact of obesity on gallstone disease, acute pancreatitis, and pancreatic cancer. Gastroenterol Clin N Am 2016;45(4):625–37.
11. Klein AP. Pancreatic cancer epidemiology: understanding the role of lifestyle and inherited risk factors. Nat Rev Gastroenterol Hepatol 2021;18(7):493–502.
12. Rawla P, Thandra KC, Sunkara T. Pancreatic cancer and obesity: epidemiology, mechanism, and preventive strategies. Clinical Journal of Gastroenterology 2019;12(4):285–91.

13. Lazarus Jv, Mark HE, Anstee QM, et al. Advancing the global public health agenda for NAFLD: a consensus statement. Nat Rev Gastroenterol Hepatol 2022;19(1):60–78.
14. Carr RM, Oranu A, Khungar V. Nonalcoholic fatty liver disease. Gastroenterol Clin N Am 2016;45(4):639–52.
15. Chalasani N, Younossi Z, Lavine JE, et al. The diagnosis and management of nonalcoholic fatty liver disease: practice guidance from the American Association for the Study of Liver Diseases. Hepatology 2018;67(1):328–57.
16. Brown GT, Kleiner DE. Histopathology of nonalcoholic fatty liver disease and nonalcoholic steatohepatitis. Metabolism: Clinical and Experimental 2016;65(8): 1080–6.
17. Kleiner DE, Makhlouf HR. Histology of nonalcoholic fatty liver disease and nonalcoholic steatohepatitis in adults and children. Clin Liver Dis 2016;20(2):293–312.
18. Powell EE, Wong VWS, Rinella M. Non-alcoholic fatty liver disease. Lancet 2021; 397(10290):2212–24.
19. Loomba R, Adams LA. Advances in non-invasive assessment of hepatic fibrosis. Gut 2020;69(7):1343–52.
20. Gerstenmaier JF, Gibson RN. Ultrasound in chronic liver disease. Insights into Imaging 2014;5(4):441–55.
21. Tamaki N, Ajmera V, Loomba R. Non-invasive methods for imaging hepatic steatosis and their clinical importance in NAFLD. Nat Rev Endocrinol 2022;18(1): 55–66.
22. Sandrin L, Fourquet B, Hasquenoph JM, et al. Transient elastography: a new noninvasive method for assessment of hepatic fibrosis. Ultrasound Med Biol 2003;29(12):1705–13.
23. Younossi ZM, Corey KE, Alkhouri N, et al. Clinical assessment for high-risk patients with non-alcoholic fatty liver disease in primary care and diabetology practices. Aliment Pharmacol Ther 2020;52(3):513–26.
24. Huang DQ, El-Serag HB, Loomba R. Global epidemiology of NAFLD-related HCC: trends, predictions, risk factors and prevention. Nat Rev Gastroenterol Hepatol 2021;18(4):223–38.
25. Shah PA, Patil R, Harrison SA. NAFLD-related hepatocellular carcinoma: the growing challenge. Hepatology 2022. https://doi.org/10.1002/HEP.32542.
26. Semmler G, Datz C, Reiberger T, Trauner M. Diet and exercise in NAFLD/NASH: Beyond the obvious. Liver Int 2021;41(10):2249–68.
27. Younossi ZM, Corey KE, Lim JK. AGA clinical practice update on lifestyle modification using diet and exercise to achieve weight loss in the management of nonalcoholic fatty liver disease: expert Review. Gastroenterology 2021;160(3): 912–8.
28. Corey KE, Rinella ME. Medical and surgical treatment options for nonalcoholic steatohepatitis. Dig Dis Sci 2016;61(5):1387–97.
29. Keating SE, Hackett DA, George J, et al. Exercise and non-alcoholic fatty liver disease: a systematic review and meta-analysis. J Hepatol 2012;57(1):157–66.
30. Simon TG, Kim MN, Luo X, et al. Physical activity compared to adiposity and risk of liver-related mortality: results from two prospective, nationwide cohorts. J Hepatol 2020;72:1062–9.
31. Hashida R, Kawaguchi T, Bekki M, et al. Aerobic vs. resistance exercise in nonalcoholic fatty liver disease: a systematic review. J Hepatol 2017;66(1):142–52.
32. Tahrani AA, Barnett AH, Bailey CJ. Pharmacology and therapeutic implications of current drugs for type 2 diabetes mellitus. Nat Rev Endocrinol 2016;12(10): 566–92.

33. Rowe IA, Wong VWS, Loomba R. Treatment candidacy for pharmacologic therapies for NASH. Clin Gastroenterol Hepatol 2022;20(6):1209–17.
34. Patton H, Heimbach J, McCullough A. AGA clinical practice update on bariatric surgery in cirrhosis: expert review. Clin Gastroenterol Hepatol 2021;19(3):436–45.
35. Camilleri M, Malhi H, Acosta A. Gastrointestinal complications of obesity. Gastroenterology 2017;152(7):1656–70.
36. Emerenziani S, Guarino MPL, Asensio LMT, et al. Role of overweight and obesity in gastrointestinal disease. Nutrients 2020;12(1). https://doi.org/10.3390/NU12010111.
37. Khakoo NS, Ioannou S, Khakoo NS, et al. Impact of obesity on inflammatory bowel disease. Curr Gastroenterol Rep 2022;24(1):26–36.
38. Khalili H, Ananthakrishnan AN, Konijeti GG, et al. Measures of obesity and risk of Crohn's disease and ulcerative colitis. Inflamm Bowel Dis 2015;21(2):361–8.
39. Jensen CB, Ängquist LH, Mendall MA, et al. Childhood body mass index and risk of inflammatory bowel disease in adulthood: a population-based cohort study. Am J Gastroenterol 2018;113(5):694–701.
40. Johnson AM, Loftus E v. Impact of obesity on the management of inflammatory bowel disease. Gastroenterol Hepatol 2020;16(7).
41. Singh S, Dulai PS, Zarrinpar A, et al. Obesity in IBD: epidemiology, pathogenesis, disease course and treatment outcomes. Nat Rev Gastroenterol Hepatol 2017;14(2):110–21.
42. Singh S, Facciorusso A, Singh AG, et al. Obesity and response to anti-tumor necrosis factor-α agents in patients with select immune-mediated inflammatory diseases: a systematic review and meta-analysis. PLoS One 2018;13(5). https://doi.org/10.1371/JOURNAL.PONE.0195123.
43. Rozich JJ, Holmer A, Singh S. Effect of lifestyle factors on outcomes in patients with inflammatory bowel diseases. Am J Gastroenterol 2020;115(6):832–40.
44. Keum NN, Giovannucci E. Global burden of colorectal cancer: emerging trends, risk factors and prevention strategies. Nat Rev Gastroenterol Hepatol 2019;16(12):713–32.
45. Dekker E, Tanis PJ, Vleugels JLA, et al. Colorectal cancer. Lancet 2019;394(10207):1467–80.
46. Zaborowski AM, Abdile A, Adamina M, et al. Characteristics of early-onset vs late-onset colorectal cancer. JAMA Surgery 2021;156(9):865.
47. Kuipers EJ, Grady WM, Lieberman D, et al. Colorectal cancer. Nat Rev Dis Prim 2015;1(1):15065.
48. Bardou M, Barkun AN, Martel M. Obesity and colorectal cancer. Gut 2013;62(6):933–47.
49. Almazeedi S, El-Abd R, Al-Khamis A, et al. Role of bariatric surgery in reducing the risk of colorectal cancer: a meta-analysis. Br J Surg 2020;107(4):348–54.
50. Schauer DP, Feigelson HS, Koebnick C, et al. Bariatric surgery and the risk of cancer in a large multisite cohort. Ann Surg 2019;269(1):95–101.
51. Bailly L, Fabre R, Pradier C, et al. Colorectal cancer risk following bariatric surgery in a nationwide study of French individuals with obesity. JAMA Surgery 2020;155(5):395.
52. Rustgi VK, Li Y, Gupta K, et al. Bariatric surgery reduces cancer risk in adults with nonalcoholic fatty liver disease and severe obesity. Gastroenterology 2021;161(1):171–84.e10.
53. Taube M, Peltonen M, Sjöholm K, et al. Long-term incidence of colorectal cancer after bariatric surgery or usual care in the Swedish Obese Subjects study. In: Taheri S, editor. PLoS One 2021;16(3):e0248550.

54. Roth AE, Thornley CJ, Blackstone RP. Outcomes in bariatric and metabolic surgery: an updated 5-year review. Current Obesity Reports 2020;9(3):380–9.

55. Nguyen NT, Varela JE. Bariatric surgery for obesity and metabolic disorders: state of the art. Nat Rev Gastroenterol Hepatol 2017;14(3):160–9.

56. Telese A, Sehgal V, Magee CG, et al. Bariatric and metabolic endoscopy: a new paradigm. Clin Transl Gastroenterol 2021;12(6):e00364.

57. Sullivan S, Edmundowicz SA, Thompson CC. Endoscopic bariatric and metabolic therapies: new and emerging technologies. Gastroenterology 2017;152(7): 1791–801.

58. Abu Dayyeh BK, Edmundowicz S, Thompson CC. Clinical practice update: expert review on endoscopic bariatric therapies. Gastroenterology 2017;152(4): 716–29.

59. Bal BS, Finelli FC, Shope TR, et al. Nutritional deficiencies after bariatric surgery. Nat Rev Endocrinol 2012;8(9):544–56.

60. Schulman AR, Thompson CC. Complications of bariatric surgery: what you can expect to see in your GI practice. Am J Gastroenterol 2017;112(11):1640–55.

61. Concors SJ, Ecker BL, Maduka R, et al. Complications and surveillance after bariatric surgery. Curr Treat Options Neurol 2016;18(1):1–12.

# Weight Stigma and Barriers to Effective Obesity Care

Rebecca M. Puhl, PhD[a,b,*]

## KEYWORDS

- Weight stigma • Attitude • Obesity • Health care • Communication • Barrier
- Stigma reduction

## KEY POINTS

- Health-care providers express weight-based stigma toward patients with obesity, who in turn perceive negative judgements, disrespectful communication, and lack of compassion from health-care providers.
- Weight stigma in health-care encounters is associated with lower patient motivation and adherence, poorer provider–patient communication, reduced quality of care, and health-care avoidance.
- Multifaceted approaches are needed to reduce stigma-related barriers in patient care.

## INTRODUCTION

Weight stigma refers to societal devaluation of people because of their body weight or body size. In North America and many Western societies, individuals with higher weight (eg, obesity) are negatively stereotyped and face prejudice and unfair treatment across many societal settings.[1,2] High rates of obesity have not tempered societal weight bias; in fact, although societal attitudes toward other commonly stigmatized groups have improved over time, there has been little improvement in weight stigma.[3] As many as 40% of adults with obesity report experiencing weight stigma and/or discrimination[4]; prevalence rates increase with body mass index (BMI), and among adults engaged in weight management over half report experiencing weight stigma.[5] At the root of this stigma are beliefs that people with obesity are personally to blame for their weight, lazy, unmotivated, lacking willpower and self-discipline, and noncompliant with treatment.[6,7] A common setting in which weight stigma has been consistently documented is health care.[6,7] Researchers have studied weight stigma in the health-care setting from the perspectives of both providers and

[a] Rudd Center for Food Policy & Health, University of Connecticut, One Constitution Plaza, Suite 600, Hartford, CT 06103, USA; [b] Department of Human Development & Family Sciences, University of Connecticut, Storrs, CT, USA
* Department of Human Development & Family Sciences, University of Connecticut, Storrs, CT.
E-mail address: Rebecca.puhl@uconn.edu

Gastroenterol Clin N Am 52 (2023) 417–428
https://doi.org/10.1016/j.gtc.2023.02.002
0889-8553/23/© 2023 Elsevier Inc. All rights reserved.

patients; this evidence highlights a complex and prevalent problem that is harmful to patient health and creates barriers for effective patient care.

## HEALTH CONSEQUENCES OF WEIGHT STIGMA

Weight stigma incurs a range of negative consequences for health and well-being. When people are negatively stereotyped, shamed, stigmatized, or treated unfairly because of their weight, these experiences increase the risk of both psychological distress and adverse physical health outcomes. Meta-analytic evidence and systematic reviews published in the last 5 years collectively illustrate the deleterious consequences of weight stigma, including depressive symptoms, anxiety, low self-esteem, poor body image, suicidality, substance use, disordered eating behaviors, increased food consumption, unhealthy weight control behaviors, reduced physical activity, increased physiological stress, weight gain, and increased risk of mortality.[8-15] Evidence of the health harms of weight stigma has led to increasing recognition of weight stigma as a public health issue,[16] and underscores the need for health-care professionals to be aware of this problem, help reduce the adverse effects of weight stigma on patient health, and support patients who face this stigma.

## CURRENT EVIDENCE OF WEIGHT STIGMA IN HEALTH CARE
### Provider Attitudes

For several decades, researchers have documented weight-biased attitudes and stereotypes among health-care professionals toward patients with obesity.[6,17] A recent meta-analysis highlights the presence of weight bias expressed by medical professionals across a range of specialty areas, including doctors, primary care physicians, nurses, dietitians, mental health professionals, occupational therapists, and exercise physiologists.[17] Provider attitudes about patients with obesity often mirror weight-based stereotypes documented in the general population (eg, attributions of laziness, low motivation, lack of willpower, individual responsibility), and evidence has found that doctors express implicit and explicit weight bias at similar levels to the general population.[18] Moreover, weight bias is present among medical students early in their training,[19] and even among professionals who specialize in obesity.[20,21] Although most research to date has emerged from the United States, weight-biased attitudes have also been documented among health-care providers in countries such as Canada,[22] Australia,[23] Germany,[24] France,[25] Poland,[26] the United Kingdom,[27] and the Netherlands.[28]

Negative provider attitudes about patients with obesity may be overtly expressed in the health-care setting. A recent survey of medical professionals found that almost of half (48%) had witnessed stigmatizing communication or behaviors by medical staff toward patients with obesity, including offensive comments, making fun of someone's appearance, and facial expressions of disgust or smirks.[26] This aligns with reports of medical trainees' observations that patients with obesity are a target of derogatory humor and negative attitudes by health-care providers (65%) and instructors (40%).[29] Other research has documented associations between higher patient BMI and lower physician respect for the patient.[30]

### Patient Perspectives

Evidence indicates that patients with obesity are aware of biased attitudes from health-care providers. Several studies suggest that adults with obesity view doctors to be one of the most common interpersonal sources of weight stigma in their lives, with approximately one-half to two-thirds reporting that they have been stigmatized about their weight from a doctor.[31–33] For patients, each increase in their BMI category is associated with approximately a 2-fold increased likelihood of perceived stigma in primary care, and a patient's history of weight stigma experiences in health care (but not their BMI) is associated with lower perceptions of physician empathy.[34] Patient reports of weight stigma from providers commonly include perceived negative judgments about their weight, disrespectful and/or insulting comments, and lack of compassion and understanding.[35–37] In line with evidence documenting provider weight biases, research documenting patient perspectives of these health-care experiences is multinational.[31] As 2 recent examples, a 2020 national Polish study of patients with obesity found that more than 80% reported experiencing weight stigma from medical professionals,[38] and a 2022 Israeli health-care study reported that 59% of patients with obesity reported frequent disrespectful experiences from providers, and 58% reported insensitive and insulting comments from providers.[37]

Patient perceptions of weight stigma by medical professionals have been studied across diverse patient care settings, such as primary care, maternity care, and obesity care.[39–41] A 2019 systematic review of qualitative studies examining patient perspectives of clinical encounters about obesity identified consistent themes of weight stigma, including patient reports of health-care providers giving banal weight loss advice, assuming that patients were eating unhealthily and/or not trying to lose weight, attributing patient symptoms to weight without a proper history or examination, and negatively judging patients.[39] A 2020 scoping review of research examining communication practices of health-care professionals with pregnant women who have obesity showed consistent patient perceptions of weight stigma from providers.[40] Collectively, this evidence consistently points to the presence of stigmatizing health-care encounters in the lived experiences of patients with obesity.

## STIGMA-INDUCED BARRIERS TO PATIENT CARE

The presence of weight stigma in the health-care setting has concerning implications for patient care and obesity treatment. Increasing evidence indicates that weight stigma can create barriers to effective care, ranging from poor patient–provider communication and reduced quality of care to poorer patient treatment outcomes and health-care avoidance (**Table 1**).

### Provider Communication and Counseling

Weight stigma may interfere with effective provider–patient communication in several ways. The words that providers use to refer to their patients' weight can be perceived by patients as shaming or stigmatizing. A recent systematic review highlights diverse patient preferences regarding the terminology that providers use to describe their weight but also points to dislike of words such as "fat" or "obese."[42] Thus, the language that providers use to communicate about weight with patients can unintentionally contribute to stigmatizing patient experiences. Beyond language, observational studies have found that physicians demonstrate less emotional rapport (such as empathic statements, reassurance, and partnership) in primary care visits with patients with higher BMI (overweight or obesity) compared with patients with lower weight.[43] Similarly, research in prenatal care suggests that providers engage in less rapport building with women of higher BMI compared with lower BMI.[44] Another study has demonstrated less patient-centered communication from providers in health-care encounters with men who have obesity compared with men with lower weight.[45] Emerging evidence also points to racial disparities in quality of provider communication with patients of higher weight, with Black/African American adults with obesity

| Table 1 | |
| --- | --- |
| **Stigma-induced barriers to patient care and potential remedies** | |
| **Stigma-Induced Barriers to Patient Care** | |
| **Provider Communication and Counseling** | **Patient Care and Outcomes** |
| • Stigmatizing, insensitive, or blaming language<br>• Negative weight-based attitudes and stereotypes<br>• Attributing causes of obesity to personal choices/control<br>• Weight-based terminology that patients dislike<br>• Lack of patient-centered communication<br>• Inadequate rapport building and lack of empathy<br>• Attributing presenting problems to weight without considering other explanations<br>• Emphasis on weight or weight loss as only goal | • Patients feel judged and blamed for their weight<br>• Patients have lower trust in providers<br>• Poorer provider-patient communication<br>• Reduced quality of patient care<br>• Inadequate medical equipment to accommodate patients of diverse body sizes<br>• Poorer patient adherence and treatment outcomes<br>• Increased clinical attrition<br>• Patient avoidance and delay of care |
| **Strategies to Reduce Weight Stigma in Health Care** | |
| • Education about the complex etiology of obesity and body weight regulation<br>• Education about weight bias and its harmful consequences on patient health and wellbeing<br>• Training to increase providers' self-awareness of personal biases about body weight<br>• Training to improve supportive, respectful, and patient-centered communication about weight-related health<br>• Inclusion of weight stigma in medical school curricula and continuing medical education<br>• Implementation of standards to ensure comprehensive teaching on obesity and nutrition in medical school<br>• Implementation of multi-faceted stigma-reduction interventions targeting healthcare providers<br>• Development of methods for certifying knowledge of weight stigma and stigma-free skills and practices<br>• Requirements of sufficient infrastructure for effective obesity care in medical facilities<br>• Efforts to ensure that broader health communication and narratives are free of stigma, bias, and blame | |

less likely than Whites to report that their providers spend enough time with them or explain things well.[46] Within pediatric are, pediatric providers express concerns about compliance in parents who have a child with obesity; parents report being aware of these judgments and in turn report feeling nervous or uncomfortable in provider interactions.[47]

Provider communication influenced by weight stigma can affect the ways that providers counsel patients about their weight-related health. For example, when treating patients with higher weight, providers may be more likely to attribute medical complaints to weight while potentially overlooking other explanations for the patient's presenting problems.[48,49] Recent experimental evidence has documented differential treatment and decision-making of higher-weight patients by health professionals, who have a tendency to focus on the patient's weight even when the patient is not seeking treatment of their weight.[50] In prenatal care, evidence has found that providers engage in less lifestyle counseling with women with high BMI (eg, asking fewer lifestyle questions and offering less lifestyle information) compared with women with lower weight.[44] It may be that provider communication is influenced by their perceptions of normative attitudes about obesity in the health-care setting. For example, among medical students, those who perceived negative attitudes about patients with obesity to be normative in medical school demonstrated poorer patient-centered behaviors and less attentiveness, responsiveness, respectfulness, and interactivity when engaging in a patient care scenario with a standardized patient with obesity.[51] Collectively, this evidence suggests that patient body weight affects the quality of communication between providers and patients.

### Patient Care and Outcomes

Weight stigma can negatively affect patient health outcomes and quality of care.[7] Studies have demonstrated that health-care providers spend less time in appointments with patients who have higher weight compared with lower weight,[52] and express less willingness to treat patients with higher weight.[41] Perceived weight stigma during medical visits is associated with lower patient motivation and compliance,[53] including reduced adherence to medications, cancer screenings, health behavior recommendations, and self-care.[54–57] The relationship between perceived weight stigma and lower patient adherence may be mediated by lower patient trust in providers and less perceived provider empathy.[55] Quality of care can be further compromised by the lack of sufficient medical equipment that is appropriately sized for patients with larger bodies.[37]

Weight-related patient outcomes and care can be affected by weight stigma in health care. In a study of 600 adults with overweight or obesity, 21% thought that their primary care provider had negatively judged them about their weight, and in turn had lower trust in their provider.[36] Further, patients who perceived weight-based judgment from providers were less likely achieve 10% or greater weight loss compared with those who did not perceive judgement from providers about their weight.[58] Among patients with obesity engaged in medical weight loss, emerging evidence indicates that clinical attrition is significantly higher for patients with greater levels of internalized weight bias.[59] Weight stigma may also have negative implications for patients undergoing bariatric surgery.[60,61] For example, perceived weight stigma from health-care providers is associated with less postsurgery dietary adherence among bariatric surgery patients.[54] Qualitative evidence has found that postsurgery patients report receiving little communication or support from their doctors, and that weight stigma is a barrier to seeking needed mental health care following bariatric surgery.[62,63]

### HealthCare Utilization and Avoidance

People are more likely to avoid or delay care if they anticipate experiencing weight stigma in a health-care encounter.[64] Women with obesity who report delaying preventive care attribute barriers of disrespectful treatment in health care, embarrassment of being weighed, negative provider attitudes, unsolicited advice to lose weight, and inadequately sized medical equipment that is too small for their bodies.[65] Decisions to avoid future care may also stem from the language that providers use to talk about patient weight. For example, one study found that approximately 20% of adults would avoid future medical appointments or seek a new doctor if they thought their provider had used stigmatizing language about their weight.[66] Recent evidence from primary care patients suggests that the relationship between patient BMI and delaying needed care or attempting to switch primary care doctors is mediated by stigma experienced in health care and lower patient-centered communication.[67] Patient BMI was also associated with lower perceived respect from providers, which in turn mediated the association between patients' reported health-care experiences and utilization.[67]

Among adults engaged in weight management, recent multinational evidence points to the role of internalized weight bias in health-care avoidance. Across 6 Western countries (Australia, Canada, France, Germany, United Kingdom, and United States), adults with higher internalized weight bias reported more health-care avoidance, as well as a lower frequency of obtaining routine medical checkups, and worse quality of health care; these patterns persisted across all countries after accounting for BMI, demographics, and experiences of weight stigma.[31] Evidence examining potential processes underlying links between weight status and health-care avoidance in women has found that this relationship can be explained by weight stigma (experienced and internalized), body-related shame and guilt, and health-care stress.[68] In particular, body-related shame in women was associated with health-care stress, which in turn contributed to health-care avoidance.[68]

## POTENTIAL REMEDIES TO REDUCE WEIGHT STIGMA IN HEALTH CARE

Societal weight stigma is difficult to change.[3] To date, most stigma reduction interventions targeting medical trainees and health-care professionals have demonstrated pessimistic findings. A 2016 review of published interventions (primarily focused on students training in professional medical and health disciplines) showed little improvements in weight bias.[69] Studies used a variety of stigma-reduction strategies, ranging from educational reading materials, lectures, and films about weight bias and the complex etiology of obesity to self-reflection activities and interactions with patients with obesity. Although some studies reported improvements in participants' knowledge about obesity and its complex etiology, participants' attitudes and levels of bias remained largely unchanged.[69] Methodological limitations of this literature (including small sample sizes, lack of control groups or long-term follow-up) underscore the need for more empirical attention to stigma-reduction strategies.

Some recent research has pointed to several avenues for stigma-reduction in medical students that show potential promise. Several studies have targeted training of medical students with structured educational interventions that involve clinical encounters with standardized patients with higher body weight. In one study, students read articles about communication and stigma before a clinical encounter with a standardized patient with obesity and completed self-reflections both before and afterwards. Findings showed short-term decreases in negative stereotyping, and long-term (1 year) improvements in empathy and confidence in counseling toward patients with obesity.[70] Another study demonstrated that direct faculty observation of medical students during a standardized patient encounter for obesity predicted improvement in students' quality of patient-centered care, using both student self-reported ratings and ratings of independent observers.[71] Most recently, a longitudinal study with 3576 medical students found that having favorable contact with patients with higher weight during medical school training was associated with improved attitudes after 4 years of medical school.[72] Additionally, positive contact experiences with higher -weight patients during medical school partially offset the effects of their negative baseline attitudes.[72]

Nevertheless, this research literature remains scattered, and the absence of definitive approaches that can effectively reduce weight stigma in health care reiterates the importance of increased studies in this area. Efforts should prioritize testing multifaceted approaches and strategies to address this complex problem, including efforts to increase self-awareness and empathy, understanding the complex causes of obesity, respectful communication, role modeling from influential peers or leaders, and sensitivity training. It will be important for these efforts to target both continuing education for established providers engaged in clinical practice and education and training of medical students. Recent evidence indicates that current United States medical schools are not adequately training medical students in obesity management or prioritizing obesity in medical education curriculum.[73] Given that education on weight stigma is much more likely to appear in obesity-related curriculum than other content areas, these findings highlight the importance of improving medical school curriculum on obesity and weight stigma.

Optimistically, there has been growing recognition and calls for efforts to address weight stigma by and within the medical community. In 2020, an international consensus statement supported by 100+ medical and scientific organizations worldwide called for the elimination of weight stigma, including prioritizing efforts to address weight stigma in the medical community.[74] Recommendations included implementing standards to ensure comprehensive teaching about obesity into standard medical school curricula; developing methods for certifying knowledge of weight stigma, its harmful effects, and stigma-free skills and practices; and requiring appropriate infrastructure for effective obesity care in medical facilities. The statement also called for broad efforts to ensure that societal messages and narratives of obesity are free from stigma.[74] Similarly, a joint consensus statement of medical professionals from the United Kingdom emphasized the importance of addressing language in efforts to reduce weight stigma in health care, calling for initiatives that increase awareness and usage of appropriate, nonstigmatizing language to promote supportive and collaborative provider–patient communication.[75] These statements have emerged alongside recent calls to action that evidence-based, patient-centered, compassionate care be accessible to all individuals seeking treatment of obesity, and that health professionals respect patient decisions about their body weight regardless of whether or not weight loss is an intended goal.[76] It will be critical to include people affected by obesity in these efforts, whose knowledge, experiences, and perspectives can inform and guide stigma-reduction initiatives and strategies to remove bias-related barriers to care. Research examining stigma-reduction priorities according to perspectives of women with obesity suggests that efforts should go farther than education about weight stigma and sensitivity training for health-care providers and medical students to also ensure that intervention and treatment programs provide services that support patients and help them cope with weight stigma and its harmful effects on their lives.[77]

## SUMMARY

Weight stigma is prevalent and has negative consequences for health and well-being. This problem is present in health care, with stigmatizing attitudes toward patients with obesity expressed by medical professionals across diverse specialties and patient care settings. Weight stigma creates barriers to effective care, including poor patient–provider communication, reduced quality of care, and health-care avoidance. Although stigma reduction interventions in health care have demonstrated pessimistic findings, there have been increasing international calls for actions to address weight stigma in the medical community. Multifaceted approaches to reduce weight stigma will be necessary and should include self-awareness and empathy, respectful communication, role modeling, sensitivity training, and knowledge of obesity etiology. Engaging people with obesity in stigma reduction efforts is critical to ensure that their experiences and perspectives inform strategies to effectively remove bias-related barriers to patient care.

## CLINICS CARE POINTS

- Recognize that weight stigma is prevalent and contributes to increased psychological distress and poor physical health for individuals with high body weight.

- Acknowledge the complex etiology of obesity and avoid attributing patients' body weight to personal choices or individual responsibility.

- Increase self-awareness of weight-based assumptions and stereotypes, and look for examples that challenge these stereotypes.

- Use patient-centered approaches like motivational interviewing to support patients in making healthy behavior changes, and engage them colloboritvely in determining goals and addressing barriers.

- Take steps to eliminate weight stigma in provider-patient interactions through increased rapport-building, supportive counseling, and patient-centered communication.

- Acknowledge that patients' previous experiences of stigma with providers may lead patients to anticipate weight stigma in health care and delay or avoid care.

- When communicating with patients about weight-related health, use respectful and sensitive language. Ask patients for their preferred term(s) to describe their weight and use their preferred terms in your communication.

- Pratice compassionate care with patients of all body sizes, and respect patient decisions about their body weight regardless of whether or not weight loss is an intended goal.

- Create a welcoming and non-stigmatizing clinic environment for patients of diverse body sizes; ensure that medical equipment, scales, patient gowns, and seating options can accommodate patients with larger body sizes.

## DISCLOSURE

R.M. Puhl has received research grants from WW and served as a consultant for Eli Lilly and Company, outside of the submitted work.

## REFERENCES

1. Pearl RL. Weight bias and stigma: Public health implications and structural solutions. Soc Issues Policy Rev 2018;12:146–82.
2. Brewis AA, Wutich A, Falletta-Cowden A, et al. Body norms and fat stigma in a global perspective. Curr Anthropol 2011;52:269–76.
3. Charlesworth TES, Banaji MR. Patterns of implicit and explicit attitudes: Long term change and stability from 2007 to 2016. Psychol Sci 2019;30:174–92.
4. Spahlholz J, Baer N, König HH, et al. Obesity and discrimination - a systematic review and meta-analysis of observational studies. Obes Rev 2016;17:43–55.
5. Puhl RM, Lessard LM, Pearl RL, et al. International comparisons of weight stigma: addressing a void in the field. Int J Obes 2021;45:1976–85.
6. Puhl RM, Heuer CA. The stigma of obesity: a review and update. Obesity 2009; 17:941–64.
7. Phelan SM, Burgess DJ, Yeazel MW, et al. Impact of weight bias and stigma on quality of care and outcomes for patients with obesity. Obes Rev 2015;16: 319–26.
8. Bidstrup H, Brennan L, Kaufmann L, et al. Internalised weight stigma as a mediator of the relationship between experienced/perceived weight stigma and biopsychosocial outcomes: a systematic review. Int J Obes 2022;46:1–9.

9. Emmer C, Bosnjak M, Mata J. The association between weight stigma and mental health: a meta-analysis. Obes Rev 2020;21:e12935.

10. Alimoradi Z, Golboni F, Griffiths MD, et al. Weight-related stigma and psychological distress: a systematic review and meta-analysis. Clin Nutr 2020;39:2001–13.

11. Wu YK, Berry DC. Impact of weight stigma on physiological and psychological health outcomes for overweight and obese adults: a systematic review. J Adv Nurs 2018;74:1030–42.

12. Pearl RL, Puhl RM. Weight bias internalization and health: a systematic review. Obes Rev 2018;19:1141–63.

13. Warnick JL, Darling KE, West CE, et al. Weight stigma and mental health in youth: a systematic review and meta-analysis. J Pediatr Psychol 2022;47:237–55.

14. Zhu X, Smith RA, Buteau E. A meta-analysis of weight stigma and health behaviors. Stigma and Health 2022;7:1–13.

15. Pearl RL, Wadden TA, Jakicic JM. Is weight stigma associated with physical activity? A systematic review. Obesity 2021;29:1994–2012.

16. Brewis A, SturtzSreetharan C, Wutich A. Obesity stigma is a globalizing health challenge. Glob Health 2018;14:20.

17. Lawrence BJ, Kerr D, Pollard CM, et al. Weight bias among health care professionals: a systematic review and meta-analysis. Obesity 2021;29:1802–12.

18. Sabin JA, Marini M, Nosek BA. Implicit and explicit anti-fat bias among a large sample of medical doctors by BMI, race/ethnicity and gender. PLoS One 2012;7:e48448.

19. Phelan SM, Dovidio JF, Puhl RM, et al. Implicit and explicit weight bias in a national sample of 4,732 medical students: the medical student CHANGES study. Obesity 2014;22:1201–8.

20. Tomiyama JA, Finch LE, Incollingo Belsky AC, et al. Weight bias in 2001 versus 2013: contradictory attitudes among obesity researchers and health professionals. Obesity 2015;23:46–53.

21. Jungnickel T, von Jan U, Engeli S, et al. Exploring the weight bias of professionals working in the field of obesity with a mobile IAT: a pilot study. Ther Adv Endocrinol Metab 2022;13. https://doi.org/10.1177/20420188221098881.

22. Alberga AS, Nutter S, MacInnis C, et al. Examining weight bias among practicing Canadian family physicians. Obes Facts 2019;12:632–8.

23. Setchell J, Watson B, Jones L, et al. Physiotherapists demonstrate weight stigma: a cross sectional survey of Australian physiotherapists. J Physiother 2014;60:157–62.

24. Sikorski C, Luppa M, Glaesmer H, et al. Attitudes of health care professionals towards female obese patients. Obes Facts 2013;6:512–22.

25. Bocquier A, Verger P, Basdevant A, et al. Overweight and obesity: knowledge, attitudes, and practices of general practitioners in France. Obes Res 2005;13:787–95.

26. Sobczak K, Leoniuk K. Attitudes of medical professionals towards discrimination of patients with obesity. Risk Manag Healthc Policy 2021;14:4169–75.

27. Swift JA, Hanlon S, El-Redy L, et al. Weight bias among UK trainee dietitians, doctors, nurses and nutritionists. J Hum Nutr Diet 2013;26:395–402.

28. van der Voorn B, Camfferman R, Seidell J.C, et al. Weight-biased attitudes about pediatric patients with obesity in Dutch healthcare professionals from seven different professions, J Child Health Care, 2023,13674935221133953. doi: 10.1177/13674935221133953.

29. Puhl RM, Luedicke J, Grilo CM. Obesity bias in training: attitudes, beliefs, and observations among advanced trainees in professional health disciplines. Obesity 2014;22:1008–15.

30. Huizinga MM, Cooper LA, Bleich SN, et al. Physician respect for patients with obesity. J Gen Intern Med 2009;24:1236–9.

31. Puhl RM, Lessard LM, Himmelstein MS, et al. The roles of experienced and internalized weight stigma in healthcare experiences: Perspectives of adults engaged in weight management across six countries. PLoS One 2021;16:e0251566.

32. Puhl RM, Brownell KD. Confronting and coping with weight stigma: an investigation of overweight and obese adults. Obesity 2006;14:1802–15.

33. Puhl RM, Himmelstein MS, Pearl RL, et al. Weight stigma among sexual minority adults: Findings from a matched sample of adults engaged in weight management. Obesity 2019;27:1906–15.

34. Ferrante JM, Seaman K, Bator A, et al. Impact of perceived weight stigma among underserved women on doctor-patient relationships. Obes Sci Pract 2016;2: 128–35.

35. Farrell E, Hollmann E, le Roux CW, et al. The lived experience of patients with obesity: a systematic review and qualitative synthesis. Obes Rev 2021;22: e13334.

36. Gudzune KA, Bennett WL, Cooper LA, et al. Patients who feel judged about their weight have lower trust in their primary care providers. Patient Educ Couns 2014; 97:128–31.

37. Sagi-Dain L, Echar M, Paska-Davis N. Experiences of weight stigmatization in the Israeli healthcare system among overweight and obese individuals. Isr J Health Policy Res 2022;11:5.

38. Sobczak K, Leoniuk K, Rudnik A. Experience of Polish patients with obesity in contacts with medical professionals. Patient Prefer Adherence 2020;14:1683–8.

39. Ananthakumar T, Jones NR, Hinton L, et al. Clinical encounters about obesity: systematic review of patients' perspectives. Clin Obes 2020;10:e12347.

40. Dieterich R, Demirci J. Communication practices of healthcare professionals when caring for overweight/obese pregnant women: a scoping review. Patient Educ Couns 2020;103:1902–12.

41. Mulherin K, Miller YD, Barlow FK, et al. Weight stigma in maternity care: women's experiences and care providers' attitudes. BMC Pregnancy Childbirth 2013; 13:19.

42. Puhl RM. What words should we use to talk about weight? A systematic review of quantitative and qualitative studies examining preferences for weight-related terminology. Obes Rev 2020;21:e13008.

43. Gudzune KA, Beach MC, Roter DL, et al. Physicians build less rapport with obese patients. Obesity 2013;21:2146–52.

44. Washington Cole KO, Gudzune KA, Bleich SN, et al. Providing prenatal care to pregnant women with overweight or obesity: Differences in provider communication and ratings of the patient-provider relationship by patient body weight. Patient Educ Couns 2017;100:1103–10.

45. Phelan SM, Lynch BA, Blake KD, et al. The impact of obesity on perceived patient-centred communication. Obes Sci Pract 2018;4:338–46.

46. Wong MS, Gudzune KA, Bleich SN. Provider communication quality: influence of patients' weight and race. Patient Educ Couns 2015;98:492–8.

47. Halvorson EE, Curley T, Wright M, et al. Weight bias in pediatric inpatient care. Acad Pediatr 2019;19:780–6.

48. Oestbye T, Taylor D, Yancy W, et al. Associations between obesity and receipt of screening mammography, Papanicolaou tests, and influenza vaccination: Results from the Health and Retirement Study (HRS) and the asset and health dynamics among the oldest old (AHEAD) study. Am J Public Health 2005;95:1623–30.

49. Mitchell RS, Padwal RS, Chuck AW, et al. Cancer screening among the over-weight and obese in Canada. Am J Prev Med 2008;35:127–32.

50. Rathbone JA, Cruwys T, Jetten J, et al. When stigma is the norm: How weight and social norms influence the healthcare we receive. J Appl Soc Psychol 2020. https://doi.org/10.1111/jasp.12689.

51. Phelan SM, Puhl RM, Burgess DJ, et al. The role of weight bias and role-modeling in medical students' patient-centered communication with higher weight stan-dardized patients. Patient Educ Couns 2021;104:1962–9.

52. Hebl MR, Xu J. Weighing the care: physicians' reactions to the size of a patient. Int J Obes Relat Metab Disord 2001;25:1246–52.

53. Hayward LE, Neang S, Ma S, et al. Discussing weight with patients with over-weight: supportive (not stigmatizing) conversations increase compliance inten-tions and health motivation. Stigma and Health 2020;5:53–68.

54. Raves DM, Brewis A, Trainer S, et al. Bariatric surgery patients' perceptions of weight-related stigma in healthcare settings impair postsurgery dietary adher-ence. Front Psychol 2016;7:1497.

55. Snyder M, Haskard-Zolnierek K, Howard K, et al. Weight stigma is associated with provider-patient relationship factors and adherence for individuals with hypo-thyroidism. J Health Psychol 2022;27:702–12.

56. Potter L, Wallston K, Trief P, et al. Attributing discrimination to weight: associations with well-being, self-care, and disease status in patients with type 2 diabetes mel-litus. J Behav Med 2015;38:863–75.

57. Maruthur NM, Bolen SD, Brancati FL, et al. The association of obesity and cervi-cal cancer screening: a systematic review and meta-analysis. Obesity 2009;17: 375–81.

58. Gudzune KA, Bennett WL, Cooper LA, et al. Perceived judgment about weight can negatively influence weight loss: a cross-sectional study of overweight and obese patients. Prev Med 2014;62:103–7.

59. Verhaak AMS, Ferrand J, Puhl RM, et al. Experienced weight stigma, internalized weight bias, and clinical attrition in a medical weight loss patient sample. Int J Obes 2022;46:1241–3.

60. Phelan SM. An update on research examining the implications of stigma for ac-cess to and utilization of bariatric surgery. Curr Opin Endocrinol Diabetes Obes 2018;25:321–5.

61. Sarwer DB, Gasoyan H, Bauerle Bass S, et al. Role of weight bias and patient-physician communication in the underutilization of bariatric surgery. Surg Obes Relat Dis 2021;17:1926–32.

62. Jumbe S, Meyrick J. Contrasting views of the postbariatric surgery experience between patients and their practitioners: a qualitative study. Obes Surg 2018; 28:2447–56.

63. Sharman M, Hensher M, Wilkinson S, et al. What are the support experiences and needs of patients who have received bariatric surgery? Health Expect 2017;20: 35–46.

64. Drury CA, Louis M. Exploring the association between body weight, stigma of obesity, and healthcare avoidance. J Am Acad Nurse Pract 2002;14:554–61.

65. Amy NK, Aalborg A, Lyons P, et al. Barriers to routine gynecological cancer screening for White and African-American obese women. Int J Obes 2006;30: 147–55.
66. Puhl R, Peterson JL, Luedicke J. Motivating or stigmatizing? Public perceptions of weight-related language used by health providers. Int J Obes 2013;37:612–9.
67. Phelan SM, Bauer KW, Bradley D, et al. A model of weight-based stigma in health care and utilization outcomes: Evidence from the learning health systems network. Obes Sci Pract 2021;8:139–46.
68. Mensinger JL, Tylka TL, Calamari ME. Mechanisms underlying weight status and healthcare avoidance in women: a study of weight stigma, body-related shame and guilt, and healthcare stress. Body Image 2018;25:139–47.
69. Alberga AS, Pickering BJ, Alix Hayden K, et al. Weight bias reduction in health professionals: a systematic review. Clin Obes 2016;6:175–88.
70. Kushner RF, Zeiss DM, Feinglass JM, et al. An obesity educational intervention for medical students addressing weight bias and communication skills using standardized patients. BMC Med Educ 2014;14:53.
71. Miller N, Angstman KB, van Ryn M, et al. The association of direct observation of medical students with patient-centered care for obesity. Fam Med 2020;52: 271–7.
72. Meadows A, Higgs S, Burke SE, et al. Social dominance orientation, dispositional empathy, and need for cognitive closure moderate the impact of empathy-skills training, but not patient contact, on medical students' negative attitudes toward higher-weight patients. Front Psychol 2017;8:1–15.
73. Butsch WS, Kushner RF, Alford S, et al. Low priority of obesity education leads to lack of medical students' preparedness to effectively treat patients with obesity: results from the U.S. medical school obesity education curriculum benchmark study. BMC Med Educ 2020;20:23.
74. Rubino F, Puhl RM, Cummings DE, et al. Joint international consensus statement for ending stigma of obesity. Nat Med 2020;26:485–97.
75. Albury C, Strain WD, Brocq SL, et al, Language Matters working group. The importance of language in engagement between health-care professionals and people living with obesity: a joint consensus statement. Lancet Diabetes Endocrinol 2020;8:447–55.
76. Cardel MI, Newsome FA, Pearl RL, et al. Patient-centered care for obesity: How health care providers can treat obesity while actively addressing weight stigma and eating disorder risk. J Acad Nutr Diet 2022;122:1089–98.
77. Puhl RM, Himmelstein MS, Gorin AA, et al. Missing the target: including perspectives of women with overweight and obesity to inform stigma-reduction strategies. Obes Sci Pract 2017;3:25–35.

# Disparities in Access and Quality of Obesity Care

Tiffani Bell Washington, MD, MPH[a],*, Veronica R. Johnson, MD[b],
Karla Kendrick, MD, MPH[c], Awab Ali Ibrahim, MD[d], Lucy Tu[e,f], Kristen Sun, BA[g],
Fatima Cody Stanford, MD, MPH, MBA, MPA[h]

## KEYWORDS

- Disparities • Access to care • Quality obesity care • Health equity • Stigma

## KEY POINTS

- We should provide adequate access to obesity care to all those affected by the disease.
- There is a need for improved obesity health policies and precision medicine to treat obesity.
- Education about obesity, including management, weight stigma, and disparities in care, should be included in the education and training of all health care professionals.
- Every patient with obesity should be offered all appropriate treatment options regardless of age, race/ethnicity, or socioeconomic status.

## INTRODUCTION

Obesity is a chronic disease and a significant public health threat predicated on complex genetic, psychological, and environmental factors. Although a chronic disease, obesity also exacerbates pre-existing conditions and may engender new ones. Obesity is associated with high mortality rates. These high mortality rates are often secondary to comorbidities such as diabetes, hypercholesterolemia, certain cancers,

Funding: National Institutes of Health NIDDK P30 DK040561 and L30 DK118710 (F.C. Stanford).
[a] Harvard T.H. Chan School of Public Health, 677 Huntington Avenue, Boston, MA 02115, USA;
[b] Department of Medicine, Division of General Internal Medicine and Geriatrics, Northwestern University Feinberg School of Medicine, Chicago, IL, USA; [c] Beth Israel Deaconess Medical Center, Harvard Medical School, Boston, MA 02115, USA; [d] Pediatric Gastroenterology, Massachusetts General Hospital and Harvard Medical School, 55 Fruit Street, Boston, MA 02114, USA; [e] Department of Sociology, Harvard College, 33 Kirkland Street, Cambridge, MA 02138, USA; [f] Department of Molecular and Cellular Biology, Harvard College, 33 Kirkland Street, Cambridge, MA 02138, USA; [g] Boston University School of Medicine, Boston, MA 02215, USA; [h] Department of Medicine- Neuroendocrine Unit, Pediatric Endocrinology, MGH Weight Center, Nutrition Obesity Research Center at Harvard, Massachusetts General Hospital, Harvard Medical School, 50 Staniford Street, Suite 430, Boston, MA 02114, USA
* Corresponding author. 3600 South College Road, Suite E, #151 Wilmington, NC 28409.
E-mail address: TiffaniBell@hsph.harvard.edu

Gastroenterol Clin N Am 52 (2023) 429–441
https://doi.org/10.1016/j.gtc.2023.02.003
0889-8553/23/© 2023 Elsevier Inc. All rights reserved.

gastro.theclinics.com

and cardiovascular disease.[1] Obesity interventions from lifestyle modifications to pharmacotherapy and metabolic and bariatric surgery have significant downstream benefits. Disparities in access and quality of obesity care worsen health inequities for vulnerable populations.

A body mass index (BMI) ≥ 30 characterizes obesity in adults, whereas a BMI ≥ 40 characterizes severe obesity. Yet, BMI is an indirect measure of adiposity, and there is variation in BMI among various ethnic groups.[2–5] Obesity is highly prevalent, with 42.4% of the US adult population with obesity and 9.2% with severe obesity. Disparities in obesity rates are significant across racial and ethnic groups, with the lowest rates of obesity in non-Hispanic Asian adults (17.5%) and highest among non-Hispanic Black (49.6%) and Hispanic (44.8%) adults, whereas non-Hispanic White adults have rates of 42.2%.[6] Individuals' socioeconomic environments impact disparities, and they are worse in areas with more negative social sentiments (ie, racism) that increase stress.[7] Obesogenic food environments are disproportionately present in areas with a larger population of racial/ethnic minorities.[8,9]

There is a tremendous stigma associated with obesity, as many believe it to be a consequence of personal behavioral choices despite its complex etiology.[10] Overwhelming data support genetic and environmental causes, but many blame individuals with obesity for their weight status.[11] Weight stigma impacts many areas of life for people living with obesity, including the quality of health care they receive. Many physicians have negative or stereotypical beliefs about patients with obesity and primarily attribute obesity to individual behaviors.[12–14] These stereotypes negatively affect the quality-of-care patients with higher BMI receive, such as a delay in prescribing recommended medications due to a higher prevalence of physician-assumed nonadherence.[15]

Individuals with higher BMI are also more likely to avoid health care due to weight stigma. Insurance policies encourage physicians to measure a patient's weight at each visit. Health guidelines require recommendations for weight loss for patients with higher BMI regardless of their visit.[16] Such policies and practices lead to worse health outcomes in non-obesity-related and obesity-related conditions.

Disparities in obesity care disproportionately impact racial and ethnic minorities and, most powerfully, Black individuals with obesity. One study showed that research conducted on predominantly White women failed to consider other groups' racialized and gendered experiences. This lack of inclusion resulted in less recruitment to weight loss programs and less weight loss through behavioral weight interventions (BWIs) for racial/ethnic minority groups than White patients.[17]

Obesity-related conditions such as hypertension and pancreatic cancer and treatments for obesity-related diseases such as sleep apnea disproportionately affect racial/ethnic minorities.[18–20] Even restrictions for treatments based on BMI (such as total knee and hip arthroplasties), which limit access to care by patients with obesity, disproportionately restrict care for racial and ethnic minorities regardless of BMI.[21] These disparities are most significant for Black Americans. Studies have found that while Black women have the highest rates of obesity, Black men have the highest mortality rates from obesity-related illnesses.[17] Such disparities highlight the need to address the existing inequities in access and quality of obesity care.

## BACKGROUND

Current evidence-based treatment options for obesity include focusing on medication and lifestyle changes.[22] For instance, nutrition-based interventions include limiting the intake of processed foods with high sugar and fat content.[23,24] Regular physical activity is another common intervention that decreases sedentary behavior.[25] Interventions such as obesity pharmacotherapy or metabolic and bariatric surgery (MBS) may be necessary for successful, long-term outcomes.[22,26]

Health disparities are preventable differences in disease burden or opportunities to achieve optimal health that socially disadvantaged populations experience.[27,28] For example, residents of low-income neighborhoods disproportionately encounter food deserts, areas where affordable, nutritious food options are scarce.[29,30]

An analysis of the National Health and Nutrition Examination (NHANES) survey from 1999 to 2016 demonstrates that Black and Hispanic children and adolescents had the highest prevalence of obesity for all years between 1999 and 2016. In the most recent survey year, the prevalence of class I obesity (mild obesity) was most significant for Black women at 25.1% compared with 13.6% for White women.[22,31,32] Altogether, these findings indicate lifetime racial disparities in obesity prevalence, apparent in early childhood and progressing through adulthood.

In addition to this unequal disease burden, access to obesity treatment varies significantly. Lifestyle intervention programs are more successful with a higher frequency of visits. Still, many treatment facilities fail to account for discrepancies in transportation access, food insecurity, and temporal restrictions (eg, the constraints of a full-time work schedule), which complicate patient adherence.[33] Thus, even if these treatment options are theoretically productive, they may be more difficult for low-income families and racial and ethnic minorities to implement in practice. Indeed, Black and Hispanic Americans lose less weight than White patients in behavioral lifestyle intervention treatments.[28]

Anti-obesity medication (AOM) is also significantly underutilized. For instance, Claridy and colleagues found the mentioned rate for anti-obesity drugs remains at 1% despite recommendations from the American Medical Association and the Endocrine Society to use AOM for long-term weight reduction.[34] This finding may be a consequence of the inadequate coverage for AOM through federal health insurance programs, which disproportionately inhibits low-income patients from pharmacotherapy access.[35] Furthermore, Black Americans are less likely than White Americans to have considered surgical interventions.[36] Often, Black Americans are less likely to be diagnosed with obesity, and therefore, less likely to be referred to metabolic and bariatric surgery centers.[28] Among adolescents with severe obesity, bariatric surgery is most often performed on White patients; moreover, while Medicaid insurance increases the use of MBS for White adolescent patients, it paradoxically decreases the use of MBS among non-White patients.[37]

The geographic distribution of obesity medicine specialists also contributes to disparate access to care. To visit a certified obesity medicine physician, the median travel time for patients in high-income counties is 9 minutes; concurrently, patients in low-income or rural counties face a median travel time of 43 minutes.[38,39] Certain patients, including low-income families and racial and ethnic minorities, are thus more likely to be treated by a physician who does not have specialized training in obesity medicine.

The outcomes of undertreatment are significant. Disparities in obesity foreshadow integral inequality in health outcomes, including disability, the standard of living, and premature mortality.[23,40] Indeed, Black and Hispanic adults with obesity have higher odds of developing obesity-related diseases, including high blood pressure, heart attack, and stroke.[24,41] Thus, obesity has a correspondingly high economic burden. In the United States, the mean annual per capita health care cost of obesity is $1160 for men and $1650 for women, with an estimated total cost of $260 billion.[25,42]

To address the obesity epidemic and prevent increasing disparity, more investigations and interventions that address access to treatment are crucial.

### Factors Contributing to Disparities in Access and Quality of Obesity Care

Stigma and discrimination toward people with obesity cause multiple harmful effects on their physical and psychological health.[43] Many often blame persons with obesity for their weight.[43–45] Some of the common harmful ideologies associated with obesity include laziness, unattractiveness, and a lack of willpower.[43–45] Such negative connotations result in lifelong discrimination in various aspects of life, including workspace, schools, and health care.[22] Self-stigma is an often overlooked factor that has substantial adverse effects on persons with obesity.[46,47] Holding negative beliefs about oneself because of weight can lead to poor quality of life, worse health outcomes (independent of obesity-related causes), and poor mental health.[48–51]

A complex relationship between obesity and socioeconomic factors creates barriers to obesity prevention and care. Low-income and minority families face additional barriers contributing to increased obesity rates, including racism, chronic stress, and even the affordability of quality food such as vegetables, fruits, and lean meats.[52–55] Low-income families might find it more challenging to dedicate time and resources to healthy meal preparation.[53,56]

The struggle for quality obesity care continues even after diagnosis. Obesity care comprises lifestyle modifications, pharmacologic therapy, and weight loss surgery.[28] Unfortunately, minority communities face significant barriers in access to many of these measures.[28,54] Unfortunately, non-Hispanic African Americans and Hispanics are more likely to face food insecurity, making it much harder to adhere to a specific diet. Increased food insecurity rates may play a role in findings that minorities lose less weight than White patients in lifestyle intervention treatments.[57]

Black patients are less likely to be diagnosed with obesity than non-Hispanic White patients. This underdiagnosis could decrease referrals to weight loss centers where weight loss medications are generally prescribed.[28] Weight loss surgery remains the most effective treatment of moderate to severe obesity. Despite this, racial and ethnic minorities have limited access to bariatric surgery.[28,37] Many believe that limited access to MBS is due to a combination of factors, including the higher likelihood of being insured by Medicare/Medicaid insurance. Medicare/Medicaid covers many minorities. Their reimbursement policies are often unfavorable for those with obesity; moreover, many of these centers are not located in areas where minorities receive their health care.[58]

Despite the common misbelief that people with obesity are primarily responsible for their weight gain, many systemic factors such as racism, stigma, and policy likely play a significant role in our obesity epidemic. Efforts to address systemic factors are critical, and these measures should target preventing and treating obesity.

## DISPARITIES IN ACCESS AND QUALITY OF OBESITY CARE: AMELIORATING FACTORS

Targeted, evidence-based strategies are needed to address obesity prevalence and obesity-specific care disparities. As certain groups, such as racial and ethnic minorities and those of lower socioeconomic status, have a higher prevalence of obesity, interventions need to address the unique challenges experienced by these populations. Lifestyle and behavioral therapy are the first lines in the treatment of obesity. Pharmacotherapy and bariatric surgery are also cornerstones of obesity treatment, with medical devices becoming more commonly used. Access to and utilization of these therapies is crucial to reducing obesity-related care disparities.

Lifestyle interventions, including promoting healthy food choices, increased physical activity, and decreased sedentary time, are more effective when incorporating behavioral strategies, such as goal setting, self-monitoring, and cognitive restricting.[59] Frequent contact or visits with trained coaches or health care providers also increases effectiveness.[33] Historically, lifestyle and behavioral interventions tailored to address social or community factors of diverse populations have had mixed results.[60,61] However, more recently, there has been more success in reaching underserved populations. High-intensity lifestyle interventions targeted at those with low socioeconomic status (SES) and racial and ethnic minorities have shown sustained success ($\geq 5\%$ weight loss at 24 months) with content tailored to the health literacy of the individual.[62] A lifestyle behavioral intervention that utilizes a personalized range, delivered through a mobile, digital platform, has also shown success ($\geq 5\%$ weight loss at 12 months) in low-income and racial and ethnic minority populations.[63] In the latter study, high engagement with digital content was cited as a positive factor in weight loss, likely due to reduced barriers to accessing content given the use of a mobile application. Combining a lifestyle intervention with home-based parent education decreased post-partum weight gain at 12 months for Black women of low SES.[64] These studies highlight the importance of highly engaging interventions tailored for specific populations and decreasing barriers to accessing information.

Pharmacologic treatment of obesity is generally underutilized, with only 1.3% of eligible patients having prescriptions for AOMs across several large health care organizations throughout the United States.[65] There are few studies examining disparities in AOM use among underserved populations. Significant differences in prescription rates among racial and ethnic groups do not appear to be lower from majority groups, though estimates trend toward Hispanic individuals having lower rates of prescriptions.[65] Another study found that less than 10% of Black and Hispanic individuals with overweight or obesity reported using weight loss medications.[66]

Notably, Hispanic, Black, and low-income individuals are more likely to lack insurance coverage and are less likely to have adequate access to primary care, which may skew the results of these studies.[67] Once obtained, there is also a lack of evidence on whether or not responses to anti-obesity medication differ significantly among different racial and ethnic groups. In a post hoc analysis of the satiety and clinical adiposity—liraglutide evidence in nondiabetic and diabetic people (SCALE) randomized control trial, Hispanic individuals achieved similar weight loss as non-Hispanic individuals.[68–70]

Bariatric surgery is one of the most effective treatments of sustained weight loss, but only 1% of eligible individuals undergo the procedure.[71] Racial and ethnic minorities and those of low income, groups most affected by obesity, are the least likely to undergo the procedure and have less weight loss when they do, compared with Whites and those of higher income.[72,73] Similarly, those without non-private insurance or insurance coverage are less likely to have the procedure.[74–76] Interestingly, no significant racial or ethnic differences in resolving obesity-related comorbid conditions, such as type 2 diabetes mellitus and hypertension post-bariatric surgery, have been found.[73] Among low-income individuals receiving Medicaid, there was an increase in bariatric surgery rates for those living in states that expanded Medicaid through the Affordable Care Act.[77]

FDA-approved medical devices, such as intragastric balloons and vagal blockade devices, have gained traction as less invasive alternatives to bariatric surgery that may augment lifestyle changes.[78–80] There is a lack of data to speculate on how feasible or effective these treatment options are for underserved groups. A US study of the dual intragastric balloon, which included racial and ethnic minorities, effectively induced weight loss. Still, they did not compare results among racial and ethnic groups.[78–81] Insurers do not typically cover medical devices and have exorbitant out-of-pocket costs, limiting their use in socioeconomically disadvantaged groups.

We must address barriers to coverage and access to care to ensure that racial and ethnic minorities and socioeconomically disadvantaged groups can obtain all available therapies to treat obesity. The use of technology may be a means to improve the dissemination of information and reach of health care organizations to these underserved populations.[82–85]

## SUMMARY

Obesity disproportionately affects racial and ethnic minorities and, most severely, Black persons with obesity.[28] Health inequities affect many populations, including historically disadvantaged populations, persons living in rural areas, people with disabilities, and marginalized racial and ethnic groups.[86] Many factors lead to this, including limited access to *quality* obesity care and socioeconomic factors, such as living in an obesogenic food environment or experiencing frequent microaggressions and racism, which can ultimately increase chronic stress and the development of obesity.[7,86]

Not surprisingly, these disparities in disease prevalence mirror similar inequality in access to quality obesity care and stem from many places, including poor access to care, inability to access quality obesity care with obesity-trained physicians and clinicians, and decreased rate of receiving official diagnosis obesity. Despite research supporting the use of lifestyle modification in addition to weight loss medications and surgery, when necessary, there is decreased utilization in persons with lower socioeconomic status or who are ethnic minorities. Some studies indicate that weight loss therapies and surgery are less effective in racial and ethnic minorities, but these disparities are likely repercussions of the unique challenges faced by minority communities[1,28]

With the growing number of individuals with obesity, there is an urgent need to address disparities in access and quality of care. Improving formal medical obesity education and health care policies that expand coverage for obesity care may also be an impactful intervention.[16,17] With the varying efficacy of different dietary or surgery interventions, precision medicine needs to have a growing role in Obesity medicine.[18]

## CLINICS CARE POINTS

### Evidence-Based Pearl #1

*Education about obesity, including management, weight stigma, and disparities in care, should be included in the education and training of all health care professionals.*

- Faculty in curricula development often cite a lack of time, knowledge, and practical guidelines as barriers to obesity education and training.[30] Current literature highlights the need to incorporate obesity education into health care professionals' curricula, given its increasing prevalence.[54,61]

- Several interventions in health care disciplines have positively impacted the competency and skills surrounding obesity treatment.[1,6,23,30]

Pitfall: Nevertheless, many graduates of health care professional schools continue to report discomfort in the management of obesity.[19,63] Inadequate preparation for the care of patients with obesity is particularly evident among primary care providers who play a vital role in the early identification and treatment of obesity[74] International and national studies indicate that physicians, among other health care providers, receive minimal education about obesity.

## Evidence-Based Pearl #2

*Every patient with obesity should be offered all appropriate treatment options regardless of age, race/ethnicity, or socioeconomic status.*

- The foundation of obesity management is lifestyle-based interventions (ie, nutrition, physical activity, and behavioral modification). The United States Preventative Services Task Force recommends patients with obesity receive intensive multi-component behavioral intervention, including multiple behavioral interventions (in either individual or group sessions), setting weight loss goals, improving diet or nutrition, physical activity sessions, addressing barriers to change, active use of self-monitoring, and strategizing on how to maintain lifestyle changes,[87]

    Pitfalls: Unfortunately, lack of health care provider knowledge[88] and insurance coverage limits some patients' ability to receive appropriate treatment. In addition, disparities exist in who receives care for the treatment of obesity, even when insurance status among individuals is the same.[12,28,37]

## Evidence-Based Pearl #3

*We should provide adequate access to obesity care to all those affected by the disease.*

- Although lack of education and training among health care professionals affects a patient's access to obesity care, geography is another barrier. Obesity disproportionally affects those living in the Midwest and Southeast of the United States.[17] With the growing number of physicians certified in obesity medicine via the American Board of Obesity Medicine (ABOM), several studies have evaluated the geographic distribution of ABOM diplomates concerning obesity prevalence.[32,67]

- Although more physicians are becoming certified in obesity medicine to provide evidence-based care,[89,90] children and adults have difficulty accessing a physician to treat their disease, though this improves adequately. Pollack and colleagues noted the population-weighted median drive time to an ABOM diplomate decreased from 28.5 minutes in 2011 to 9.95 minutes in 2019.[59]

- This decrease in driving time does not consider race/ethnicity, distrust of medical care, financial restraints, transportation concerns, or cost of living.[66] In addition, those with severe obesity candidates for MBS may not have access to surgery due to geographic location.[91]

## Areas for future research and treatment options

With the growing number of individuals with obesity, there is a continued need to address disparities in access and quality of care. With the increased popularity of the ABOM board certification examination, we propose greater emphasis and additional resources for obesity in education and training programs.[18,34]

- *Improved obesity health policies*: In addition, the development of health care policies to expand coverage for obesity care would allow more patients to obtain adequate treatment of their disease. The Treat and Reduce Obesity Act (TROA) was initially introduced in 2013 to the Congress but has yet to pass. With the passage of this bill, effective treatment options will be available to all those with obesity at a lower cost.[92] TROA is one tool that could help reduce health inequities.

- *A need for Precision medicine*: Current literature also highlights disparities in response among different obesity treatment modalities.[93] For example, some dietary interventions are more effective in specific racial and ethnic groups. Likewise, distinct differences are noted in how patients respond to anti-obesity pharmacotherapy or surgical procedures. Precision medicine needs to have a growing role in obesity medicine.

## CONFLICT OF INTEREST DISCLOSURES (INCLUDES FINANCIAL DISCLOSURES)

The authors have no conflicts of interest to disclose.

## REFERENCES

1. Bischoff SC, Boirie Y, Cederholm T, et al. Towards a multidisciplinary approach to understanding and managing obesity and related diseases. Clin Nutr 2017;36(4): 917–38.
2. Hudda MT, Nightingale CM, Donin AS, et al. Patterns of childhood body mass index (BMI), overweight and obesity in South Asian and black participants in the English National child measurement programme: effect of applying BMI adjustments standardizing for ethnic differences in BMI-body fatness associations. Int J Obes 2018;42(4):662–70.
3. Stanford FC, Lee M, Hur C. Race, Ethnicity, Sex, and Obesity: Is It Time to Personalize the Scale? Mayo Clin Proc 2019;94(2):362–3.
4. Yarlagadda S, Townsend MJ, Palad CJ, et al. Coverage of obesity and obesity disparities on American Board of Medical Specialties (ABMS) examinations. J Natl Med Assoc 2021;113(5):486–92.
5. Mastrocola MR, Roque SS, Benning LV, et al. Obesity education in medical schools, residencies, and fellowships throughout the world: a systematic review. Int J Obes 2020;44(2):269–79.
6. Hales CM, Carroll MD, Fryar CD, et al. Prevalence of obesity and severe obesity among adults: the United States, 2017-2018. NCHS Data Brief 2020;360:1–8.
7. Park HJ, Francisco SC, Pang MR, et al. Exposure to anti-black lives matter movement and obesity of the black population. Soc Sci Med 2021;114265:1–9.
8. Bower KM, Thorpe RJ, Rhode C, et al. The intersection of neighborhood racial segregation, poverty, and urbanicity and its impact on food store availability in the United States. Prev Med 2014;58:33–9.
9. Kwate NO, Yau C-Y, Loh J-M, et al. Inequality in obesigenic environments: fast food density in New York City. Health Place 2009;15(1):364–73.
10. Kyle TK, Dhurandhar EJ, Allison DB. Regarding obesity as a disease: evolving policies and their implications. Endocrinol Metab Clin North Am 2016;45(3): 511–20.
11. Tylka TL, Annunziato R, Burgard D, et al. The weight-inclusive versus weight-normative approach to health: evaluating the evidence for prioritizing well-being over weight loss. J Obes 2014;2014:983495.
12. Foster GD, Wadden TA, Makris AP, et al. Primary care physicians' attitudes about obesity and its treatment. Obes Res 2003;11(10):1168–77.
13. Price JH, Desmond SM, Krol RA, et al. Family practice physicians' beliefs, attitudes, and practices regarding obesity. Am J Prev Med 1987;3(6):339–45.
14. Tomiyama AJ, Finch LE, Belsky ACI, et al. Weight bias in 2001 versus 2013: contradictory attitudes among obesity researchers and health professionals. Obesity 2015;23(1):46–53.
15. Huizinga MM, Bleich SN, Beach MC, et al. Disparity in physician perception of patients' adherence to medications by obesity status. Obesity 2010;18(10): 1932–7.
16. Mensinger JL, Tylka TL, Calamari ME. Mechanisms underlying weight status and healthcare avoidance in women: A study of weight stigma, body-related shame and guilt, and healthcare stress. Body Image 2018;25:139–47.

17. Carr LTB, Bell C, Alick C, et al. Responding to health disparities in behavioral weight loss interventions and COVID-19 in black adults: recommendations for health equity. J Racial Ethn Health Disparities 2022;9(3):739–47.

18. Cohen SM, Howard JJM, Jin MC, et al. Racial disparities in surgical treatment of obstructive sleep apnea. OTO Open 2022;6(1). 2473974X221088870.

19. Batayeh B, Shelton R, Factor-Litvak P, et al. Racial disparities in avoidant coping and hypertension among midlife adults. J Racial Ethn Health Disparities 2022; 10(1):410–7.

20. Twohig PA, Butt MU, Gardner TB, et al. Racial and gender disparities among obese patients with pancreatic cancer: a trend analysis in the United States. J Clin Gastroenterol 2022. https://doi.org/10.1097/MCG.0000000000001688.

21. Carender CN, DeMik DE, Elkinset JM, et al. Are body mass index cutoffs creating racial, ethnic, and gender disparities in eligibility for primary total hip and knee arthroplasty? J Arthroplasty 2022;37(6):1009–16.

22. Johnson VR, Acholonu NO, Dolan AC, et al. Racial disparities in obesity treatment among children and adolescents. Curr Obes Rep 2021;10(3):342–50.

23. Ard JD, Miller G, Kahan S. Nutrition interventions for obesity. Med Clin North Am 2016;100(6):1341–56.

24. Kerr JA, Loughman A, Knox A, et al. Nutrition-related interventions targeting childhood overweight and Obesity: A narrative review. Obes Rev 2019; 20(Suppl 1):45–60.

25. de Lannoy L, Cowan T, Fernandez A, et al. Physical activity, diet, and weight loss in patients recruited from primary care settings: An update on obesity management interventions. Obes Sci Pract 2021;7(5):619–28.

26. Nguyen NT, Varela JE. Bariatric surgery for obesity and metabolic disorders: state of the art. Nat Rev Gastroenterol Hepatol 2017;14(3):160–9.

27. Division of Population Health, N.C.f.C.D.P.a.H.P. *Health Disparities*. The United States has become increasingly diverse in the last century. According to the 2010 U.S. Census, approximately 36 percent of the population belongs to a racial or ethnic minority group. Though health indicators such as life expectancy and infant mortality have improved for most Americans, some minorities experience a disproportionate burden of preventable disease, death, and disability compared with non-minorities. 2017. Available at: https://www.cdc.gov/aging/ disparities/index.htm#:~:text=Health%20disparities%20are%20preventable% 20differences,other%20population%20groups%2C%20and%20communities. Accessed March 16, 2022.

28. Byrd AS, Toth AT, Stanford FC. Racial disparities in obesity treatment. Curr Obes Rep 2018;7(2):130–8.

29. Ghosh-Dastidar B, Cohen D, Hunter G, et al. Distance to store, food prices, and obesity in urban food deserts. Am J Prev Med 2014;47(5):587–95.

30. Anekwe CV, Jarrell A, Townsend M, et al. Socioeconomics of obesity. Curr Obes Rep 2020;9(3):272–9.

31. Skinner AC, Ravanbakht SN, Skelton JA, et al. Prevalence of obesity and severe obesity in US Children, 1999-2016. Pediatrics 2018;141(3).

32. Gudzune K.A., Johnson V.R., Bramante C.T., et al., Geographic availability of physicians certified by the american board of obesity medicine relative to obesity prevalence, *Obesity*, 27(12), 2019, 1958–1966.

33. Webb VL, Wadden TA. Intensive lifestyle intervention for obesity: principles, practices, and results. Gastroenterology 2017;152(7):1752–64.

34. Claridy M.D., Czepiel K.S., Bajaj S.S., et al., Treatment of obesity: pharmacotherapy trends of office-based visits in the United States From 2011 to 2016, *Mayo Clin Proc*, 96 (12), 2021, 2991–3000.

35. Gomez G, Stanford FC. US health policy and prescription drug coverage of FDA-approved medications for the treatment of obesity. Int J Obes 2018;42(3): 495–500.

36. Wee CC, Huskey KW, Bolcic-Jankovic D, et al. Sex, race, and consideration of bariatric surgery among primary care patients with moderate to severe obesity. J Gen Intern Med 2014;29(1):68–75.

37. Perez NP, Westfal ML, Stapleton SM, et al. Beyond insurance: race-based disparities in the use of metabolic and bariatric surgery for the management of severe pediatric obesity. Surg Obes Relat Dis 2020 Mar;16(3):414–9.

38. Pollack C.C., Onega T., Edmond J.A., et al., A national evaluation of geographic accessibility and provider availability of obesity medicine diplomates in the United States between 2011 and 2019, *Int J Obes*, 46 (3), 2022, 669–675.

39. Townsend MJ, Reddy N, Stanford FC. Geography and equity: expanding access to obesity medicine diplomate care. Int J Obes 2022;46(3):447–8.

40. Flegal KM, Kit BK, Orpana H, et al. Association of all-cause mortality with overweight and obesity using standard body mass index categories: a systematic review and meta-analysis. JAMA 2013;309(1):71–82.

41. Zhang H, Rodriguez-Monguio R. Racial disparities in the risk of developing obesity-related diseases: a cross-sectional study. Ethn Dis 2012;22(3):308–16.

42. Pratt CA, Loria CM, Arteage SS, et al. A systematic review of obesity disparities research. Am J Prev Med 2017;53(1):113–22.

43. Puhl RM, Latner JD. Stigma, obesity, and the health of the nation's children. Psychol Bull 2007;133(4):557–80.

44. Puhl R, Brownell KD. Bias, discrimination, and obesity. Obes Res 2001;9(12): 788–805.

45. Puhl RM, Heuer CA. Obesity stigma: important considerations for public health. Am J Public Health 2010;100(6):1019–28.

46. Wu YK, Berry DC. Impact of weight stigma on physiological and psychological health outcomes for overweight and obese adults: A systematic review. J Adv Nurs 2018;74(5):1030–42.

47. Hilbert A, Braehler E, Haeuser W, et al. Weight bias internalization, core self-evaluation, and health in overweight and obese persons. Obesity 2014;22(1):79–85.

48. Ramos Salas X, Forhan M, Caulfield T, et al. Addressing internalized weight bias and changing damaged social identities for people living with obesity. Front Psychol 2019;10:1409.

49. Pearl RL, White MA, Grilo CM. Weight bias internalization, depression, and self-reported health among overweight binge eating disorder patients. Obesity 2014; 22(5):E142–8.

50. Lear SA, Gasevic D, Schuurman N. Association of supermarket characteristics with the body mass index of their shoppers. Nutr J 2013;12:117.

51. Cooksey-Stowers K, Schwartz MB, Brownell KD. Food swamps predict obesity rates better than food deserts in the United States. Int J Environ Res Public Health 2017;14(11).

52. Block JP, Scribner RA, DeSalvo KB. Fast food, race/ethnicity, and income: a geographic analysis. Am J Prev Med 2004;27(3):211–7.

53. Darmon N, Drewnowski A. Does social class predict diet quality? Am J Clin Nutr 2008;87(5):1107–17.

54. Aaron DG, Stanford FC. Is obesity a manifestation of systemic racism? A ten-point strategy for study and intervention. J Intern Med 2021;290(2):416–20.
55. Harris JL, Frazier W III, Kumanyika S, et al. Increasing disparities in unhealthy food advertising targeted to Hispanic and Black youth.
56. Dubowitz T., Acevedo-Garcia D., Lindsay A.C., et al., Lifecourse, immigrant status and acculturation in food purchasing and preparation among low-income mothers, *Public Health Nutr*, 10 (4), 2007, 396–404.
57. Berkowitz S.A., Berkowitz T.S.Z., Meigs J.B., et al., Trends in food insecurity for adults with cardiometabolic disease in the United States: 2005-2012, *PLoS One*, 12 (6), 2017, e0179172.
58. Wallace AE, Young-Xa Y, Hartley D, et al. Racial, socioeconomic, and rural-urban disparities in obesity-related bariatric surgery. Obes Surg 2010;20(10):1354–60.
59. Burgess E, Hassmen P, Welvaert M, et al. Behavioural treatment strategies improve adherence to lifestyle intervention programmes in adults with obesity: a systematic review and meta-analysis. Clin Obes 2017;7(2):105–14.
60. Taveras EM, Marshall R, Sharifi M, et al. Comparative effectiveness of clinical-community childhood obesity interventions: a randomized clinical trial. JAMA Pediatr 2017;171(8):e171325.
61. Ard JD, Carson TL, Shikany JM, et al. Weight loss and improved metabolic outcomes amongst rural African American women in the Deep South: six-month outcomes from a community-based randomized trial. J Intern Med 2017;282(1): 102–13.
62. Katzmarzyk P.T., Martin C.K., Newton R.L., et al., Weight loss in underserved patients - a cluster-randomized trial, *N Engl J Med*, 383 (10), 2020, 909–918.
63. Bennett GG, Steinberg D, Askew S, et al. Effectiveness of an app and provider counseling for obesity treatment in primary care. Am J Prev Med 2018;55(6): 777–86.
64. Haire-Joshu D., Cahill A.G., Stein R.I., et al., Randomized controlled trial of home-based lifestyle therapy on postpartum weight in underserved women with overweight or obesity, *Obesity*, 27 (4), 2019, 535–541.
65. Saxon D.R., Iwamoto S.J., Mettenbrink C.J., et al., Anti-obesity medication use in 2.2 million adults across eight large health care organizations: 2009-2015, *Obesity*, 27 (12), 2019, 1975–1981.
66. Burroughs VJ, Nonas C, Sweeney CT, et al. Self-reported weight loss practices among African American and Hispanic adults in the United States. J Natl Med Assoc 2010;102(6):469–75.
67. Buchmueller TC, Levy HG. The ACA's impact on racial and ethnic disparities in health insurance coverage and access to care. Health Aff 2020;39(3):395–402.
68. O'Neil PM, Garvey WT, Gonzalez-Campoy JM, et al. Effects of liraglutide 3.0 mg on weight and risk factors in hispanic versus non-hipanic populations: subgroup analysis from scale randomized trials. Endocr Pract 2016;22(11):1277–87.
69. Osei-Assibey G., Adi Y., Kyrou I., et al., Pharmacotherapy for overweight/obesity in ethnic minorities and White Caucasians: a systematic review and meta-analysis, *Diabetes Obes Metab*, 13 (5), 2011, 385–393.
70. Egan BM, White K. Weight loss pharmacotherapy: brief summary of the clinical literature and comments on racial differences. Ethn Dis 2015;25(4):511–4.
71. *Estimate of bariatric surgery numbers, 2011-2020*. American Society for Metabolic and Bariatric Surgery. (2022). Available at: https://asmbs.org/resources/estimate-of-bariatric-surgery-numbers. Accessed March 12, 2023.
72. Hecht L.M., Pester B., Braciszewski J.M., et al., Socioeconomic and racial disparities in bariatric surgery, *Obes Surg*, 30(6), 2020, 2445–2449.

73. Zhao J., Samaan J.S., Abboud Y., et al., Racial disparities in bariatric surgery postoperative weight loss and co-comorbiditysolution: a systematic review, *Surg Obes Relat Dis*, 17(10), 2021, 1799–1823.
74. Bhogal S.K., Reddigan J.I., Rotstein O.D., et al., Inequity to the utilization of bariatric surgery: a systematic review and meta-analysis, *Obes Surg*, 25(5), 2015, 888–899.
75. Martin M, Beekley A, Kjorstad R, et al. Socioeconomic disparities in eligibility and access to bariatric surgery: a national population-based analysis. Surg Obes Relat Dis 2010;6(1):8–15.
76. Santry H.P., Lauderdale D.S., Cagney K.A., et al., Predictors of patient selection in bariatric surgery, *Ann Surg*, 245(1), 2007, 59–67.
77. Brooks E.S., Bailey E.A., Mavroudis C.L. et al., The effects of the affordable care act on utilization of bariatric surgery, *Obes Surg*, 31(11), 2021, 4919–4925.
78. Ponce J, Woodman G, Swain J, et al. The reduce pivotal trial: a prospective, randomized controlled pivotal trial of a dual intragastric balloon for the treatment of obesity. Surg Obes Relat Dis 2015;11(4):874–81.
79. Genco A, Lopez-Nava G, Wahlen C, et al. Multi-centre European experience with intragastric balloon in overweight populations: 13 years of experience. Obes Surg 2013;23(4):515–21.
80.. Sarr MG, Billington CJ, Brancatisano R, et al. The empower study: randomized, prospective, double-blind, multicenter trial of vagal blockade to induce weight loss in morbid obesity. Obes Surg 2012;22(11):1771–82.
81. Ikramuddin S, Blackstone RP, Brancatisano A, et al. Effect of reversible intermittent intra-abdominal vagal nerve blockade on morbid obesity: the ReCharge randomized clinical trial. JAMA 2014;312(9):915–22.
82. Joseph R.P., Keller C., Adams M.A., et al., Print versus a culturally-relevant Facebook and text message delivered intervention to promote physical activity in African American women: a randomized pilot trial, *BMC Wom Health*, 15, 2015, 30.
83. Marcus B.H., Dunsinger S.I., Pekmezi D., et al., Twelve-month physical activity outcomes in Latinas in the Seamos Saludables trial, *Am J Prev Med*, 48(2), 2015, 179–182.
84. Lohse B., Belue R., Smith S., et al., About Eating: an online program with evidence of increased food resource management skills for low-income women, *J Nutr Educ Behav*, 47 (3), 2015, 265–272.
85. King AC, Bickmore TW, Campero MI, et al. Employing virtual advisors in preventive care for underserved communities: results from the COMPASS study. J Health Commun 2013;18(12):1449–64.
86. Newsome FA, Gravlee CC, Cardel MI. Systemic and environmental contributors to obesity inequities in marginalized racial and ethnic groups. Nurs Clin North Am 2021;56(4):619–34.
87. Bomberg EM, Palzer EF, Rudser KD, et al. Anti-obesity medication prescriptions by race/ethnicity and use of an interpreter in a pediatric weight management clinic. Ther Adv Endocrinol Metab 2022;13. 20420188221090009.
88. Bray G.A., Heisel W.E., Afshin A., et al., The science of obesity management: an endocrine society scientific statement, *Endocr Rev*, 39 (2), 2018, 79–132.
89. Gudzune KA, Wickham EP 3rd, Schmidt SL, et al. Physicians certified by the American Board of Obesity Medicine provide evidence-based care. Clin Obes 2021;11(1):e12407.
90. Stanford FC, Kyle TK. Why food policy and obesity policy are not synonymous: the need to establish clear obesity policy in the United States. Int J Obes 2015;39(12):1667–8.

91. Butsch WS, Kushner RF, Alford S, et al. Low priority of obesity education leads to lack of medical students' preparedness to effectively treat patients with obesity: results from the U.S. medical school obesity education curriculum benchmark study. BMC Med Educ 2020;20(1):23.

92. Bajaj S.S., Jain B., Kyle T.K., et al., Overcoming congressional inertia on obesity requires better literacy in obesity science, *Obesity*, 30 (4), 2022, 799–801.

93. Dietz WH, Burr LA, Hall K, et al. Management of obesity: improvement of health-care training and systems for prevention and care. Lancet 2015;385(9986): 2521–33.

# Obesity Management in Children and Adolescents

Gunther Wong, BS[a,b,c,d], Gitanjali Srivastava, MD[a,b,c,d],*

## KEYWORDS

- Pediatric obesity • Medical weight loss • Weight management
- Comprehensive obesity care • Bariatric surgery • Adjuvant obesity medication

## KEY POINTS

- Obesity in the pediatric population is increasing in the United States and globally.
- Childhood obesity predisposes to shorter life spans and increased risk for comorbid cardiometabolic and psychosocial disorders.
- Intensive health behavior and lifestyle treatment is recommended for all children with obesity.
- Pharmacologic and surgical interventions are safe and effective in children whose clinical picture warrants them.

## INTRODUCTION/HISTORY/DEFINITIONS/BACKGROUND

### Introduction

Obesity in children and adolescents is a significant public health issue with a high prevalence in many high-income countries, as well as increasing prevalence in low-income and middle-income countries.[1] Childhood obesity is associated with multiple cardiometabolic and psychosocial comorbidities, including dysglycemia, hypertension, dyslipidemia, nonalcoholic fatty liver disease (NAFLD), metabolic syndrome, and increased risk for intrapersonal and interpersonal problems.[2,3] Additionally, childhood obesity is associated with continued obesity in adulthood and decreased expected life span.

### Epidemiology

The increasing rates of childhood obesity worldwide highlight the importance of effective clinical diagnosis and treatment. The global age-standardized prevalence of obesity between 1975 and 2016 increased from 0.7% to 5.6% in girls and from

ᵃ Department of Medicine, Division of Diabetes, Endocrinology & Metabolism, Vanderbilt University School of Medicine, Nashville, TN, USA; ᵇ Department of Surgery, Vanderbilt University School of Medicine; ᶜ Department of Pediatrics, Vanderbilt University School of Medicine; ᵈ Vanderbilt Weight Loss Center, Vanderbilt University Medical Center, Thompson Lane, Suite 22200, Nashville, TN 37204, USA
* Corresponding author. Vanderbilt Weight Loss Center, Vanderbilt University Medical Center, Thompson Lane, Suite 22200, Nashville, TN 37204.
*E-mail address:* gitanjali.srivastava@vumc.org

Gastroenterol Clin N Am 52 (2023) 443–455
https://doi.org/10.1016/j.gtc.2023.03.011
0889-8553/23/© 2023 Elsevier Inc. All rights reserved.

0.9% to 7.8% in boys. The prevalence of obesity is highest in the Polynesia, Micronesia, the Middle East and North Africa, the Caribbean, and the United States, with each of these regions having a childhood obesity rate greater than 20%.[4] Among age subgroups in the United States, there has been a dramatic increase in obesity rates in the last 30 years. Between 1988 and 2018, obesity rates in the 2 to 5-year age group increased from 7.2% to 13.7%; in the 6 to 11-year age group increased from 11.3% to 19.3%; and in the 12 to 19-year age group increased from 10.5% to 20.9%.[5,6] In the United States, childhood obesity also has substantial racial and ethnic differences, with African American and Hispanic children having a higher obesity prevalence compared with children of White race.[7] The nature of the COVID-19 global pandemic may also be contributing to recent increases in childhood obesity. A study of multiple pediatric cohorts in the United States found greater body mass index (BMI) increases in the period of the COVID-19 pandemic compared with earlier years.[8]

## Causes

The etiology of obesity in the pediatric population and its recent increase in prevalence is multifactorial. Genetic studies indicate that heritability of adiposity ranges from 40% to 75%.[9] Meta-analysis of genetic obesity studies has found at least 97 loci associated with BMI.[10] One strongly associated loci is the FTO (fat mass and obesity associated) gene on chromosome 16. Homozygous carriers of the risk variant of FTO have 1.67 times increased odds of obesity compared with nonrisk carriers.[11] Additionally, FTO risk variants may account for 22% of common obesity.[12] Preclinical models have shown that FTO is associated with energy metabolism and adipose tissue homeostasis, potentially through epitranscriptomic marking and RNA processing.[13]

There are several known monogenic and syndromic forms of obesity. In children with early-onset, severe obesity, or adults with a lifetime history of obesity, monogenic or syndromic causes should be suspected. Syndromic causes of obesity include the following:

- Prader-Willi syndrome caused by absent expression of paternal genes on chromosome 15q11.2-q13. This syndrome is characterized by severe hypotonia in early childhood, delayed development, and hyperphagia that lead to early-onset obesity.[14]
- Bardet-Biedl syndrome, a ciliopathy resulting in hyperphagia, obesity, retinitis pigmentosa and retinal dystrophy, polydactyly, hypogonadism, and severe developmental delay.[15,16]
- Pseudohypoparathyroidism, or Albright hereditary osteodystrophy, caused by end-organ resistance to PTH that results in short stature, hyperphagia, obesity, round facies, brachydactyly, and skeletal abnormalities.[15]
- Patients with WAGR (Wilms tumor, aniridia, genitourinary abnormalities, and intellectual disability) syndrome with an alteration to the brain-derived neurotrophic factor (BDNF) gene.[17]
- ROHHAD (rapid onset obesity with hypothalamic dysfunction, hypoventilation, and autonomic dysregulation).[15]
- Obesity-hypotonia or Cohen syndrome caused by mutation in the COH1/VPS13 B gene that leads to altered facies, microcephaly, hypotonia, developmental delay, myopia, and truncal obesity.[17]

Important monogenic causes of obesity include the following:

- Leptin, the protein coded by the *lep* or obese (*ob*) gene. Leptin is a peptide hormone that plays a role in satiety and hunger signaling in the brain, and the maintenance of energy homeostasis.[18] Deficiencies in leptin receptor (LEPR) are associated with monogenic obesity.[19]

- Proopiomelanocortin (POMC), a hypothalamic hormone, and its receptor, melanocortin 4 receptor (MC4R), which activate satiety signals in the brain.[19,20]

Other monogenic causes include mutations in SH2B1, NTRK2, SIM1, GNAS, and PCSK1.[17,21,22] These genes provide potential therapeutic targets. One such therapeutic is setmelanotide, a Food and Drug Administration (FDA) approved MC4R agonist for children aged 6 years and older who have obesity-causing variants in POMC, PCSK1, or LEPR.[19]

Environmental factors also play a significant role in the development of childhood obesity. Sedentary lifestyles and caloric intake exceeding needs are important modifiable risk factors for the development of obesity. In particular, high glycemic index foods, including sugar-sweetened beverages such as fruit juice or soda are correlated with increased rates of childhood obesity.[23] Additionally, the increase in recreational media devices, such as television, smartphones, and video games, has been attributed to the increasing prevalence of childhood obesity.[24–27] Sleep is another important modifiable risk factor for childhood obesity. Increased sleep during childhood and later school start times are correlated with lower childhood BMI.[28–30] In children who require their use, obesogenic medications such as glucocorticoids, antipsychotics, and antiepileptics can all predispose childhood weight gain.[31]

Social determinants of health, such as race, ethnicity, and socioeconomic status, are highly correlated with incidence of childhood obesity. Children with obesity are more likely to come from households of lower socioeconomic status.[32] The mechanism of this relationship is complex; children from financially disadvantaged households are more likely to have reduced health education and increased stress and emotional turmoil compared with children from financially advantaged households. High-stress environments, increased cortisol levels, and early development of obesity-associated mental health conditions such as depression and anxiety are all mechanisms in which socioeconomic status can affect childhood obesity.[32,33] Race is also a predictor of childhood obesity; in the United States, Hispanic, Native American, and African American children have greater rates of childhood obesity, often independent of other social determinants of health.[34,35]

## DISCUSSION
### Observation/Assessment/Evaluation

BMI is the most used tool to assess levels of body fat, defined as follows:

$$BMI = \frac{weight\ (kg)}{height^2\ (m^2)}$$

There is no perfect measure of body fat level, and all measures should be considered in conjunction with the full patient clinical presentation, including genetic background, level of activity, and fat distribution. However, BMI has been shown to correlate well with body fat mass and comorbid health conditions.[36–39] Because distributions of muscle, skeletal mass, and body fat change through childhood and adolescence, absolute BMI is an inappropriate metric to define obesity in childhood. Instead, percentile cutoffs are appropriate. The American Academy of Pediatrics (AAP) recommends 2 cutoff points: a BMI of less than 85th percentile is considered low risk and a BMI of greater than 95th percentile is high risk and the threshold for obesity. BMI between 85th and 95th percentiles can be considered overweight (**Table 1**). A BMI greater than 120% above the 95th percentile for age is considered severe obesity.[39] For example, a 10-year-old boy with BMI of 23 would be considered in the obese category, whereas an 18-year-old boy with the same BMI would be considered healthy weight (**Fig. 1**).

In addition to BMI assessment, which should be conducted at least annually, a thorough history and physical examination is essential to the evaluation of childhood obesity. Important aspects of the patient history include[39] the following:

- Assessment of behavior and lifestyle, including diet, level of activity, and amount of television and other screen media time.
- Duration and quality of sleep.
- Family history, particularly of parental obesity or obesity-related comorbidities.
- The presence of mental health conditions that may predispose or be comorbid with obesity (ie, depression, anxiety).

Techniques that may facilitate nonstigmatizing discussion of obesity include asking permission to discuss weight, using nonlabeling phrases such as "child with obesity," and using neutral words for obesity (eg, unhealthy weight, gaining too much weight for age).[39]

A complete review of systems and physical examination is also important to identify weight-related comorbidities or the presence of syndromic obesity (**Tables 2** and **3**). Common weight-related comorbidities that should be screened for include[39] the following:

- Asthma, which has increased prevalence in obese children.[40]
- Gastrointestinal disorders, including NAFLD, gallstones, gastroesophageal reflux disease (GERD), and constipation.
- Endocrine disorders, particularly type 2 diabetes mellitus (T2DM), polycystic ovarian syndrome (PCOS), and Cushing syndrome. All female adolescents with obesity should be evaluated for menstrual irregularities and signs of hyperandrogenism to assess for PCOS.[39]
- Idiopathic intracranial hypertension.
- Cardiovascular disorders, including hypertension and dyslipidemia.
- Mental health comorbidities, including anxiety, depression, and eating disorders.

**Table 1**
**Weight loss goals per age and BMI**

| BMI Category | 2–5 y | 6–11 y | 12–18 y |
|---|---|---|---|
| Healthy Weight 5th–84th percentile | Maintain weight | Maintain weight | Maintain weight |
| Overweight/(−) no risk factors 85th–94th percentile | Maintain weight | Maintain weight | Maintain weight |
| Overweight/(+) risk factors 85th–94th percentile | Maintain weight or slow weight gain | Maintain weight | Maintain weight or gradual weight loss |
| Obesity 95th–99th percentile | Maintain weight | Gradual weight loss of 1 lb/mo | Weight loss up to 2 lbs/wk |
| Severe obesity ≥99th percentile | Acceptable to lose up to 1 lb/mo if BMI >21 | Weight loss of 2 lbs/wk | Weight loss up to 2 lbs/wk |

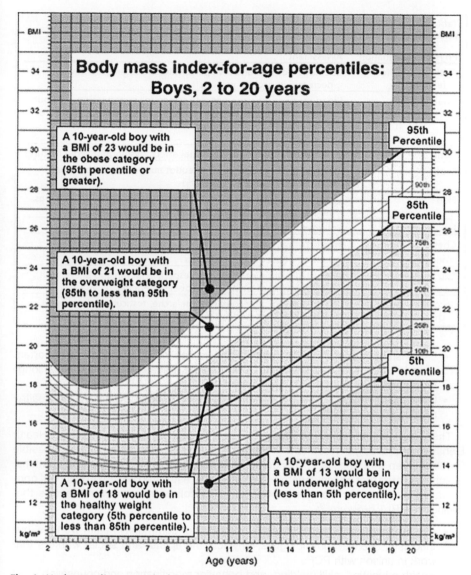

**Fig. 1.** Understanding growth charts and BMI percentile categories in children.

- Musculoskeletal disorders, including tibia vara and slipped capital femoral epiphysis (SCFE), both of which are increased in prevalence among children with obesity.

Among children with BMI greater than 85th percentile, additional laboratory tests are indicated, including glucose, liver function tests, and lipid panels (**Table 4**).

### Treatment

The following goals of obesity treatment are multifactorial[38].

- Decreased BMI percentile.
- Control or reversal of weight-related comorbidities.

**Table 2**
**Physical examination findings in childhood obesity**

| Physical Examination | Assessment |
|---|---|
| Anthropometric features | Calculation of BMI and BMI percentiles based on growth curve, decreases in growth velocity |
| Vital signs | Blood pressure measurements to screen for hypertension, rule out "white coat" hypertension, repeat BP measurements on several occasions, which are required to diagnose hypertension in children |
| General | Body fat distribution, psychosocial affect, dysmorphic facial features |
| Eyes | CN VI paralysis, papilledema (pseudotumor cerebri), abnormally shaped eyes (syndromic obesity) |
| Skin | Acanthosis nigricans (insulin resistance), keratosis pilaris, skin tags, intertrigo, acne, hirsutism (PCOS), violaceous striae |
| Neck/thyroid | Enlarged tonsils causing obstruction, thyromegaly, goiter |
| Chest | Heart rhythm, wheezing |
| Abdomen | Palpation of liver size, tenderness |
| Extremities | Abnormal gait, joint tenderness especially at hip and knees, foot pain, bowing of tibia (Blount disease), edema, polydactyly |
| Secondary sexual characteristics | Tanner staging, gynecomastia, thelarche, testicular enlargement, microphallus, precocious puberty |

- Establishment of permanent healthy lifestyle habits. This outcome is important even in the absence of significant BMI change, because of the potential long-term benefits of behavioral modification.
- Emotional health, including improved self-esteem, body positivity, and healthy relationship with food.

The American Academy of Pediatrics now recommends that Intensive Health Behavior and Lifestyle Treatment (IHBLT) should be initiated as quickly as possible for all children with obesity.[39] This guideline differs from previous recommendations, which stipulated that obesity treatment be gradually escalated based on failure of conservative measures or worsening obesity.[38] The following are several factors that define an IHBLT program[39]:

- A multidisciplinary treatment team consisting of community health workers, nutritionists, exercise physiologists, physical therapists, and social workers that work in unison with PCPs.
- Health education, skill building, and behavior modification and counseling.
- A high "dose" of intervention, with a target of greater than 26 hours of engagement during a 3 to 12-month period. Greater engagement has been shown to be correlated with superior BMI loss and resolution of comorbidities.

Besides greater engagement, there are several characteristics of IHBLT that have been shown to facilitate superior results.

- Face-to-face engagement. There is a greater body of evidence to support the effectiveness of face-to-face engagement. Although telemedicine and mobile tools offer opportunities for greater reach of care, more research is required to show their effectiveness.
- Family-based engagement. Intervention that includes the parents and family are superior to those only targeting the child (eg, school-based).

**Table 3**
Review of systems for weight-related problems in childhood obesity

| Symptoms | Possible Cause | Concerns/Comments |
|---|---|---|
| Sad mood, loss of interest, school avoidance, poor self-esteem, poor school performance | Peer victimization, depression, anxiety | Concern for worsening obesity |
| Shortness of breath, wheezing or cough | Asthma | Exacerbation of asthma and weight gain |
| Ambiguous abdominal recurrent pain | Nonalcoholic fatty liver disease (though patients can be asymptomatic) | May progress to steatohepatitis, cirrhosis; note elevation of aspartate aminotransferase or alanine aminotransferace (AST/ALT) more than 60 U/L on more than 2 occasions or persistent elevation for 6 mo needs pediatric GI referral |
| Encopresis, fecal soiling, abdominal distension | Constipation | May be associated with irregular eating patterns |
| Right upper quadrant pain or epigastric pain | Gallbladder disease | Consider need for cholecystectomy if symptoms recur or worsen |
| Heartburn, dysphagia | Gastroesophageal reflux disease | May be associated with irregular eating patterns |
| Irregular menses, acne, hirsutism | Polycystic ovarian syndrome | Concern for insulin resistance, infertility, T2DM |
| Primary amenorrhea | Polycystic ovarian syndrome, Prader-Willi syndrome | Association with infertility or worsening obesity |
| Hip pain, thigh pain or waddling gait | Slipped capital femoral epiphysis | Association with hip deformity and dysfunction, worsening obesity; evaluate with hip X-rays |
| Knee pain/foot pain | Blount disease (bowing of tibia), flat feet, sprains, fractures | Association with decreased physical activity and worsening obesity; evaluate with knee-X-rays |
| Polyuria, polydipsia, unexpected weight loss | Type 2 diabetes mellitus | Concern for insulin resistance, worsening glucose control, renal involvement |
| Sleep problems<br>Loud snoring or apnea<br>Daytime sleepiness or restlessness<br>Nocturnal enuresis | Obstructive sleep apnea | Association with poor sleep efficiency, poor attention, poor academic performance, pulmonary hypertension (HTN), right ventricular hypertrophy (RVH), food cravings, or difficulty with satiety |
| Smoke smell from clothes | Tobacco use as form of weight loss | Increased cardiovascular risk |

Table 4
Laboratory tests for evaluation of childhood overweight and obesity

| | Overweight[a] | Obesity[b] |
| --- | --- | --- |
| Age <10 y | Lipids every 2 y | Lipids every 2 y |
| Age >10 y with no risk factors | Lipids every 2 y | Lipids every 2 y plus: ALT/AST, fasting glucose |
| Age >10 y with risk factors (eg, hypertension, smoking, family hx of diabetes, stroke, or CVD) | Lipids every 2 y plus: ALT/AST, fasting glucose | Lipids every 2 y plus: ALT/AST, fasting glucose |

[a] BMI 85 to 94th percentile.
[b] BMI ≥ 95th percentile.
*Data from* Refs.[49–53]

- Multicomponent engagement. A strong IHBLT program should incorporate multiple approaches, including addressing nutrition, fitness, mental health, and parenting.

IHBLT programs often exist in larger cities and within academic medical centers. Access to IHBLT programs is not universal in the United States, and significant inequities exist based on geographic are, demographics, socioeconomic status, and insurance. If IHBLT is not available or feasible, primary care providers should seek to incorporate available local programs and resources. Although not yet supported by randomized clinical trials, the AAP offers several behavioral recommendations primary care providers can offer to children with obesity[39] as follows:

- Reduction of sugar-sweetened beverages.
- Following the United States Department of Agriculture (USDA) MyPlate recommendations (choosemyplate.gov).
- Sixty minutes of daily moderate physical activity.
- Limit screen time and other sedentary behavior.
- Avoid skipping breakfast.
- The 5-2-1-0 system (**Table 5**).
- Encouraging sufficient sleep.

## Pharmacologic Intervention

In addition to behavior and lifestyle changes, there are several options for pharmacotherapy for the treatment of pediatric obesity. Pharmacotherapy should only be initiated as an adjunct to behavior and lifestyle changes and a thorough discussion of medication risks and benefits should be undertaken. Pharmacologic options that are FDA-approved include the following:

Table 5
5-2-1-0 message for children

| | 5-2-1-0 Message for all Children |
| --- | --- |
| 5 | At least 5 servings of fruits and vegetables daily |
| 2 | No more than 2 h of television or screen time (remove TV/computer from bedroom; no screen time for children <2 y) |
| 1 | At least 1 h of physical activity daily |
| 0 | Zero sugary drinks, more water and low-fat milk |

- Glucagon-like-peptide receptor antagonists (GLP-1RAs). Two medications in this class are FDA-approved for the treatment of obesity in children aged 12 years and older: liraglutide and semaglutide. In clinical trials, 43.3% of patients receiving liraglutide had BMI change of greater that 5%, and 26.1% of patients had BMI change of 10%, compared with 18.7% and 8.1%, respectively, in the placebo group.[41] Semaglutide is a recently approved GLP-1RA, which appears in clinical trials to facilitate substantially greater weight loss in adolescents than other antiobesity medications.[42]
- Orlistat, an inhibitor of fat absorption, approved for children aged 12 years and older.[43]
- Setmelanotide, a MC4R agonist approved for individuals with POMC, LEPR, or PCSK1 deficiencies, is approved for children aged 6 years and older.[19]
- Phentermine/topiramate, approved for children aged 12 years and older.[44]
- Phentermine alone, which is approved for short-course therapy (<3 months) in children aged 16 years and older.

Several medications are sometimes prescribed off-label for obesity.

- Metformin. Although a systematic review found that Metformin resulted in a modest reduction in BMI, these results were heterogenous across populations and clinical trials, with its benefits still uncertain.[45]
- Lisdexamfetamine. This medication is FDA approved for the treatment of attention-deficit/hyperactivity disorder (ADHD) in the pediatric population aged 6 years and older. It is used off-label for the treatment of obesity comorbid with binge-eating disorder, although clinical trials indicating its effectiveness or safety in this usage do not yet exist.[39,46]
- Other GLP-1RAs.

Implementation of these medications should be undertaken at a dedicated pediatric weight management center with comprehensive services, including dieticians, behavioral health services, and exercise counseling.

### Metabolic and Bariatric Surgery

Metabolic and bariatric surgery has been shown in clinical trials to be safe in the pediatric population and produces durable weight loss and comorbidity improvement.[47]

| Table 6 Recommended selection criteria for adolescent bariatric surgery | |
|---|---|
| BMI ≥35 kg/m² [Class 2 Obesity or ≥120th of the 95th BMI Percentile for Age/Gender] plus an Obesity-Related Medical Comorbidity | BMI ≥40 kg/m² [Class 3 Obesity or ≥140th of 95th BMI Percentile for Age/Gender Irrespective of Medical Comorbidity] |
| Examples of medical comorbidities: T2DM Moderate-Severe OSA (AHI >15 events/h) Pseudotumor cerebri Severe steatohepatitis Mild OSA (≥5 events/h) HTN Insulin resistance Prediabetes Dyslipidemia Impaired quality of life or ADLs | |

Additionally, evidence shows that adolescents have a higher probability of remission of cardiometabolic risk factors such as T2DM and HTN compared with adults after undergoing surgery, suggesting that early intervention may alleviate the cumulative effect of chronic obesity.[39]The American Academy of Pediatrics and the American Society for Metabolic and Bariatric Surgery recommend consideration of bariatric surgery in children whose BMI is greater than 140% of the 95th BMI percentile for age, or greater than 120% of the 95th BMI percentile for age with the presence of an obesity-related medical comorbidity (**Table 6**).[48]

## SUMMARY

Obesity in the pediatric population is increasing in the United States and worldwide. Obesity in this population is associated with comorbid cardiometabolic and psychosocial disorders, continued obesity into adulthood, and decreased life span. Although there are well-researched genetic and syndromic causes of pediatric obesity, increasing rates can also be attributed to public health, lifestyle, and behavioral factors. Regular, annual BMI screening of adolescents is important to monitor body fat levels. Thorough history and physical examination are necessary to identify comorbid conditions. For children with obesity or who are overweight with risk factors or related comorbidities, IHBLT should be initiated as quickly as possible. For patients without access to IHBLT, PCPs should incorporate available local resources and provide sound behavioral and lifestyle recommendations. For patients requiring adjunctive therapy, there are several options for pharmacologic therapy, including recently approved GLP-1RAs that seem to offer superior weight loss results in clinical trials compared with other antiobesity medications. For patients meeting the criteria for metabolic and bariatric surgery, these procedures facilitate significant reduction in BMI and resolution of comorbidities with a similar safety profile to adults receiving the procedure. Ultimately, obesity is a chronic, multifactorial disease that requires longitudinal treatment over multiple domains.

## CLINICS CARE POINTS

- Obesity is increasing worldwide. The global age-standardized prevalence of obesity between 1975 and 2016 increased from 0.7% to 5.6% in girls and from 0.9% to 7.8% in boys.

- Social determinants of health can both increase incidence of childhood obesity and decrease access to effective care.

- The heritability of obesity may be anywhere from 40% to 75%. Future research may drive additional therapeutics based on genetic causes, such as the use of setmelanotide in patients with POMC, PCSK1, and LEPR deficiencies.

- Annual BMI screening and thorough history and physical are necessary to identify childhood obesity and screen for comorbidities.

- Among children above the 85th percentile for BMI, additional screening of lipids, glycemic levels, and liver enzymes is indicated (see **Table 4**).

- IHBLT should be initiated immediately for children with obesity. The AAP no longer recommends a tiered approach to treatment based on failed conservative measures or increasing severity.

- Pharmacologic options are available for patients requiring adjunctive treatment.

- Metabolic and bariatric surgery is safe and effective for patients meeting treatment criteria (see **Table 6**).

## DISCLOSURES

G. Srivastava reports advisory/consultant fees from Novo Nordisk and Rhythm, outside the submitted article. G. Srivastava is a Diplomate of the American Board of Obesity Medication.

## REFERENCES

1. Jebeile H, Kelly AS, O'Malley G, et al. Obesity in children and adolescents: epidemiology, causes, assessment, and management. Lancet Diabetes Endocrinol 2022;10(5):351–65.
2. Daniels SR, Arnett DK, Eckel RH, et al. Overweight in children and adolescents: pathophysiology, consequences, prevention, and treatment. Circulation 2005; 111(15):1999–2012.
3. Small L, Aplasca A. Child Obesity and Mental Health: A Complex Interaction. Child Adolesc Psychiatr Clin N Am 2016;25(2):269–82.
4. NCD-RisC, NRFC. Worldwide trends in body-mass index, underweight, overweight, and obesity from 1975 to 2016: a pooled analysis of 2416 population-based measurement studies in 128·9 million children, adolescents, and adults. Lancet 2017;390(10113):2627–42.
5. Ogden CL, Fryar CD, Martin CB, et al. Trends in Obesity Prevalence by Race and Hispanic Origin-1999-2000 to 2017-2018. JAMA 2020;324(12):1208–10.
6. Ogden CL, Flegal KM, Carroll MD, et al. Prevalence and trends in overweight among US children and adolescents, 1999-2000. JAMA 2002;288(14):1728–32.
7. Skinner AC, Ravanbakht SN, Skelton JA, et al. Prevalence of Obesity and Severe Obesity in US Children, 1999-2016. Pediatrics 2018;(3):141. https://doi.org/10.1542/peds.2017-3459.
8. Knapp EA, Dong Y, Dunlop AL, et al. Changes in BMI During the COVID-19 Pandemic. Pediatrics 2022;(3):150. https://doi.org/10.1542/peds.2022-056552.
9. Loos RJ. The genetics of adiposity. Curr Opin Genet Dev 2018;50:86–95.
10. Locke AE, Kahali B, Berndt SI, et al. Genetic studies of body mass index yield new insights for obesity biology. Nature 2015;518(7538):197–206.
11. Frayling TM, Timpson NJ, Weedon MN, et al. A common variant in the FTO gene is associated with body mass index and predisposes to childhood and adult obesity. Science 2007;316(5826):889–94.
12. Dina C, Meyre D, Gallina S, et al. Variation in FTO contributes to childhood obesity and severe adult obesity. Nat Genet 2007;39(6):724–6.
13. Zhao X, Yang Y, Sun BF, et al. FTO and obesity: mechanisms of association. Curr Diab Rep 2014;14(5):486.
14. Cassidy SB, Schwartz S, Miller JL, et al. Prader-Willi syndrome. Genet Med 2012; 14(1):10–26.
15. Koves IH, Roth C. Genetic and Syndromic Causes of Obesity and its Management. Indian J Pediatr 2018;85(6):478–85.
16. Forsyth R, Gunay-Aygun M. Bardet-Biedl Syndrome Overview. 2003 Jul 14 [updated 2023 Mar 23]. In: Adam MP, Mirzaa GM, Pagon RA, et al, editors. GeneReviews® [Internet]. Seattle (WA): University of Washington, Seattle; 1993–2023; 1993.
17. Kostovski M, Tasic V, Laban N, et al. Obesity in Childhood and Adolescence, Genetic Factors. Pril (Makedon Akad Nauk Umet Odd Med Nauki) 2017;38(3): 121–33.
18. Obradovic M, Sudar-Milovanovic E, Soskic S, et al. Leptin and Obesity: Role and Clinical Implication. Front Endocrinol 2021;12:585887.

19. Clement K, van den Akker E, Argente J, et al. Efficacy and safety of setmelanotide, an MC4R agonist, in individuals with severe obesity due to LEPR or POMC deficiency: single-arm, open-label, multicentre, phase 3 trials. Lancet Diabetes Endocrinol 2020;8(12):960–70.

20. Yu K, Li L, Zhang L, et al. Association between MC4R rs17782313 genotype and obesity: A meta-analysis. Gene 2020;733:144372.

21. Mendes de Oliveira E, Keogh JM, Talbot F, et al. Obesity-Associated. N Engl J Med 2021;385(17):1581–92.

22. Stijnen P, Ramos-Molina B, O'Rahilly S, et al. PCSK1 Mutations and Human Endocrinopathies: From Obesity to Gastrointestinal Disorders. Endocr Rev 2016;37(4): 347–71.

23. Ebbeling CB, Feldman HA, Chomitz VR, et al. A randomized trial of sugar-sweetened beverages and adolescent body weight. N Engl J Med 2012; 367(15):1407–16.

24. Hancox RJ, Milne BJ, Poulton R. Association between child and adolescent television viewing and adult health: a longitudinal birth cohort study. Lancet 2004; 364(9430):257–62.

25. Epstein LH, Roemmich JN, Robinson JL, et al. A randomized trial of the effects of reducing television viewing and computer use on body mass index in young children. Arch Pediatr Adolesc Med 2008;162(3):239–45.

26. Falbe J, Rosner B, Willett WC, et al. Adiposity and different types of screen time. Pediatrics 2013;132(6):e1497–505.

27. Stettler N, Signer TM, Suter PM. Electronic games and environmental factors associated with childhood obesity in Switzerland. Obes Res 2004;12(6):896–903.

28. Jiang F, Zhu S, Yan C, et al. Sleep and obesity in preschool children. J Pediatr 2009;154(6):814–8.

29. Altenburg TM, Chinapaw MJ, van der Knaap ET, et al. Longer sleep–slimmer kids: the ENERGY-project. PLoS One 2013;8(3):e59522.

30. Gariepy G, Janssen I, Sentenac M, et al. School Start Time and the Healthy Weight of Adolescents. J Adolesc Health 2018;63(1):69–73.

31. Kumar S, Kelly AS. Review of Childhood Obesity: From Epidemiology, Etiology, and Comorbidities to Clinical Assessment and Treatment. Mayo Clin Proc 2017; 92(2):251–65.

32. Williams AS, Ge B, Petroski G, et al. Socioeconomic Status and Other Factors Associated with Childhood Obesity. J Am Board Fam Med 2018;31(4):514–21.

33. Hemmingsson E. Early Childhood Obesity Risk Factors: Socioeconomic Adversity, Family Dysfunction, Offspring Distress, and Junk Food Self-Medication. Curr Obes Rep 2018;7(2):204–9.

34. Rogers R, Eagle TF, Sheetz A, et al. The Relationship between Childhood Obesity, Low Socioeconomic Status, and Race/Ethnicity: Lessons from Massachusetts. Child Obes 2015;11(6):691–5.

35. Isong IA, Rao SR, Bind MA, et al. Racial and Ethnic Disparities in Early Childhood Obesity. Pediatrics 2018;141(1). https://doi.org/10.1542/peds.2017-0865.

36. Pietrobelli A, Faith MS, Allison DB, et al. Body mass index as a measure of adiposity among children and adolescents: a validation study. J Pediatr 1998; 132(2):204–10.

37. Freedman DS, Khan LK, Dietz WH, et al. Relationship of childhood obesity to coronary heart disease risk factors in adulthood: the Bogalusa Heart Study. Pediatrics 2001;108(3):712–8.

38. Barlow SE, Committee E. Expert committee recommendations regarding the prevention, assessment, and treatment of child and adolescent overweight and obesity: summary report. Pediatrics 2007;120(Suppl 4):S164–92.
39. Hampl SE, Hassink SG, Skinner AC, et al. Clinical Practice Guideline for the Evaluation and Treatment of Children and Adolescents With Obesity. Pediatrics 2023. https://doi.org/10.1542/peds.2022-060640.
40. Ford ES. The epidemiology of obesity and asthma. J Allergy Clin Immunol 2005; 115(5):897–909 [quiz: 910].
41. Kelly AS, Auerbach P, Barrientos-Perez M, et al. A Randomized, Controlled Trial of Liraglutide for Adolescents with Obesity. N Engl J Med 2020;382(22):2117–28.
42. Weghuber D, Barrett T, Barrientos-Perez M, et al. Once-Weekly Semaglutide in Adolescents with Obesity. N Engl J Med 2022;387(24):2245–57.
43. Chanoine JP, Hampl S, Jensen C, et al. Effect of orlistat on weight and body composition in obese adolescents: a randomized controlled trial. JAMA 2005; 293(23):2873–83.
44. Dhillon S. Phentermine/Topiramate: Pediatric First Approval. Paediatr Drugs 2022;24(6):715–20.
45. Masarwa R, Brunetti VC, Aloe S, et al. Efficacy and Safety of Metformin for Obesity: A Systematic Review. Pediatrics 2021;147(3). https://doi.org/10.1542/peds.2020-1610.
46. Guerdjikova AI, Blom TJ, Mori N, et al. Lisdexamfetamine in Pediatric Binge Eating Disorder: A Retrospective Chart Review. Clin Neuropharmacol 2019; 42(6):214–6.
47. Inge TH, Jenkins TM, Xanthakos SA, et al. Long-term outcomes of bariatric surgery in adolescents with severe obesity (FABS-5+): a prospective follow-up analysis. Lancet Diabetes Endocrinol 2017;5(3):165–73.
48. Eisenberg D, Shikora SA, Aarts E, et al. American Society for Metabolic and Bariatric Surgery (ASMBS) and International Federation for the Surgery of Obesity and Metabolic Disorders (IFSO): Indications for Metabolic and Bariatric Surgery. Surg Obes Relat Dis 2022;18(12):1345–56.
49. Daniels SR, Greer FR, Co Nutrition. Lipid screening and cardiovascular health in childhood. Pediatrics 2008;122(1):198–208.
50. Krebs NF, Himes JH, Jacobson D, et al. Assessment of child and adolescent overweight and obesity. Pediatrics 2007;120(Suppl 4):S193–228.
51. Horsely L. AP Clinical Report on Lipid Screening in Children. Am Fam Physician 2009;703–5.
52. Adolescents EPoIGfCHaRRiCa, National Heart Ln, and Blood Institute. Expert panel on integrated guidelines for cardiovascular health and risk reduction in children and adolescents: summary report. Pediatrics 2011;128(Suppl 5):S213–56.
53. Pratt JSA, Browne A, Browne NT, et al. ASMBS pediatric metabolic and bariatric surgery guidelines. Surg Obes Relat Dis 2018;14(7):882–901.

# Dietary Supplements for Weight Loss

Steven B. Heymsfield, MD

## KEYWORDS

- Overweight • Obesity • Diet • Prescription medicine

## KEY POINTS

- Dietary supplements for weight loss, consumed by millions of Americans who are overweight and obese, are regulated by the Federal Drug Administration as foods and not drugs.
- The weight loss efficacy of these products, supported largely by "structure-function" claims on their labels, is at best minimal as established by in-depth systematic reviews and meta-analyses.
- While generally safe, dietary supplements for weight loss are known to be associated with adverse reactions; some products have hidden pharmacologically active ingredients that may pose risks to some people.
- People with overweight and obesity who plan to embark on a weight loss program should be educated by their physicians on the current status of dietary supplements and guided toward more effective currently available measures including lifestyle approaches, pharmacologic options, and bariatric surgical treatments.

## INTRODUCTION

Several questions arise when considering dietary supplements for weight loss: are any of those currently on the market effective, and if so, are they safe? What thresholds should we use for judging their efficacy and safety? The answers to these questions are still evolving and pose one of the great challenges facing contemporary drug regulators across the globe. This review will examine these questions that are relevant to almost all practitioners who manage patients with obesity.

## HISTORY

Dietary supplements trace their origin to secret remedies developed by medicine makers during the late seventeenth century.[1] The English crown granted "letters patent" to these formulations that soon became popular in the American colonies. Patent

Pennington Biomedical Research Center, Louisiana State University System, 6400 Perkins Road, Baton Rouge, LA 70808, USA
*E-mail address:* steven.heymsfield@pbrc.edu

Gastroenterol Clin N Am 52 (2023) 457–467
https://doi.org/10.1016/j.gtc.2023.03.010
0889-8553/23/© 2023 Elsevier Inc. All rights reserved.

**gastro.theclinics.com**

medicines introduced by American entrepreneurs proliferated and became a thriving industry during the 18th century.[1] The "golden age" of patent medicines followed in the 19th century as these products promised miracle cures while conventional medicine continued with medieval practices such as bloodletting and purgatives.[1,2]

### Creation of the Food and Drug Administration

Despite their popularity in the 19th century, patent medicines were not without serious side effects and questionable efficacy. Increasing the recognition of patent medicine evils led Colliers Weekly to launch a series of essays exposing this largely corrupt industry in 1905.[3] The muckraker Samuel Hopkins Adams authored the first of his now classic Colliers series "The Great American Fraud" on October 7th, 1905[4] (**Fig. 1**). Hopkins Adams reported to readers that "Gullible America will spend this year some 75 millions dollars in the purchase of patent medicines. In consideration of this sum it will swallow huge quantities of alcohol, an appalling amount of opiates and narcotics, a wide assortment of varied drugs ranging from powerful and dangerous heart depressants to insidious liver stimulants; and far in excess of other ingredients, undiluted fraud".

Momentum created by the writings of other muckrakers, including The Jungle in 1905 by Upton Sinclair,[5] contributed to the passage of the original Pure Food and Drugs Act by Congress and signed into law by President Theodore Roosevelt in 1906.[6] The 1906 law prohibited interstate commerce in the "manufacture, sale, or transportation of adulterated or misbranded or poisonous or deleterious food, drugs,

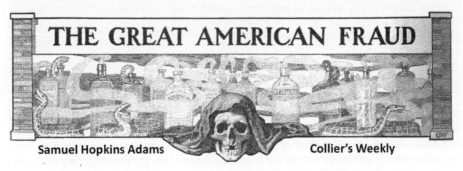

**THE GREAT AMERICAN FRAUD**

Samuel Hopkins Adams    Collier's Weekly

| October 7th, 1905 | I. The Great American Fraud |
| October 28th, 1905 | II. Peruna and the "Bracers" |
| November 18th, 1905 | III. Liquozone |
| December 2nd, 1905 | IV. The Subtle Poisons |
| January 13th, 1906 | V. Preying on the Incurables |
| February 17th, 1906 | VI. The Fundamental Fakes |
| November 4th, 1905 | VII. The Patent Medicine Conspiracy Against the Freedom of the Press |

**Fig. 1.** Samuel Hopkins Adams classic series on the "Great American Fraud" that contributed to the passage of the Pure Food and Drugs Act in 1905. This series and legislative actions that followed paved the way for the creation of the FDA. (*Modified from* Adams SH. The Great American Fraud. Collier's Weekly. 1905; with permission.)

| Table 1 | |
|---|---|
| **Federal drug administration obesity drug guidance** | |
| Target Population | BMI >27 kg/m² plus a weight-related comorbidity or BMI >30 kg/m² |
| Primary analysis | Intention to treat population |
| Phase 3 clinical trial Size and duration | ≥4500 Overweight and obese subjects studied for at least 1 y |
| Efficacy criteria | Mean placebo-subtracted weight loss ≥5% or proportion of drug-treated subjects who lose ≥5% of baseline body weight is ≥ 35% and approximately double the proportion who lose ≥5% in the placebo group |
| Secondary end points | Blood pressure and pulse, lipoprotein lipids, fasting glucose and insulin, hemoglobin $A_{1c}$ in diabetics, quality of life, waist circumference |

Abbreviation: BMI, body mass index.

medications, and liquors." Several years later, in 1912, congress passed the Sherley Amendment that outlawed labeling medicines with false medical claims aimed at deceiving consumers.[7] The Food, Drug, and Insecticide Administration's name was changed to the Food and Drug Administration (FDA) under a 1930 agricultural appropriations act.[6,7] Additional amendments and instituted regulations over the decades that followed gradually tightened the prescription drug approval process.[6,7] Today the FDA has rigorous safety and efficacy standards for the approval of new weight loss medicines (**Table 1**).[8] As of 2022, 5 prescription drugs meeting the criteria outlined in the table are currently approved by the FDA for the treatment of people with overweight and obesity.[9]

In 1972 the FDA set in place regulations guiding the sale of pharmaceutical products without a physician's prescription. Regulations guiding the approval of over-the-counter (OTC) products are complex, but in general can follow a conventional prescription drug approval pathway or rely on a "monograph" that details dosages and labeling requirements of established active ingredients.[10] Only one OTC weight loss product is presently approved for sale in the United States.[11,12]

The FDA also approves "devices" for weight loss and today one ingestible product in pill form is "cleared" for marketing in the United States.[13] Medical devices are cleared by the FDA if a manufacturer can show that their product is "substantially equivalent to another (similar) legally marketed device" that has FDA clearance or approval.[14] That is, the manufacturer has to show that their device is equally safe and effective and works in the same manner as a currently approved device. Purchase of this FDA-cleared device requires a prescription.

After considering OTC products and prescription medicines and devices there now remain between 50,000 and 80,000 dietary supplements on the market, many of which are targeted to consumers who are overweight or obese. That's a 10 to 20-fold increase in marketed dietary supplements from 1994.[15] Yearly expenditures on dietary supplements in 1994 were $4 billion and now exceed $50 billion,[16] $2 billion of which is for weight loss products. Over 15% of US adults have used a dietary supplement for weight loss.[17]

By the late 1980s and early 1990s pressure was increasing on congress and the FDA to regulate the dietary supplement industry. Intense industry lobbying led to a compromise bill in 1994, the Dietary Supplement Health and Education Act (DSHEA).[18] Dietary supplements according to the traditional FDA definition included essential nutrients such as vitamins and minerals. The 1990 Nutrition Labeling and Education Act expanded the dietary supplement definition to include herbs or similar nutritional substances.[19] DSHEA further expanded the definition of dietary supplements in 1994 to include.[20]

- Products (other than tobacco) that are intended to supplement the diet that bears or contains one or more of the following dietary ingredients: a vitamin, a mineral, an herb or other botanical, an amino acid, a dietary substance for use by man to supplement the diet by increasing the total daily intake, or a concentrate, metabolite, constituent, extract, or combinations of these ingredients;
- Are intended for ingestion in pill, capsule, tablet, or liquid form;
- Are not represented for use as a conventional food or as the sole item of a meal or diet; and
- Include products such as an approved new drug, certified antibiotic, or licensed biologic that was marketed as a dietary supplement or food before approval, certification, or license (unless the Secretary of Health and Human Services waives this provision).

The 1994 law thus cast a very wide net when defining dietary supplements, keeping the door open to myriad weight loss formulations. A critical feature of DSHEA is the regulations guiding what statements are permissible on the product label. Specifically, the label must.

- State that the product is a "dietary supplement" or the word "dietary" can be replaced by the name of the key ingredient;
- Provide a complete listing of ingredients and serving size information;
- Give relevant safety information;
- And importantly, if the supplement bears a claim to affect the structure or function of the body, a claim of general well-being, or a claim of a benefit related to a classical nutrient deficiency disease, the label must include "This statement has not been evaluated by the Food and Drug Administration. This product is not intended to diagnose, treat, cure, or prevent any disease."

The labels present on almost all dietary supplements for weight loss include structure/function claims. For example, a product with caffeine that increases energy expenditure might include on the label "boosts metabolism". However, dietary supplement labels cannot state that respective products will "treat, cure, or prevent obesity". Unlike prescription drugs for weight loss, under DSHEA FDA does not have the authority to approve dietary supplements for safety and effectiveness or their labeling before they are sold in stores or online.[20] Regulatory actions can, however, be taken by the FDA or Federal Trade Commission when a manufacturer makes unsubstantiated weight loss claims. The FDA has the authority to inspect dietary supplement manufacturing facilities to confirm that companies are meeting all manufacturing and labeling requirements.

### 2022 Pending Legislation

As of 2022 congress was considering the Durbin-Braun Dietary Supplement Bill or "Dietary Supplement Listing Act".[21] This legislation would require companies to register their products with the FDA, list ingredients, and provide a copy of the label that includes structure/function claims. A publicly searchable database of listed products would be made available by the FDA. While this legislation would be a step forward, Cohen and colleagues[22] argue that the Durbin-Braun Bill fails to fully protect consumers: the FDA would not have a mechanism to confirm a product's actual ingredients versus label claims and some misleading health claims will still go unchecked. Registration of products might give consumers the false impression that the FDA has established their purity, safety, and health benefits.[22]

Almost 3 centuries have passed since patent medicines arrived on American shores. Pharmaceutical companies emerged over that time period and with them came regulatory agencies such as the FDA. Only 7 prescription and OTC weight loss products have passed through the FDA's rigorous approval process and are on the market today. Dietary supplements are the direct descendants of patent medicines with the modest regulatory framework put in place with DSHEA. The question imposed on us as clinicians and investigators is to thus establish if any dietary supplements for weight loss are effective and safe.

## EFFICACY

Rigorous testing is required by the FDA before prescription drugs or devices can be marketed. By contrast, dietary supplements for weight loss can be marketed without prior FDA evaluations. Sometimes studies of products are published that describe their safety and efficacy, although these reports often have limitations that include small sample sizes, lack of randomization and double blinding according to rigorous criteria, failure to set a primary end point with power size calculations, use of unacceptable statistics to analyze data, lack of control of confounding lifestyle factors, short duration, and many other specious practices that make their interpretation difficult. This has left the scientific and clinical communities with limited options for establishing product and ingredient safety and efficacy. There are, however, several credible sources of information on dietary supplements. First, the FDA maintains an Office of Dietary Supplement Programs that publishes a Dietary Supplement and Products and Ingredients List[23] and a Dietary Supplement Ingredient Advisory List[24] on the web. Second, the National Institutes of Health maintains an Office of Dietary Supplements that publishes extensive ingredient fact sheets and updates on topics related to supplements.[17,25] Lastly, systematic reviews and meta-analyses have been published that specifically examine dietary supplements for weight loss. Several of these publications in peer review journals provide a good overview of the current status of dietary supplements for weight loss.

Pittler and Ernst published systematic reviews of dietary supplements for weight loss in 2004 and 2005.[26,27] The authors included only randomized double-blind trials along with previous systematic reviews and meta-analyses. Supplement ingredients included chitosan, chromium picolinate, Ephedra sinica, Garcinia cambogia, glucomannan, guar gum, hydroxy-methylbutyrate, plantago psyllium, pyruvate, yerba maté, and yohimbe. Only one group of products showed promise as a weight loss aid, those containing ephedrine or botanical sources of ephedrine. The same year, in 2004, the FDA banned all ephedra-containing dietary supplements after receiving reports of 18,000 adverse events and several high-profile deaths.[28] Pittler and Ernst concluded that "None of the reviewed dietary supplements can be recommended for over-the-counter use."

Onakpoya from the same group reported a "systematic review of systematic reviews" in 2011.[29] The articles collected by the authors included systematic reviews of a specific food supplement or combination supplement for reducing body weight. Nine systematic reviews met the author's rigorous inclusion criteria. The 9 reviewed articles led the author's to again conclude that "the existing systematic reviews of clinical trials testing the efficacy of food supplements in reducing body weight fail to provide good evidence that any of these preparations generate clinically relevant weight loss without undue risks."

Batsis and colleagues recently conducted an extensive systematic review of dietary supplements and alternative therapies for weight loss that was published in 2021.[30] Their review was accompanied by a commentary by Kidambi and colleagues.[31] Over 20,504 citations were reviewed by Batsis and colleagues that included 1,743 full-text articles reporting the efficacy of 14 dietary supplements. Only 52 studies were considered sufficiently low risk of bias and thus could be reviewed in support of efficacy. Sixteen of these studies (31%) reported significant pre/post-between-group differences (range: 0.3 kg, 4.93 kg) in weight change. The authors concluded that their review did not "support strong, high-quality evidence of efficacy for any of the products". As noted in earlier reviews, the authors point out that the "considerable heterogeneity in trial design, bias, efficacy, and duration, suggests a need to develop trials accounting for methodological flaws."

These representative reviews are consistent in their findings that currently available dietary supplements for weight loss have no or very modest weight loss efficacy. Can a weight loss efficacy expectation be set for dietary supplements? We can gain perspective on that question by reviewing orlistat, the only nonprescription weight medicine now approved by the FDA for OTC purchase. One-year weight loss for orlistat in carefully conducted randomized trials is about 4% above placebo.[32] Clinically meaningful weight loss with lifestyle measures or medications is usually considered about 5% above placebo levels over the longer term of months or years.[32] We thus have a framework within which to judge dietary supplement weight loss efficacy. A supplement that produces less than 4% to 5% weight loss in carefully conducted longer term studies would not be expected to have meaningful clinical benefits.

## SAFETY

Emergency department visits for adverse events related to dietary supplements are well known. Geller and colleagues estimated that dietary supplements accounted for over 20,000 visits and 2,000 yearly hospitalizations based on a representative 2004 to 2013 emergency department sample.[33] The recent death of a US Representative's wife attributed to a dietary supplement containing mulberry leaf highlights these risks.[34] Mulberry leaf purportedly can "curb cravings", "lower blood sugar", and "help in reducing obesity".[34-36] The congressman's wife was reported to have "just joined a gym" and was "carefully dieting".[36]

The FDA monitors adverse event reports and complaints received from industry, health care professionals, and consumers related to dietary supplement products.[37] Enforcement actions can be taken by the FDA for unsafe products that can be recalled or removed from the market. Adverse events can be reported to the FDA through the Safety Reporting Portal at www.safetyreporting.hhs.gov, a local FDA Consumer Complaint Coordinator (www.fda.gov/consumer-complaint-coordinators), or by calling FDA's SAFEFOOD Information Line at 1 to 888-SAFEFOOD (1–888–723–3366).

Product adulteration with active drugs is also well established and consumers can consult with the FDAs Health Fraud Product Database (https://www.fda.gov/consumers/health-fraud-scams/health-fraud-product-database)[38] to check on specific supplements. Between 2007 and 2019 almost 1000 products tested by the FDA included either hidden ingredients or hazardous substances; one-third of these products were for weight loss.[38] White reported in 2022 that dietary supplements for weight loss were the second most commonly adulterated products, behind that of supplements for sexual enhancement.[39] Sibutramine, a weight loss drug removed by the FDA from the market for adverse cardiovascular events, was the most commonly detected adulterant; others included phenolphthalein and fluoxetine.

Some products include third-party certification seals on their labels.[40] These labels from credible independent testing groups confirm that product manufacturing and storage facilities are compliant with "GMP" (Good Manufacturing Practices), and that the product contains the ingredients reported on the label.

## DISCUSSION

All of the evidence published in peer-reviewed journals up to now supports the position that dietary supplements for weight loss are at best minimally effective and in some cases carry risks through allergic reactions, drug interactions, and adulteration. Additionally, there are financial costs associated with purchase of dietary supplements and these expenses can be relatively large for low-income patients. The balance thus tips in favor of not recommending dietary supplements for weight loss when another modern lifestyle, pharmacologic, and surgical treatments are an option. Whether dietary supplements might in some way facilitate weight loss when combined with lifestyle measures remains unknown but a testable hypothesis. The search for bioactive compounds that promote meaningful weight loss and that can be defined as dietary supplements continues worldwide across academic and industry laboratories.

What explains the enduring, and even increasing, popularity of dietary supplements for weight loss? Two interacting factors determine the magnitude of an individual's embrace of dietary supplements for weight loss, susceptibility, and exposure to misinformation.[41] At the patient level we live in a culture awash with bias against people with obesity[42] and constant admonitions by health practitioners and federal organizations to lose weight if you suffer from excess adiposity. Susceptibility is amplified by commonly held patient views[43]: *dichotomous thinking* lumping dietary supplements into the good/healthy versus bad/unhealthy category; and contributing to that cognitive construct, "*natural*" and "*botanical*" ingredients are perceived as inherently healthy and safe. Older adults, lack of analytical thinking, and right-wing political orientation are consistent findings in studies of people susceptible to misinformation.[41] Patent medicines and now their descendants dietary supplements have as their market people with these kinds of vulnerabilities for whom conventional medical treatments have no or limited efficacy, are out of reach because of cost, or an inability to find expert guidance in weight control efforts.

These patient characteristics and conditions are often the substrate for unscrupulous marketers of dietary supplements and some cases the progenitors are major food companies. Promotional materials for dietary supplements that lure people with overweight and obesity into purchasing products using false or misleading claims have changed little over the past century (**Fig. 2**). The internet and television are flooded with this kind of misinformation, hucksters with a veneer of professionalism tout products that have no or weak efficacy,[44] and regulatory agencies such as the FDA and Federal Trade Commission have limited capabilities to reel them in. Baron and Ejnes recently weighed in on the role of physicians spreading misinformation on social media, posing the question "do right and wrong answers still exist in medicine?".[45] What is perceived as medically "true" is "increasingly crowdsourced" and often follows nontraditional scientific methods.

Patient susceptibility and exposure to misinformation do not always translate to "infection". According to van der Linden,[41] "immunization" against misinformation begins with providing patients "facts" such as those presented in this review. Warning

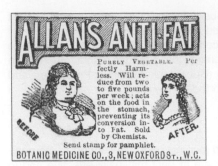

**1897**

**1947**

**2022**

**Fig. 2.** Advertisement for a patent medicine published in 1897 and another one 5 decades later in 1947[48] (*upper panels*). A 2022-email to the author promoting a dietary supplement for weight loss. Ads like these promote "harmless" and fast weight loss, often without the need to diet or exercise. The email text makes classic structure-function claims (eg, fat blocker, serotonin increase) but does not associate the multiple ingredients with treating or curing obesity as is mandated by the FDA.

against "myths" (eg, weight loss is possible using dietary supplements even without dieting or exercise) comes next. In a recent study, Roozenbeek and colleagues[46] found that exposing the manipulation technique to participants in their study "inoculated" them, making them more skeptical of misinformation. Van der Linden suggests ending the discussion with patients by reinforcing the facts.[41] Successful patient-physician conversations must overcome inherent cognitive biases of which Harris and colleagues[47] identified 6 (eg, Visceral…"Excessive emotional involvement of the clinician" in a patient relationship) that tended to influence clinical approaches to dietary supplements.

## SUMMARY

Modern dietary supplements for weight loss are the descendants of patent medicines that have passed through a coarse filter that excludes banned ingredients on the one hand and approved FDA products on the other. No single supplemental ingredient or combination of ingredients is recognized at this point by the scientific community as having clinically relevant efficacy. Moreover, some products pose risks to patients through several pathways, including the inclusion of hidden bioactive pharmaceuticals known to produce weight loss. People with obesity are recognized as susceptible hosts and infection with misinformation is pervasive leading to a vast supplement market with thousands of products that continue to grow. Increasing attention is being directed at "inoculation" approaches that immunize patients to false claims of ingredient and product benefit. Many laboratories in academia and industry continue the search for dietary supplements that can promote or facilitate safe and effective sustained weight loss.

## FUNDING

This work was partially supported by National Institutes of Health NORC Center Grants P30DK072476, Pennington Biomedical Research Center, and P30DK040561, Harvard Medical School, United States.

## CONFLICT OF INTEREST

S.B. Heymsfield reports his role on the Medical Advisory Boards of Tanita Corporation, Amgen, and Medifast; he is also an Amazon Scholar.

## REFERENCES

1. Young JH. The toadstool millionaires; a social history of patent medicines in America before Federal regulation. Princeton, N.J.: Princeton University Press; 1961.
2. National Museum of American History Behring Center. Balm of America: Patent Medicine Collection. Available at: https://americanhistory.si.edu/collections/object-groups/balm-of-america-patent-medicine-collection/history. Accessed September 9, 2022.
3. Collier's Weekly and Patent Medicines. J Am Med Assoc 1905;XLV(11):793–4. https://doi.org/10.1001/jama.1905.02510110049008.
4. Adams S.H., The great American fraud, 1905, Collier's Weekly, Springfield, OH.
5. Sinclair U. The Jungle. New York: Doubleday, Page & company; 1906.
6. U.S. Food & Drug Administration. Milestones in U.S. Food and Drug Law. Available at: https://www.fda.gov/about-fda/fda-history/milestones-us-food-and-drug-law. Accessed September 9, 2022.
7. U.S. Food & Drug Administration. Milestones of Drug Regulation in the United States. Available at: https://www.fda.gov/media/109482/download#: ~ :text=1912% 20Congress%20enacts%20the%20Sherley,a%20standard%20difficult%20to% 20prove. Accessed September 9, 2022.
8. Colman E. Food and Drug Administration's Obesity Drug Guidance Document: a short history. Circulation 2012;125(17):2156–64.
9. FDA-Approved Drugs to Treat Overweight and Obesity. J Psychosoc Nurs Ment Health Serv 2022;60(8):7–8.
10. PEW Research Center. Regulation of Over-the-Counter Drug Products Should Be Streamlined. [Fact Sheet]. 2017; Available at: https://www.pewtrusts.org/en/research-and-analysis/fact-sheets/2017/03/regulation-of-over-the-counter-drug-products-should-be-streamlined#: ~ :text=How%20are%20OTC%20drugs% 20regulated,and%20population%20before%20marketing%20them. Accessed September 9, 2022.
11. Cignarella A, Busetto L, Vettor R. Pharmacotherapy of obesity: An update. Pharmacol Res 2021;169:105649.
12. GSK. alli Product Info & Usage. 2022; Available at: https://www.myalli.com/about/product-use/. Accessed September 9, 2022.
13. Plenity for weight management. Med Lett Drugs Ther 2021;63(1624):77–8.

14. Greenway FL, Aronne LJ, Raben A, et al. A Randomized, Double-Blind, Placebo-Controlled Study of Gelesis100: A Novel Nonsystemic Oral Hydrogel for Weight Loss. Obesity 2019;27(2):205–16.

15. Mishra S, Stierman B, Gahche JJ, et al. Dietary Supplement Use Among Adults: United States, 2017-2018. NCHS Data Brief 2021;399:1–8.

16. Dick Durbin United States Senator Illinois. Durbin applauds inclusion of important dietary supplement provisions in bipartisan senate committee's FDA user fee package. Press Release. 2022; Available at: https://www.durbin.senate.gov/newsroom/press-releases/durbin-applauds-inclusion-of-important-dietary-supplement-provisions-in-bipartisan-senate-committees-fda-user-fee-package. Accessed September 9, 2022.

17. National Institutes of Health (NIH) Office of Dietary Supplements (ODS). Dietary Supplements for Weight Loss: Fact Sheet for Health Professionals. 2022. Available at: https://ods.od.nih.gov/factsheets/WeightLoss-HealthProfessional/. Accessed September 9, 2022.

18. 103rd United States Congress. Dietary Supplement Health and Education Act of 1994. Public Law 103-417. 103rd Congress. 1994. Available at: https://ods.od.nih.gov/About/DSHEA_Wording.aspx. Accessed September 9, 2022.

19. Wikipedia contributors. Nutrition Labeling and Education Act of 1990. 2022; Available at: https://en.wikipedia.org/w/index.php?title=Nutrition_Labeling_and_Education_Act_of_1990&oldid=1102251787. Accessed September 9, 2022.

20. Wikipedia contributors. Dietary Supplement Health and Education Act of 1994. 2022; Available at: https://en.wikipedia.org/wiki/Dietary_Supplement_Health_and_Education_Act_of_1994. Accessed September 9, 2022.

21. (2021-2022). tUSC. S.4090 - Dietary Supplement Listing Act of 2022. 2022; Available at: https://www.congress.gov/bill/117th-congress/senate-bill/4090/text Accessed September 9, 2022.

22. Cohen PA, Avorn J, Kesselheim AS. Institutionalizing Misinformation - The Dietary Supplement Listing Act of 2022. N Engl J Med 2022;387(1):3–5.

23. U.S. Food & Drug Administration. Dietary Supplement Products & Ingredients. 2022; Available at: https://www.fda.gov/food/dietary-supplements/dietary-supplement-products-ingredients. Accessed September 9, 2022.

24. U.S. Food & Drug Administration. Dietary Supplement Ingredient Advisory List. 2022; Available at: https://www.fda.gov/food/dietary-supplement-products-ingredients/dietary-supplement-ingredient-advisory-list. Accessed September 9, 2022.

25. National Institutes of Health (NIH) Office of Dietary Supplements (ODS). Office of Dietary Supplements Homepage. Available at: https://ods.od.nih.gov/. Accessed September 9, 2022.

26. Pittler MH, Ernst E. Dietary supplements for body-weight reduction: a systematic review. Am J Clin Nutr 2004;79(4):529–36.

27. Pittler MH, Ernst E. Complementary therapies for reducing body weight: a systematic review. Int J Obes 2005;29(9):1030–8.

28. Shekelle PG, Hardy ML, Morton SC, et al. Efficacy and safety of ephedra and ephedrine for weight loss and athletic performance: a meta-analysis. JAMA 2003;289(12):1537–45.

29. Onakpoya IJ, Wider B, Pittler MH, et al. Food supplements for body weight reduction: a systematic review of systematic reviews. Obesity 2011;19(2):239–44.

30. Batsis JA, Apolzan JW, Bagley PJ, et al. A Systematic Review of Dietary Supplements and Alternative Therapies for Weight Loss. Obesity 2021;29(7):1102–13.

31. Kidambi S, Batsis JA, Donahoo WT, et al. Dietary supplements and alternative therapies for obesity: A Perspective from The Obesity Society's Clinical Committee. Obesity 2021;29(7):1095–8.
32. Yanovski SZ, Yanovski JA. Long-term drug treatment for obesity: a systematic and clinical review. JAMA 2014;311(1):74–86.
33. Geller AI, Shehab N, Weidle NJ, et al. Emergency Department Visits for Adverse Events Related to Dietary Supplements. N Engl J Med 2015;373(16):1531–40.
34. Chung C. Death of rep. Tom McClintock's wife tied to white mulberry leaf. The New York Times 2022. Available at: https://www.nytimes.com/2022/08/25/us/lori-mcclintock-death-white-mulberry-leaf.html. Accessed September 9, 2022.
35. Lim HH, Yang SJ, Kim Y, et al. Combined treatment of mulberry leaf and fruit extract ameliorates obesity-related inflammation and oxidative stress in high fat diet-induced obese mice. J Med Food 2013;16(8):673–80.
36. Young S. Congressman's Wife Died After Taking Herbal Remedy Marketed for Diabetes and Weight Loss. 2022; Available at: https://khn.org/news/article/tom-lori-mcclintock-death-herbal-remedy-diabetes-weight-loss-white-mulberry/. Accessed September 9, 2022.
37. U.S. Food & Drug Administration. How to report a problem with dietary supplements. 2022; Available at: https://www.fda.gov/food/dietary-supplements/how-report-problem-dietary-supplements. Accessed September 9, 2022.
38. U.S. Food & Drug Administration. Health Fraud Product Database. 2022; Available at: https://www.fda.gov/consumers/health-fraud-scams/health-fraud-product-database. Accessed September 9, 2022.
39. White CM. Continued Risk of Dietary Supplements Adulterated With Approved and Unapproved Drugs: Assessment of the US Food and Drug Administration's Tainted Supplements Database 2007 Through 2021. J Clin Pharmacol 2022; 62(8):928–34.
40. Dietary Supplements Quality Collaborative (DSQC). Dietary Supplements Quality Collaborative (DSQC) Homepage. 2021; Available at: https://www.dsqcollaborative.org/. Accessed September 9, 2022.
41. van der Linden S. Misinformation: susceptibility, spread, and interventions to immunize the public. Nat Med 2022;28(3):460–7.
42. Rubino F, Puhl RM, Cummings DE, et al. Joint international consensus statement for ending stigma of obesity. Nat Med 2020;26(4):485–97.
43. Ubel PA. Why Too Many Vitamins Feels Just About Right. JAMA Intern Med 2022; 182(8):791–2.
44. Christensen J, Wilson J. Congressional hearing investigates Dr. Oz 'miracle' weight loss claims. 2014; Available at: https://www.cnn.com/2014/06/17/health/senate-grills-dr-oz. Accessed September 9, 2022.
45. Baron RJ, Ejnes YD. Physicians Spreading Misinformation on Social Media - Do Right and Wrong Answers Still Exist in Medicine? N Engl J Med 2022;387(1):1–3.
46. Roozenbeek J, van der Linden S, Goldberg B, et al. Psychological inoculation improves resilience against misinformation on social media. Sci Adv 2022;8(34): eabo6254.
47. Harris IM, Danner CC, Satin DJ. How Does Cognitive Bias Affect Conversations With Patients About Dietary Supplements? AMA J Ethics 2022;24(5):E368–75.
48. Young JH. The Medical Messiahs: Chapter 13. 2002; Available at: https://quackwatch.org/hx/mm/13-2/. Accessed September 9, 2022.

# Developing Effective Strategies for Obesity Prevention

Sophia V. Hua, PhD, MPH[a],*, Caroline E. Collis, BA[b],
Jason P. Block, MD, MPH[c]

## KEYWORDS

- Obesity prevention • Nutrition policy • Beverage tax • Calorie labeling
- Nutrition assistance programs

## KEY POINTS

- Nutrition policies are intended to improve diet quality and decrease rising obesity prevalence.
- Evidence shows that beverage taxes and recent nutritional changes to the Special Supplemental Nutrition Program for Women, Infants, and Children, the National School Lunch Program, and School Breakfast Program are all policies that can encourage healthier consumption. Calorie labeling of prepared foods is associated with modest declines in calories purchased from ready-to-eat foods.
- In cost-effectiveness analyses, beverage taxes, calorie labeling, and changes to federal nutrition assistance programs are projected to be cost-saving or cost-efficient in decreasing the increase in obesity prevalence.
- Multiple policies acting in concert are more likely to be successful than single policies.

## INTRODUCTION

Obesity is a population-wide health crisis, and prevention strategies need to work in conjunction with—and extend beyond—clinical treatment to support a comprehensive approach to address the obesity epidemic.

In this article, we will review several nutrition policies that have been evaluated in the United States, including beverage taxes, food and beverage labeling, and changes to food assistance programs such as the Supplemental Nutrition Assistance Program

[a] Department of Nutrition, Harvard T.H. Chan School of Public Health, 665 Huntington Avenue, Boston, MA 02115, USA; [b] Department of Population Medicine, Harvard Pilgrim Health Care Institute, 401 Park Drive, Suite 401, Boston, MA, USA; [c] Department of Population Medicine, Harvard Pilgrim Health Care Institute, Harvard Medical School, 401 Park Drive, Suite 401, Boston, MA, USA
* Corresponding author. Department of Nutrition, Harvard T.H. Chan School of Public Health, 665 Huntington Avenue, Building II, Boston, MA 02115, USA.
*E-mail address:* sophiahua@fas.harvard.edu

Gastroenterol Clin N Am 52 (2023) 469–482
https://doi.org/10.1016/j.gtc.2023.03.013
0889-8553/23/© 2023 Elsevier Inc. All rights reserved.

(SNAP), Special Supplemental Nutrition Program for Women, Infants, and Children (WIC), the National School Lunch Program (NSLP), and the School Breakfast Program (SBP). We also present some international evaluations of similar policies enacted across the world. Several other obesity prevention policies have been discussed as strategies to improve diet and prevent excess weight gain, including restrictions in food marketing or advertising and restrictions on the types of food that can be offered in kid's meals or in checkout counters at retail food stores, among others. Because these policies either have not been introduced in the United States (eg, advertising restrictions) or have not yet been fully evaluated (eg, kid's meal policies), we do not discuss them in this article. We also do not discuss policies intended to promote physical activity.

## CURRENT EVIDENCE
### Beverage and Food Taxes

Consumption of sugary beverages and ultra-processed foods is associated with weight gain.[1,2] Although governments have historically enacted food and beverage sales taxes to generate revenue, more recently, taxes have been used to discourage unhealthy consumption by raising the prices of unhealthy products and decreasing demand (**Fig. 1**). In the United States, these obesity prevention taxes have mostly been levied on sugary beverages; other countries have also introduced taxes to disincentivize the purchase of unhealthy snack foods.

### Types of taxes
There are several types of beverages taxes used (**Fig. 2**).

- Sales taxes are levied directly on the consumer with revenue collected by the government. In the United States, customers typically only see these prices when the item is paid for because the price of the item does not include the sales tax. In other countries, these types of taxes are reflected in the actual price of the item. In this article, we do not address these taxes because they are usually very small and not implemented with the purpose of promoting public health. Existing evidence suggests that these small taxes have limited effect on demand.
- Excise taxes are paid for by manufacturers or distributors in a manner that leads to an increase in the actual price of the item.
  - *Specific excise taxes* are taxes based on quantity (eg, 1 cent-per-ounce).
  - *Ad valorem excise taxes* are taxes in which a certain percentage of the product's price is taxed (eg, 18% of the price).
- Value-added taxes are taxes levied at each stage of production and ultimately are added to the price of the item.

### Food taxes
Most of the evidence for the taxation of unhealthy foods comes from Mexico, which implemented an 8% nonessential energy-dense food tax in 2014. As predicted, the

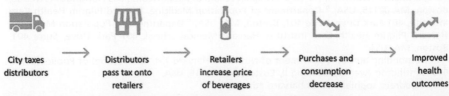

| City taxes distributors | → | Distributors pass tax onto retailers | → | Retailers increase price of beverages | → | Purchases and consumption decrease | → | Improved health outcomes |

**Fig. 1.** Causal model for beverage taxes and health. The effect of beverage taxes on health outcomes requires several intermediate steps, including the effect of taxes on the price of items and the resulting effects on purchases, consumption, and health.

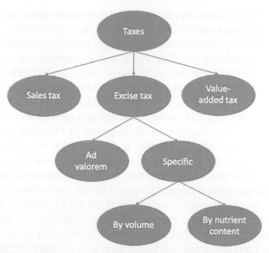

**Fig. 2.** Types of taxes. To raise revenue and improve health, several types of taxes have been used on beverages. More recently, specific excise taxes have been used in the United States.

increased price of taxed foods such as cakes and chips resulted in households buying less taxed foods both immediately and 2 years post-implementation.[3,4] Although Denmark passed a saturated fat tax in 2011, the government repealed it by the end of 2012, preventing the opportunity to fully evaluate this type of tax.[5]

### Beverage taxes—evidence from the United States
By 2022, seven cities in the United States had enacted sugary drink-specific excise taxes ranging from 1 to 2 cents per ounce. Of the seven cities, only Philadelphia's tax includes artificially-sweetened beverages in addition to sugar-sweetened beverages. The Navajo Nation also enacted a 2% sales tax on sugary drinks as part of a broader junk food tax. Currently, there are no state-level excise taxes on sugary beverages, and several states have passed prohibitions on further beverage taxes from being passed at the local level for at least some designated period.[6]

Evaluations of citywide taxes in Berkeley, CA; Philadelphia, PA; Oakland, CA; Boulder, CO; and Seattle, WA, have consistently shown that beverage taxes increased the price of taxed beverages. The tax pass-through amount varied according to the city and the store type, with some instances of undershifting, such as in supermarkets; overshifting also has been identified, such as in drug stores[7–9] (**Box 1**).

These beverage taxes would do little for public health without some effect on behavior. Health impact evaluations of these taxes have consistently documented

| Box 1 | |
| **Definition of terms** | |
| **Term** | **Definition** |
| Tax pass-through | The extent the tax is passed onto consumers through increased prices |
| Undershifting | The price increase of taxed goods is <100% of the tax |
| Overshifting | The price increase of taxed goods is >100% of the tax |
| Cross-border shopping | Purchases that are made outside of the city as a result of a tax in the city |

decreased purchasing of taxed beverages after tax implementation. Although cross-border shopping occurred in some cities such as Philadelphia (25% of the decrease in Philadelphia was offset by cross-border shopping)[8] and Oakland (46% offset),[10] not all cities have demonstrated this (eg, Seattle[11]), and the amount of cross-border shopping does not completely offset the decrease in purchased volume.

A few longitudinal studies have examined the effect of taxes over time on beverage purchasing in a cohort of individuals, and the results are not perfectly consistent. One study that relied on collecting food retail receipts from participants in Philadelphia and Baltimore (comparison city) found that participants in Philadelphia purchased 12.5 fewer ounces of taxed beverages per day 6 months after the tax was implemented compared with participants in Baltimore during the same time.[12] At 12 months post-tax, the differences attenuated. Another study in Philadelphia used consumption surveys to examine household consumption of taxed beverages in Philadelphia and surrounding counties (comparison) before and 10 to 11 months after the tax was implemented. These researchers found that while children had no change in consumption, adult participants in Philadelphia were consuming 10 to 11 fewer sodas a month after the tax compared with participants in surrounding counties.[13] More longitudinal research, with large enough samples to detect small differences, is needed to determine how individuals change their behaviors over time in response to a beverage tax and the effect that these taxes have on weight outcomes.

Taken together, these studies in the United States' context show that (1) beverage taxes increase the cost of taxed beverages, and (2) the subsequent decrease in the volume purchased of taxed beverages is both sustained and robust even in cities with documented cross-border shopping. Evidence on effects of consumption of sugary drinks is still incomplete, with some evidence for reduction among adults.

### Beverage taxes—evidence from non-US countries

Internationally, a similar picture emerges. Research on the effect of beverage taxes in Mexico (1 peso per liter), Chile (18% ad valorem), France (0.07 euro per liter), and Barbados (10% ad valorem in 2015, 20% ad valorem starting 2022) has found that prices of sugary beverages have increased after taxes were levied.[14–17] According to a recent meta-analysis pooling 46 estimates for 18 different tax policies, the average tax pass-through was 82%.[18]

The effect of taxes on the sales of sugary beverages varied with the level of taxation.[19,20] In France, the tax of 0.07 euro per liter led to an approximately 8% price increase for sodas, which resulted in limited effects. In contrast, Mexico's tax of 1 peso per liter led to an approximately 11% price increase for sodas and was associated with an 8% decrease in purchasing of taxed beverages per household.[17,19,21] Research from the United Kingdom, which taxes on a two-tiered system based on the amount of sugar in a 100 mL beverage serving, found that the amount of sugar purchased declined after the tax, even though the volume of sugary drinks purchased did not.[22] This finding could be an indication of supply-side changes in the amount of sugar in items, rather than solely changes in consumer demand.

### Summary

Beverage taxes are a powerful public health tool to disincentivize consumers from purchasing sugary beverages. Cost-effectiveness analysis of beverage taxes in the United States project that these policies will prevent cases of childhood obesity and will be cost-saving, especially because they raise revenue.[23] That increased revenue, often millions of dollars per year, can be invested in the community. The Berkeley, CA, beverage tax, for example, has earmarked funds for nutrition education and efforts to reduce sugary drink consumption.[24] Mexico's government used funds to increase clean water access in schools.[25] Further research is underway to determine whether these taxes have had any impact on health outcomes, an important future direction of research in this area.

### Calorie labeling in retail food environments

One of the most expansive obesity prevention policies implemented in the last several decades was the requirement that chain food establishments post calorie counts on menus. This policy was first implemented in the New York City (NYC) in 2008. Because of the rapid growth in popularity of these policies in other cities and states, the restaurant industry eventually supported a federal law that would require a uniform standard across the United States. Included in the 2010 Patient Protection and Affordable Care Act, the federal calorie labeling law required that all chains with $\geq 20$ establishments post calories on menus, menu boards, or labels on products (eg, packaged sandwiches in retail food stores). The policy includes most retail food chains, including restaurants and supermarkets, with exceptions for institutional food settings (eg, schools and nursing facilities). The policy was not fully implemented until 2018.

Myriad studies have evaluated labeling, with most studies in laboratory settings. A large meta-analysis in 2015 found that calorie labeling was associated with an 18-kcal reduction in calorie content of purchased meals but with significant heterogeneity of treatment effects.[26] Among six controlled studies conducted in restaurant settings, the average calorie reduction was 7 kcal, a nonsignificant finding.

Very few studies have been conducted in real-world retail food establishments with large enough samples to detect small differences. Bollinger and colleagues investigated the effect of calorie labeling in Starbucks before and after the April 2018 implementation of the NYC calorie labeling ordinance.[27] Researchers had data available from all store transactions (>100 million) in NYC (222 intervention restaurants) and Boston and Philadelphia (94 control restaurants) from January 2018 through February 2019. Calorie labeling was associated with a 6% average reduction in overall calories purchased in NYC versus Boston/Philadelphia restaurants. Calories purchased from beverages did not decline; the overall reduction in calories was driven by a decline in food calories purchased (14%, or 14 kcal decline). People purchasing larger calorie meals ($\geq 250$ kcal) had a much greater reduction in calorie content after labeling. Rather than purchasing fewer calories per item, three-quarters of the decline in calories resulted from customers purchasing fewer items after versus before labeling. Profitability did not decrease after labeling. The restaurant customers surveyed appeared to integrate calorie content more in their purchasing decisions after labeling compared with prior.

Petimar and colleagues have investigated calorie labeling effects at both chain fast-food restaurants and supermarkets. The research team first examined all transactions (nearly 50 million) from 104 fast-food restaurants in Louisiana, Mississippi, and Texas that were part of a large national chain that implemented labeling a year before the federal requirement.[28] The study period included 2 years of data pre-labeling (2015–2017) and 2 years after (2017–2019). After labeling, calories purchased declined immediately with a slow rise thereafter, such that the calorie content of meals was 4.7% lower (73 kcal) on average at the end of the post-labeling period, with larger declines for sides (vs entrees and beverages) (**Fig. 3**). Sugar, fat, and sodium content also declined post-labeling. Much of the reductions was from a decline in items per transaction.

In their subsequent study of calorie labeling of prepared foods sold in supermarkets, a growing segment of the *ready-to-eat* food market, Petimar and colleagues

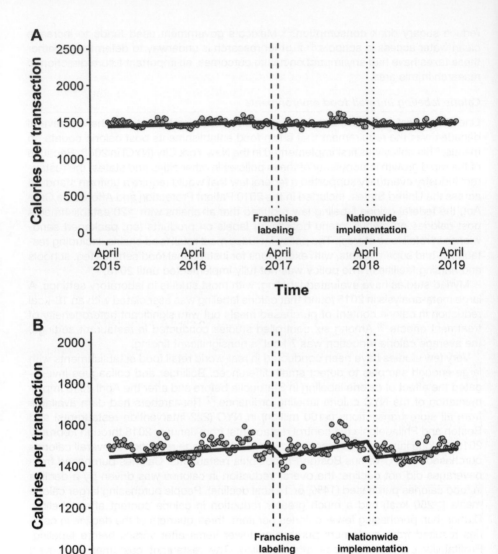

**Fig. 3.** (*A*) Calorie labeling effects on calories purchased in fast-food restaurants. After the implementation of calorie labeling in a large fast-food chain, calories purchased declined by 4.7% (73 kcal) by the end of the study period. (*B*) Same as (*A*) but magnified to see level and trend changes more easily. (*From* Petimar J, Zhang F, Rimm EB, et al. Changes in the calorie and nutrient content of purchased fast food meals after calorie menu labeling: A natural experiment. PLoS Med. Jul 2021;18(7):e1003714; with permission.)

examined all transactions at a New England regional supermarket chain with 173 stores.[29] With data for 2 years before and 7 months following labeling (also implemented in April 2017, 1 year before the requirement), they found a 5.1% reduction in average calorie content of purchased prepared bakery items (9.8 kcal) and an

11% reduction for deli items (17.2 kcal); no change was evident for entree items. As with the fast-food study, most of the reduction was from a decline in the number of items purchased per transaction. No substitution to packaged food items, not subject to labeling, was apparent after labeling, with calories purchased from these items also declining slightly (though to a lesser extent than prepared items).

Calorie labeling is very low cost compared with other obesity prevention policies. A prior cost-effectiveness study of calorie labeling, using estimates with lower calorie reductions than found in recent quasi-experimental studies, was consistent with either a cost-saving or relatively low cost of the intervention.[23] However, more research still needs to be done to explore the varied effects of the policy on diverse populations. Although the studies above found calorie reductions in both high- and low-income neighborhoods,[29] surveys have found that lower-income customers recognize and use calorie information less often.[30] Harm also should be further explored, such as the possibility that calorie posting could increase the risk of disordered eating behaviors. No consistent evidence has demonstrated this, but more work should be done to confirm this. Further, very few studies have been done on full-service of sit-down restaurants.

### Summary

Calorie labeling is associated with small reductions in calorie content of meals or purchases, mostly from a reduction in items purchased. Some customers, but clearly not all, are noticing and acting on this information. The impact of such small calorie reductions, though, is not clear. Information such as calorie posting seems necessary but not sufficient to affect population weight and health outcomes.

### Federal nutrition programs

Federal nutrition programs aim to address both food insecurity and obesity in the United States (**Box 2**).

| Box 2 | | |
|---|---|---|
| **A sample of federal nutrition programs in the United States** | | |
| **Program Name** | **Description** | **Nutritional Standards?** |
| Supplemental Nutrition Assistance Program (SNAP) | Benefits provided to low-income families to purchase food at stores (not restaurants) | No |
| Special Supplemental Nutrition Program for Women, Infants, and Children (WIC) | Benefits for food, health care, and nutrition education provided to low-income pregnant and postpartum women, to infants, and to children ≤5 y of age | Yes, based on the Dietary Guidelines for Americans (DGA) |
| National School Lunch Program (NSLP) and School Breakfast Program (SBP) | Meal program that provides low cost/free meals to students in public schools, nonprofit private schools, and some childcare institutions. Some school districts provide these meals free of charge to any student while others may require proof of low-income | Yes, based on the DGA |

### Supplemental Nutrition Assistance Program

Supplemental Nutrition Assistance Program (SNAP) is a poverty reduction program that successfully alleviates food insecurity among its participants.[31] Beyond educational programs linked to SNAP, very few changes to promote healthier dietary consumption have been integrated into the program. The United States Department of Agriculture Healthy Incentives Pilot (USDA HIP; 2011–2012) was a federal demonstration project that provided a 30% rebate on fruit and vegetable purchases made with SNAP dollars to 7500 households. Analyses of before and after surveys from over 2000 participants showed that those randomized to the HIP group consumed about a quarter cup more fruits and vegetables than those in the non-HIP group.[32] Separately, the Double Up Food Bucks program, which is administered by the Fair Food Network in over 25 states with federal grants, matches the number of SNAP dollars spent on fresh produce. SNAP recipients participating in the program who spend $10 on fresh produce, for example, receive an additional $10 to spend on more fresh produce. Although no study has examined long-term consumption data, studies analyzing supermarket scanner data have shown that this program increases the amount of fresh produce purchased among SNAP participants.[33,34]

Moving beyond just incentives, Harnack and colleagues examined how incentives alone, restrictions on purchasing sugary beverages or junk food with benefits, and the combination of the two would affect purchasing behavior among participants who are SNAP-eligible in a randomized controlled trial.[35] Participants who had both the 30% financial incentive to purchase fresh produce and restrictions on what they could buy with SNAP dollars purchased fewer total calories (−96 calories/day from baseline; Control: +80 calories/day from baseline), fewer discretionary calories (−64 calories/day from baseline; Control: +13 calories/day from baseline), more fruit (+0.4 servings/day from baseline; Control: 0 servings/day from baseline), and had improved Healthy Eating Index scores when compared with the control group over 12 weeks. Thus far, SNAP has not allowed restrictions on purchase of sugary beverages and junk food. However, cost-effectiveness analyses suggest that implementing restrictions and financial incentives to eat healthier may ultimately be cost-saving.[36]

Separate from healthy eating, it is not clear whether SNAP participation is associated with increased body weight as the program is currently structured. Longitudinal studies have found no associations with childhood obesity,[37–39] and positive associations with obesity in adult women but not men.[40]

### Special Supplemental Nutrition Program for Women, Infants, and Children

In 2009, WIC revised its food packages for the first time in nearly 30 years to better reflect recommendations from the Dietary Guidelines for Americans (DGA). Changes included expanding whole grain options; reducing the amount of milk (requiring low-fat or skim), cheese, eggs, and fruit juice; and offering cash value incentives to purchase additional fruits and vegetables. These revisions led to modest improvements in dietary quality, with increases in low-fat dairy intake, whole grains, and fruit consumption among mothers and children.[41] In Los Angeles, Chaparro and colleagues were able to track the growth of children from three groups: (1) those who participated in WIC before the food package revisions; (2) those who participated both before and after; and (3) those who only participated after.[42] They found that children who received only the revised packages had healthier growth trajectories through age 4 than children who only received the old packages. In another research, models suggest that the recent decrease in obesity prevalence (−0.34% points per year) among 2–4-year-olds may have been in part due to changes to the WIC package.[43]

Consistent with these findings, other studies have found that youth ≤5 years who spent more time enrolled in WIC have healthier diets than those who spent less time,[44–46] and that WIC participation does not lead to unhealthy weight gain.[39,42]

### National School Lunch Program and School Breakfast Program

The NSLP was implemented in 1946 in part as a national security measure after many were unable to enroll in the military during World War II due to diet-related illnesses. Twenty years later, the SBP was established. The intent of these programs, which provided food assistance to 30 million students before 2020 and many more since, was to deliver adequate nutrition to students. In the past few decades, there have been efforts to increase the nutritional value of the provided meals given the rising prevalence of childhood obesity. The 2010 Healthy, Hunger-Free, Kids Act (HHFKA) overhauled the nutritional standards of these programs, requiring increases in provision of fruits, vegetables, and whole grains and limits on calories, sodium, and trans fat. These policies affected the SBP, NSLP, and foods sold on the premises (ie, competitive foods).

The HHFKA has been evaluated, including six studies that were included in a comprehensive systematic review of school nutrition programs.[47] Of the six studies, three with a low risk for bias found that the selection of fruit increased after implementation of the HHFKA standards. When measuring actual consumption using plate waste and visual estimation techniques, one study found no differences in fruit, vegetable, or whole grain consumption before versus after implementation; in contrast, two of the studies documented increased vegetable and overall entree consumption after HHFKA implementation. These results alleviated some concerns that children would waste more foods with healthier offerings and were concordant with other studies evaluating similar non-HHFKA interventions.

The competitive food provisions of HHFKA have been less extensively evaluated, though studies conducted before HHFKA demonstrated that excess consumption of these foods was associated with overall poor dietary quality. The overall cost-effectiveness of HHFKA, especially the provisions on competitive foods, has been projected to lower the number of cases of obesity substantially over 10 years and to be either cost-effective or cost-saving.[23]

### Summary

The US government invests billions of dollars across these federal nutrition programs to ensure millions of food-insecure Americans have access to affordable food. Changes implemented to WIC, NSLP, and SBP in the last two decades have demonstrated efforts toward alignment with the DGA so that participants have the ability to purchase healthier foods. The current evidence suggests that federal nutrition programs with nutritional guidelines in place promote healthier diets and may help prevent weight gain.

## DISCUSSION

This article has demonstrated that some policies can affect dietary choices and perhaps body weight; however, single policies are likely not strong enough to have a lasting effect on body weight and health. Other countries have tried more comprehensive approaches. As an example, to combat the increasing prevalence of obesity, the Chilean government implemented the Law of Food Labeling and Advertising in 2016. These regulations were comprehensive and sweeping in scope, touching upon front-of-package labeling, child-directed marketing, and sales of unhealthy foods in schools. Evaluations of these interventions have shown declines in the household purchase of calories, sodium, and sugar.[48]

Although obesity prevention policies can improve diet quality, they are not expected to decrease the prevalence of obesity. Instead, if effective, they would decrease the rate of rise in obesity prevalence compared with the counterfactual of no policy. Hall and colleagues estimated that only a 7 kcal increase in per capita daily calories was responsible for the rapidly rising obesity prevalence from 1978 to 2005.[49] Reversing this rapid rise would only require an average per capita daily reduction of this calorie amount. In contrast, reversing population obesity prevalence to what it was in the late 1970s would require a reduction of 220 kcal/person/day.

In addition to the lack of obesity prevalence reduction, policies are difficult to evaluate. First, researchers typically do not have available, large-scale, representative data on health outcomes (or even true consumption) to help determine effects. Second, policies that are implemented in large geographic areas preclude evaluating the effects of a policy compared with a control group (such as with national calorie labeling). Those implemented in smaller areas, on the other hand, often lack available data on health outcomes (such as comparisons of policies implemented in cities/states compared with control cities/states) because no such data are routinely collected in enough quantity in small geographic areas before and after policies are implemented. To determine effects on health outcomes, researchers rely on cost-effectiveness analyses that link together multiple datasets. Cost-effectiveness analyses are still pending for calorie labeling; for all other policies discussed in this article (ie, beverage taxes, adding nutritional guidelines to SNAP, and adding nutrition standards for competitive foods sold in schools), analyses have demonstrated these policies to be either cost-saving or cost-effective.

## SUMMARY

Overweight and obesity affect most of the Americans, and clinical guidance must be supplemented by policies that address diet quality and caloric intake at the population level. Beverage taxes, calorie labeling, and nutritional changes to federal nutrition programs are all steps the US government has taken to disincentivize unhealthy choices. To improve upon current policies and to enact new ones will require cross-sector collaboration and the political will to make lasting changes.

## CLINICS CARE POINTS

- Beverage taxes decrease purchases of sugary drinks, with data on consumption still incomplete.
- Calorie labeling of prepared foods is associated with mildly reduced calorie content of purchases.
- Federal nutrition assistance programs with restrictions on what can be purchased or offered lead to healthier diets.

## DISCLOSURE

Dr S.V. Hua is supported by the NIH National Research Service Award (T32 DK 007703). Ms C.E. Collis and Dr J.P. Block are supported by a grant from the National Institute of Diabetes and Digestive and Kidney Disorders (R01 DK115492, PI: Block).

The content of this article is solely the responsibility of the authors and does not necessarily represent the official views of the NIH, United States.

## REFERENCES

1. Hall KD, Ayuketah A, Brychta R, et al. Ultra-Processed Diets Cause Excess Calorie Intake and Weight Gain: An Inpatient Randomized Controlled Trial of Ad Libitum Food Intake. Cell Metab 2019;30(1):226.
2. Malik VS, Pan A, Willett WC, et al. Sugar-sweetened beverages and weight gain in children and adults: a systematic review and meta-analysis. Am J Clin Nutr 2013;98(4):1084–102.
3. Taillie LS, Rivera JA, Popkin BM, et al. Do high vs. low purchasers respond differently to a nonessential energy-dense food tax? Two-year evaluation of Mexico's 8% nonessential food tax. Prev Med 2017;105S:S37–42.
4. Batis C, Rivera JA, Popkin BM, et al. First-Year Evaluation of Mexico's Tax on Nonessential Energy-Dense Foods: An Observational Study. PLoS Med 2016; 13(7):e1002057.
5. Stafford N. Denmark cancels "fat tax" and shelves "sugar tax" because of threat of job losses. BMJ Br Med J (Clin Res Ed) 2012;345:e7889.
6. Crosbie E, Pomeranz JL, Wright KE, et al. State Preemption: An Emerging Threat to Local Sugar-Sweetened Beverage Taxation. Am J Public Health 2021;111(4): 677–86.
7. Leider J, Li Y, Powell LM. Pass-through of the Oakland, California, sugar-sweetened beverage tax in food stores two years post-implementation: A difference-in-differences study. PLoS One 2021;16(1):e0244884.
8. Roberto CA, Lawman HG, LeVasseur MT, et al. Association of a Beverage Tax on Sugar-Sweetened and Artificially Sweetened Beverages With Changes in Beverage Prices and Sales at Chain Retailers in a Large Urban Setting. JAMA 2019;321(18):1799–810.
9. Jones-Smith JC, Pinero Walkinshaw L, Oddo VM, et al. Impact of a sweetened beverage tax on beverage prices in Seattle, WA. Econ Hum Biol 2020;39: 100917.
10. Leger PT, Powell LM. The impact of the Oakland SSB tax on prices and volume sold: A study of intended and unintended consequences. Health Econ 2021; 30(8):1745–71.
11. Powell LM, Leider J. Impact of a sugar-sweetened beverage tax two-year post-tax implementation in Seattle, Washington, United States. J Public Health Policy 2021;42(4):574–88.
12. Lawman HG, Bleich SN, Yan J, et al. One-year changes in sugar-sweetened beverage consumers' purchases following implementation of a beverage tax: a longitudinal quasi-experiment. Am J Clin Nutr 2020;112(3):644–51.
13. Cawley J, Frisvold D, Hill A, et al. The impact of the Philadelphia beverage tax on purchases and consumption by adults and children. J Health Econ 2019;67: 102225.
14. Alvarado M, Kostova D, Suhrcke M, et al. Trends in beverage prices following the introduction of a tax on sugar-sweetened beverages in Barbados. Prev Med 2017;105S:S23–5.
15. Cuadrado C, Dunstan J, Silva-Illanes N, et al. Effects of a sugar-sweetened beverage tax on prices and affordability of soft drinks in Chile: A time series analysis. Soc Sci Med 2020;245:112708.

16. Caro JC, Corvalan C, Reyes M, et al. Chile's 2014 sugar-sweetened beverage tax and changes in prices and purchases of sugar-sweetened beverages: An observational study in an urban environment. PLoS Med 2018; 15(7):e1002597.

17. Capacci S, Allais O, Bonnet C, et al. The impact of the French soda tax on prices and purchases. An ex post evaluation. PLoS One 2019;14(10): e0223196.

18. Andreyeva T, Marple K, Marinello S, et al. Outcomes Following Taxation of Sugar-Sweetened Beverages: A Systematic Review and Meta-analysis. JAMA Netw Open 2022;5(6):e2215276.

19. Colchero MA, Rivera-Dommarco J, Popkin BM, et al. In Mexico, Evidence Of Sustained Consumer Response Two Years After Implementing A Sugar-Sweetened Beverage Tax. Health Aff 2017;36(3):564–71.

20. Alvarado M, Unwin N, Sharp SJ, et al. Assessing the impact of the Barbados sugar-sweetened beverage tax on beverage sales: an observational study. Int J Behav Nutr Phys Act 2019;16(1):13.

21. Colchero MA, Salgado JC, Unar-Munguia M, et al. Changes in Prices After an Excise Tax to Sweetened Sugar Beverages Was Implemented in Mexico: Evidence from Urban Areas. PLoS One 2015;10(12):e0144408.

22. Pell D, Mytton O, Penney TL, et al. Changes in soft drinks purchased by British households associated with the UK soft drinks industry levy: controlled interrupted time series analysis. BMJ 2021;372:n254.

23. Gortmaker SL, Wang YC, Long MW, et al. Three Interventions That Reduce Childhood Obesity Are Projected To Save More Than They Cost To Implement. Health Aff (Millwood) 2015;34(11):1932–9.

24. Map and Chart the Movement. Healthy Food America. Updated 2019. 2022. Available at: https://www.healthyfoodamerica.org/map. Accessed June 10, 2022.

25. Carriedo A, Koon AD, Encarnacion LM, et al. The political economy of sugar-sweetened beverage taxation in Latin America: lessons from Mexico, Chile and Colombia. Global Health 2021;17(1):5.

26. Long MW, Tobias DK, Cradock AL, et al. Systematic review and meta-analysis of the impact of restaurant menu calorie labeling. Am J Public Health 2015;105(5): e11–24.

27. Bollinger B, Leslie P, Sorensen A. Calorie Posting in Chain Restaurants. Am Econ J Econ Pol 2011;3(1):91–128.

28. Petimar J, Zhang F, Rimm EB, et al. Changes in the calorie and nutrient content of purchased fast food meals after calorie menu labeling: A natural experiment. PLoS Med 2021;18(7):e1003714.

29. Petimar J, Grummon AH, Zhang F, et al. Assessment of Calories Purchased After Calorie Labeling of Prepared Foods in a Large Supermarket Chain. JAMA Intern Med 2022. https://doi.org/10.1001/jamainternmed.2022.3065.

30. Chen R, Smyser M, Chan N, et al. Changes in awareness and use of calorie information after mandatory menu labeling in restaurants in King County, Washington. Am J Public Health 2015;105(3):546–53.

31. Mabli J, Ohls J. Supplemental Nutrition Assistance Program Participation Is Associated with an Increase in Household Food Security in a National Evaluation. J Nutr 2015;145(2):344–51.

32. Olsho LE, Klerman JA, Wilde PE, et al. Financial incentives increase fruit and vegetable intake among Supplemental Nutrition Assistance Program

participants: a randomized controlled trial of the USDA Healthy Incentives Pilot. Am J Clin Nutr 2016;104(2):423–35.

33. Rummo PE, Noriega D, Parret A, et al. Evaluating A USDA Program That Gives SNAP Participants Financial Incentives To Buy Fresh Produce In Supermarkets. Health Aff 2019;38(11):1816–23.

34. Steele-Adjognon M, Weatherspoon D. Double Up Food Bucks program effects on SNAP recipients' fruit and vegetable purchases. BMC Publ Health 2017; 17(1):946.

35. Harnack L, Oakes JM, Elbel B, et al. Effects of Subsidies and Prohibitions on Nutrition in a Food Benefit Program: A Randomized Clinical Trial. JAMA Intern Med 2016;176(11):1610–8.

36. Mozaffarian D, Liu J, Sy S, et al. Cost-effectiveness of financial incentives and disincentives for improving food purchases and health through the US Supplemental Nutrition Assistance Program (SNAP): A microsimulation study. PLoS Med 2018; 15(10):e1002661.

37. Schmeiser MD. The impact of long-term participation in the supplemental nutrition assistance program on child obesity. Health Econ 2012;21(4): 386–404.

38. Fan M, Jin Y. The Supplemental Nutrition Assistance Program and Childhood Obesity in the United States: Evidence from the National Longitudinal Survey of Youth 1997. American Journal of Health Economics 2015;1(4):432–60.

39. Lee MM, Kinsey EW, Kenney ELUS. Nutrition Assistance Program Participation and Childhood Obesity: The Early Childhood Longitudinal Study 2011. Am J Prev Med 2022;63(2):242–50.

40. Gibson D. Food stamp program participation is positively related to obesity in low income women. J Nutr 2003;133(7):2225–31.

41. Schultz DJ, Byker Shanks C, Houghtaling B. The Impact of the 2009 Special Supplemental Nutrition Program for Women, Infants, and Children Food Package Revisions on Participants: A Systematic Review. J Acad Nutr Diet 2015;115(11): 1832–46.

42. Chaparro MP, Crespi CM, Anderson CE, et al. The 2009 Special Supplemental Nutrition Program for Women, Infants, and Children (WIC) food package change and children's growth trajectories and obesity in Los Angeles County. Am J Clin Nutr 2019;109(5):1414–21.

43. Daepp MIG, Gortmaker SL, Wang YC, et al. WIC Food Package Changes: Trends in Childhood Obesity Prevalence. Pediatrics 2019;143(5). https://doi.org/10.1542/peds.2018-2841.

44. Weinfield NS, Borger C, Au LE, et al. Longer Participation in WIC Is Associated with Better Diet Quality in 24-Month-Old Children. J Acad Nutr Diet 2020; 120(6):963–71.

45. Borger C, Paolicelli CP, Sun B. Duration of Special Supplemental Nutrition Program for Women, Infants, and Children (WIC) Participation is Associated With Children's Diet Quality at Age 3 Years. Am J Prev Med 2022;62(6): e343–50.

46. Anderson CE, Martinez CE, Ritchie LD, et al. Longer WIC participation duration is associated with higher diet quality at age 5 years. J Nutr 2022. https://doi.org/10.1093/jn/nxac134.

47. Cohen JFW, Hecht AA, Hager ER, et al. Strategies to Improve School Meal Consumption: A Systematic Review. Nutrients 2021;(10):13. https://doi.org/10.3390/nu13103520.

48. Taillie LS, Bercholz M, Popkin B, et al. Changes in food purchases after the Chilean policies on food labelling, marketing, and sales in schools: a before and after study. Lancet Planet Health 2021;5(8):e526–33.

49. Grummon AH, Taillie LS. Supplemental Nutrition Assistance Program participation and racial/ethnic disparities in food and beverage purchases. Public Health Nutr 2018;21(18):3377–85.

# Moving?

## Make sure your subscription moves with you!

To notify us of your new address, find your **Clinics Account Number** (located on your mailing label above your name), and contact customer service at:

**Email: journalscustomerservice-usa@elsevier.com**

**800-654-2452** (subscribers in the U.S. & Canada)
**314-447-8871** (subscribers outside of the U.S. & Canada)

**Fax number: 314-447-8029**

**Elsevier Health Sciences Division**
**Subscription Customer Service**
**3251 Riverport Lane**
**Maryland Heights, MO 63043**

*To ensure uninterrupted delivery of your subscription, please notify us at least 4 weeks in advance of move.

Printed and bound by CPI Group (UK) Ltd, Croydon, CR0 4YY

03/10/2024

01040471-0003